Developments in Cardiovascular Medicine

VOLUME 123

The titles published in this series are listed at the end of this volume.

Occult Atherosclerotic Disease
Diagnosis, Assessment and Management

edited by

ABDUL-MAJEED SALMASI
Department of Cardiology, Central Middlesex Hospital, London, UK

and

ANDREW N. NICOLAIDES
Irvine Laboratory for Cardiovascular Investigation and Research, St. Mary's Hospital, London, UK

KLUWER ACADEMIC PUBLISHERS
DORDRECHT / BOSTON / LONDON

Library of Congress Cataloging-in-Publication Data

Occult atherosclerotic disease : diagnosis, assessment, and management / edited by Abdul-Majeed Salmasi and Andrew N. Nicolaides.
p. cm. -- (Developments in cardiovascular medicine ; v. 123)
Includes index.
ISBN 0-7923-1188-4 (HB : alk. paper)
1. Atherosclerosis. 2. Cerebrovascular disease. 3. Coronary heart disease. I. Salmasi, Abdul-Majeed. II. Nicolaides, Andrew N. III. Series.
[DNLM: 1. Arteriosclerosis. 2. Atherosclerosis. 3. Carotid Artery Diseases. 4. Coronary Diseases. W1 DE997VME v. 123 / WG 550 015]
RC692.028 1991
616.1'36--dc20
DNLM/DLC
for Library of Congress 91-7042

ISBN 0-7923-1188-4

Published by Kluwer Academic Publishers,
P.O. Box 17, 3300 AA Dordrecht, The Netherlands.

Kluwer Academic Publishers incorporates
the publishing programmes of
D. Reidel, Martinus Nijhoff, Dr W. Junk and MTP Press.

Sold and distributed in the U.S.A. and Canada
by Kluwer Academic Publishers.
101 Philip Drive, Norwell, MA 02061, U.S.A.

In all other countries, sold and distributed
by Kluwer Academic Publishers Group
P.O. Box 322, 3300 AH Dordrecht, The Netherlands.

Printed on acid-free paper

Table of contents

PART FIVE: Occult atherosclerotic disease of the renal and mesenteric arteries

PART SIX: New techniques, combined lesions and prevention

List of contributors

ABDUL-KADIR ABDULLA MB, ChB
Formerly Senior Registrar
Department of Pathology
The National Heart Hospital
Westmoreland Street
London W1
UK

PAUL S. VAN BEMMELEN MD
Department of Surgery
University of Washington
Seattle
Washington 98115
USA

JESAIA BENHORIN MD
The Heiden Department of Cardiology
Bikur Cholim Hospital
Haddasah Medical School
Hebrew University
Jerusalem
Israel

PETER F. COHN MD
Professor of Medicine
Cardiology Division
State University of New York
Health Sciences Centre
Stony Brook
New York 11794
USA

MARY PAULA COLGAN MD, RVT
Director of the Vascular Laboratories
Department of Vascular Surgery
St. James' Hospital
James' Street
Dublin 8
Republic of Ireland

JACK COLLIN MA, MD, FRCS
Consultant Surgeon and Reader in Surgery
Nuffield Department of Surgery
John Radcliffe Hospital
University of Oxford
Headington
Oxford OX3 9DU
UK

ROBERT S. ELKELES FRCP
Consultant Physician
St. Mary's Hospital
Praed Street
London W2 1NY
UK

MARY ELLIS BSc
Department of Surgery
Charing Cross and Westminster Hospital Medical School
Fulham Palace Road
London W6 8RF
UK

ASEEL N. FATTAH MB, ChB, MRCPath
Consultant Histopathologist
Queen Elizabeth II Hospital
Howlands
Welwyn Garden City
Hertfordshire
UK

F. GERRY R. FOWKES PhD, FRCPE, FFCM
Reader in Community Medicine
Usher Institute
Medical School
Teviot Place
Edinburgh EH8 9AG
Scotland

ROGER M GREENHALGH MA, MD, MChir, FRCS
Professor and Head of Department of Surgery
Charing Cross and Westminster Hospital Medical School
Fulham Palace Road
London W6 8RF
UK

MICHAEL J GRIGG FRACS
Senior Lecturer and Vascular Surgeon
Alfred Hospital
Monash University
Melbourne
Australia

THOMAS S. HATSUKAMI MD
Department of Surgery
University of Washington
Seattle
Washington 98115
USA

JAEKYEONG HEO MD, FCCP
Philadelphia Heart Institute
Presbyterian Medical Centre of Philadelphia
39th & Market Streets
Philadelphia
Pennsylvania 19104
USA

RICHARD S. HOULSTON PhD
Department of Clinical Genetics
The Royal Free Hospital
Pond Street, Hampstead
London NW3
UK

STEVE E. HUMPHRIES PhD
Professor of Genetics
The Charing Cross Sunley Research Centre
Charing Cross Hospital
Lurgan Avenue
London W6 8LW
UK

ABDULMASSIH S. ISKANDRIAN MD, FACC, FACP, FCCP
Clinical Professor of Medicine
University of Pennsylvania
Co-Director, Philadelphia Heart Institute
Presbyterian Medical Centre of Philadelphia
39th & Market Streets
Philadelphia, Pennsylvania 19104
USA

SUSAN LAING MA, PhD
Lecturer
Department of Surgery
Charing Cross and Westminster Hospital Medical School
Fulham Palace Road
London W6 8RF
UK

CHE SAM LO PhD
Hospital Scientist
Department of Medicine
Monash Medical Centre
Prince Henry's Hospital
Melbourne
Australia

CHRISTOPHER J. MATHIAS MB BS, D PHIL, FRCP
Professor of Neuro vascular Medicine
St. Mary's Hospital
Praed Street
London W2 1NY
Director of the Autonomic Investigation Unit
University Department of Clinical Neurology
Institute of Neurology and National Hospital for Nervous diseases
Queen Square
London
UK

P GEOFFREY MATTHEWS MB, BS, PhD, FRACP, DDU
Department of Vascular Medicine
Monash Medical Centre
Melbourne
Australia

PETER MAZEIKA MRCP
Department of Clinical Cardiology
Hammersmith Hospital
Royal Postgraduate Medical School
Du Cane Road
London W12 OHS
UK

DERMOT J. MOORE MD, FRCSI
Department of the Vascular Surgery
St. James' Hospital
James' Street
Dublin 8
Republic of Ireland

VASKAR MUKERJI MD
Associate Professor of Medicine
Division of Cardiology
1E-65 Health Sciences Centre
Columbia
Missouri 65212
USA

KENNETH A MYERS MS, FACS, FRACS, DDU
Professor and Head of Department of Vascular Surgery
Monash Medical Centre
Melbourne
Australia

ANDREW N. NICOLAIDES MS, FRCS
Professor of Vascular Surgery
Director, Irvine Laboratory for Cardiovascular Investigation and Research
St. Mary's Hospital
Praed Street
London W2 1NY
UK

PETROS NIHOYANNOPOULOS MD
Senior Lecturer in Cardiology, Honorary Consultant Cardiologist and Director of the Echocardiography Laboratory
Clinical Cardiology
Hammersmith Hospital
Du Cane Road
London W12 OHS
UK

BRENT M. PARKER MD
Professor of Medicine
Division of Cardiology
Health Sciences Centre
Columbia
Missouri 65212
USA

RICHARD G. PETTY MSc, MD, MRCP
Consultant Physician
Section of Vascular Biology
MRC Clinical Research Centre
Northwick Park Hospital
Watford Road
Harow
Middlesex HAI 3UJ
UK

SOPHIE C. RENTON FRCS
Vascular Surgeon
Irvine Laboratory For Cardiovascular Investigation and Research
St. Mary's Hospital
Praed Street
London W2 1NY
UK

ABDUL-MAJEED SALMASI MD, PhD, FACA
Department of Cardiology
Central Middlesex Hospital
London NW10
UK

GREGOR D. SHANIK MD, M.Ch., FRCSI, FRCS
Professor of the Vascular Surgery
St. James' Hospital
James' Street
Dublin 8
Republic of Ireland

SHLOMO STERN MD, FACC
Professor of Medicine
The Heiden Department of Cardiology
Bikur Cholim Hospital
Haddasah Medical School
Hebrew University
Jerusalem
Israel

D EUGENE STRANDNESS Jr. MD, FACS
Professor of Surgery
Department of Surgery
University of Washington
Seattle
Washington 98115
USA

DAN TZIVONI MD, FACC
Professor of Medicine
The Heiden Department of Cardiology
Bikur Cholim Hospital
Haddasah Medical School
Hebrew University
Jerusalem
Israel

MARK L WAHLQVIST B Med Sc, MD (Adelaide), MD(Uppsala), FRACP, FAIFST, FACN
Professor of Medicine
Monash University
Prince Henry's Hospital
Melbourne
Australia

Preface

Occult atherosclerotic diseases impose great challenges in the cardiovascular practice. Although their pathology is not much different from that of the overt group of diseases, the clinical approach to their diagnoses remains a puzzle. This has mainly emerged as a result of the problems faced in trying to pick up the vulnerable subjects from among the general public. More definitive candidates to be evaluated are those belonging to one of the high risk groups. There are no statistical figures available on the incidence of occult atherosclerotic disease in the "non risky" general public and this is definitely an area that needs further investigation.

Atherosclerotic disease whether they are in the cerebral, coronary, renal or lower limb arteries are theoretically interrelated because the basic pathological changes are usually similar. However there still remain some differences which are mainly due to variation in the flow pattern in the arteries. Thus it will be important clinically and from the management point of view to investigate for the presence of occult disease in other arteries if an atherosclerotic disease in a certain artery has been discovered. This approach is of a great significance especially from the preventive point of view in order to avoid catastrophic events which may have resulted from pathology in the other region.

The purpose of this book is to highlight various aspects of atherosclerotic disease. It discusses the epidemiology, diagnosis and management of each group of diseases in addition to the clinical approach of diagnosing combined lesions. Obviously the prevention of these illnesses is a subject that received a good deal of attention in this book.

PART ONE

Pathophysiological considerations

1. The cell biology of atherosclerosis

RICHARD G. PETTY[1]

Atherogenesis is a complex multi-factorial process, involving endothelial cell damage or dysfunction, mononuclear cell adhesion, lipid accumulation and myointimal cell proliferation.

Cell and molecular biology of the vessel wall

The walls of large arteries consist of three layers: intima, media and adventitia. The intima comprises a single layer of endothelial cells overlying a continuous basement membrane composed of type IV collagen and structural glycoproteins. The media is composed of smooth muscle cells surrounded by a matrix composed of types I and III collagen, elastin, and glycoproteins. The outer layer is the adventitia composed of fibroblasts, adipocytes, mast cells, collagens, lipids and glycoproteins. Extracellular matrix forms a major portion of the media and the adventitia, and its precise composition varies at different stages of the development of atherosclerosis, and the synthesis of these matrix molecules is thought to reflect the state of differentiation of arterial smooth muscle cells. Three families of proteoglycans have been identified in blood vessels, including proteoglycans enriched in chondroitin, dermatan and heparan sulphates although the location of each varies at different sites in the vessel wall [1]. Endothelial cells synthesise and secrete both heparan sulphate and dermatan sulphate containing proteoglycans, while vascular smooth muscle cells primarily synthesise and secrete chondroitin sulphate and dermatan sulphate proteoglycans, with considerably less heparan sulphate proteoglycan.

1. I am grateful to Dr Jeremy Pearson for reading the manuscript and for many helpful comments, and Dr Amanda Tomlinson for drawing Figure 1.1.

A.-M. Salmasi and A. N. Nicolaides (eds.), Occult Atherosclerotic Disease, 3–17.

Endothelial cell biology

Endothelial cells form the lining of blood vessels, and are intimately concerned in maintaining thromboresistance. The pathophysiology of the vascular endothelium, [2] which has been recently reviewed will be summarised briefly.

The vascular endothelium is highly specialised and has central roles in the maintenance of vascular tone and permeability, in the regulation of leukocyte 'traffic', and in the modulation of haemostasis and thrombosis (Table 1.1). It is one cell thick, and constitutes a dynamic interface between the blood and the rest of the body.

Table 1.1. Functions of the vascular endothelium

Maintenance of thromboresistance
Maintenance of selective permeability
Modulation of leukocyte interactions with the tissues
Integration and transduction of blood-borne signals
Regulation of inflammatory and immune reactions
Regulation of vascular tone
Regulation of vascular growth

The basement membrane on which endothelial cells rest *in vivo* not only anchors the latter within the vessel wall, but also provides a secondary barrier to the exchange of fluid, protein and the formed elements of the blood with the extravascular space. It is a complex structure containing collagens, elastin, laminin, fibronectin, thrombospondin, microfilaments, and at least three types of proteoglycan. Endothelial cells are responsible for the synthesis of these membrane components [3], and the formed matrix acts reciprocally to modulate the growth, proliferation and phenotypic expression of the endothelium [4]. Unstimulated platelets do not normally adhere to intact endothelial cells. However, exposure of the basement membrane, for instance by removal or contraction of endothelial cells, leads to rapid adhesion of platelets which may further aggregate and degranulate if organised collagen fibrils are also exposed.

The maintenance of thromboresistance involves a balance between pro- and anti-coagulant activities by vascular endothelial cells (Table 1.2). Adhesion of platelets to the subendothelium, particularly at high shear rates, is critically dependent on von Willebrand factor (vWF). Endothelial cells synthesise, store and secrete this glycoprotein, both into plasma, and the extracellular matrix. Von Willebrand factor is a co-factor which cross-links platelets to the subendothelium, in addition to its role in the circulation as a carrier for factor VIII [5].

Endothelial cells fail to initiate coagulation by the intrinsic pathway, but once the coagulation cascade has been triggered, endothelial cells (like

Table 1.2. The haemostatic/thrombotic balance of endothelial cells

Anticoagulant	Procoagulant
Prostacyclin	Platelet-activating factor
Heparin-like molecules	Coagulation factors
Thrombomodulin	Tissue factor
Tissue plasminogen activator	Tissue plasminogen activator inhibitor
Ecto-ADPase	von Willebrand factor

blood platelets) serve to localise and greatly promote prothrombin activation by providing an organised surface with receptors for factors Xa, IXa, Va and thrombin [6].

In common with other tissue cells, endothelium has the capacity to express tissue factor (thromboplastin) and, hence, to initiate the extrinsic pathway. Unlike them, however, this factor VII binding activity is present only when endothelial cells are perturbed by a variety of stimuli, of which the best characterised are thrombin, bacterial lipopolysaccharides and cytokines [7, 8].

Endothelium is the major site for two anticoagulant reactions involving thrombin. In the first of these it is responsible *in vivo* for the binding of thrombin, and catalysing its inactivation by circulating antithrombin, which is also expressed at the endothelial cell luminal surface [9]. This reaction, which occurs only slowly in solution unless enhanced by heparin, is probably accelerated *in vivo* by the presence of heparin-like glycosaminoglycans on the surface of the endothelium. The second reaction is due to the binding of thrombin by a specific endothelial cell surface protein, thrombomodulin, which dramatically increases the ability of thrombin to activate proteolytically the circulating anticoagulant protein C [10]. Endothelial cells further contribute to this process by synthesising and secreting protein S, the co-factor for protein C activity [11].

Resolution of a fibrin clot is due to plasminogen activators, of which two types exist; urokinase which activates plasminogen in the fluid phase, and tissue type (t-PA), which is active only when bound to fibrin. Although endothelial cells in culture can secrete both forms, it is clear that release into the blood stream is acutely stimulated *in vivo* by venostasis or by agonists such as vasopressin or noradrenaline, and is only of endothelial cell-derived t-PA [12]. The regulation of fibrinolytic activity secreted by endothelium is complex and not yet fully understood. Studies *in vitro* have shown that thrombin directly induces t-PA release, but have as yet failed to demonstrate vasopressin- or noradrenaline-induced release. In addition, the major circulating fast acting t-PA inhibitor, plasminogen activator inhibitor 1 (PAI-1), is concurrently synthesised and released by endothelium. Interestingly, cytokines upregulate PAI-1 but not t-PA secretion by endothelial cells, thus providing an additional element in the shift towards procoagulant activity induced by these agents [12].

As already mentioned, endothelial cells are intrinsically non-thrombogenic – unstimulated platelets will not adhere to them. The adhesion of stimulated platelets to endothelial cells is powerfully inhibited by prostacyclin (PGI_2). This labile arachidonic acid metabolite is transiently synthesised and secreted by endothelium in response to a variety of agonists, notably including thrombin, bradykinin, adenosine diphosphate (ADP) and adenosine triphosphate (ATP) [13]. Thus mediators generated in plasma during coagulation and platelet aggregation induce a response from undamaged endothelium to limit the size of a forming thrombus. PGI_2 inhibits platelet stimulation by activating adenylate cyclase, and is additionally a powerful vasodilator in several vascular beds, acting by the same mechanism on vascular smooth muscle [14]. Endothelium-derived relaxing factor (EDRF) – another highly labile endothelial cell product released in response to similar stimuli – has been shown to interact synergistically with PGI_2 to inhibit platelet function [15].

Aggregating platelets release ATP and ADP, which both induce EDRF and PGI_2 release from endothelium. ADP is pro-aggregatory, recruiting platelets into the developing platelet plug. Endothelial cells possess nucleotide ectoenzymes which are responsible for the inactivation of these vasoactive metabolites, producing adenosine, (an inhibitor of platelet aggregation), which is then cleared from the circulation by uptake into endothelial cells and erythrocytes. Thus a series of interactions between adenosine metabolites and endothelium regulates vascular tone and platelet function [16].

Neutrophils adhere to endothelial cells preferentially. The blood pool of neutrophils is in dynamic equilibrium between freely circulating cells and a high proportion that is temporarily adherent to endothelium. Upregulation of this adhesive interaction, and of subsequent neutrophil emigration, is the mechanism by which inflammatory response is initiated. This can be achieved both by stimulation of the neutrophil, particularly by chemotactic agents, and by alteration of EC properties [17]. The most dramatic example of the latter is the development of greatly enhanced adhesiveness for neutrophils by cytokine- or lipopolysaccharide-treated endothelium. This is due to the novel surface expression of at least one specific endothelium-leukocyte adhesion molecule (ELAM-1). Macrophage-released cytokines may also increase leukocyte adherence to endothelial cells, and is probably of importance in the development of the atherosclerotic process (see below).

Smooth muscle cells biology

Smooth muscle cells are the only cell type present in the arterial media. In the normal young adult the major part of the cytoplasm is occupied by myofilaments located primarily towards the periphery of the cell. There are three types of these myofilaments; the vast majority are the thin type and consist of different types of actin, mysoin-containing thick filaments and intermediate filaments consisting of varying ratios of desmin and vimentin. In the rat, 51% of aortic medial cells contain vimentin only, while 48% contain both vimentin and desmin, and only 1% contain desmin alone. By contrast, fibroblasts contain only vimentin filaments [18].

Smooth muscle cells are responsible for maintaining vascular tone by contracting and relaxing, and vascular integrity by proliferation and synthesis of extracellular matrix [19].

Vascular smooth muscle cells exist in one of two phenotypes: either contractile or synthetic. In the latter, the numerous myofilament bundles are largely replaced by large amounts of rough endoplasmic reticulum, Golgi apparatus and free ribosomes. In practice most vascular smooth muscle cells show characteristics of both phenotypes. The cell phenotype can be modulated by cell interactions, alterations to extracellular matrix, or in response to other signals such as hormones. In particular, heparin and other glycosaminoglycans may control such phenotypic changes. When the smooth muscle cell is stimulated to migrate and proliferate it becomes more active synthetically, as well as becoming more responsive to stimuli causing cell proliferation.

Smooth muscle cells are the major cellular component in the mature atherosclerotic plaque and are primarily synthetic in character [20]. It had originally been thought that fibroblasts were the main cell type present in advanced atherosclerotic lesions, but the advent of electron microscopy and of immunohistochemical methods successfully differentiated these modified smooth muscle cells from other cell types which could contribute to the cellular components of the plaque [20]. Modifed smooth muscle cells are a major cell type trapping and processing cholesterol-rich lipids which enter the arterial lumen and are retained in the vessel wall. In addition, modified smooth muscle cells of the synthetic phenotype are responsibe for the production of extracellular matrix which is involved in the localization of low density lipoproteins (LDL) in the vessel wall. There is evidence that there may be important changes in arterial smooth muscle cells as they become incorporated into the atherosclerotic plaque, with probable monoclonal transformation of these cells [21].

The cellular pathology of atherosclerosis

The fatty streak is the earliest lesion of atherosclerosis, and appears to be a ubiquitous lesion. It is marked by the subendothelial aggregation of 'foam cells' whose cytoplasm is filled with lipid droplets, mostly free cholesterol and cholesteryl esters. This flat, lipid-rich area is commonly found even in children and also contains macrophages and some smooth muscle [22]. It is present in up to 10% of the aorta in children as young as 10 years, but in most situations it does not progress and can be regarded as a benign lesion. Particularly in children, the fatty streak is not necessarily found at sites where atherosclerotic plaque will develop later, with the exception of the coronary vessels, where fatty streaks are found in the precise locations where plaque is expected to develop. In studies on non-human hypercholesterolaemic primates, fatty streak-like lesions were the earliest to develop, and many of the advanced lesions of atherosclerosis occured at sites where fatty streaks were originally present [23]. So it would seem that fatty streaks are universal in occurrence and distribution, but only evolve into fibrous plaques in certain locations, and in predisposed individuals. Studies in which monoclonal antibodies were used as markers of macrophages and smooth muscle cells, have indicated that most foam cells are of macrophage origin in the fatty streak, and of smooth muscle cells origin in more advanced lesions [24]. T cells are also present in the fatty streak [25], but there is little extracellular lipid.

The fibrous plaque is found in more advanced atherosclerotic lesions and is made up of intimal smooth muscle cells surrounded by connective tissue matrix components, and variable amounts of intracellular and extracellular lipid. On the luminal surface this lesion is usually covered by a dense fibrous cap containing smooth muscle and connective tissue.

Accumulation of cholesterol within the arterial wall is an important characteristic of developing atherosclerotic lesions. In early lesions, cholestryl esters are found in foam cells in the intima. These foam cells may be modified macrophages [26] or smooth muscle cells [27]. They derive from macrophages by VLDL uptake, and perhaps also by way of LDL modification, which is recognized and taken up the acetyl-LDL receptor. The precise pathways by which foam cells are formed from smooth muscle cells remain unclear. Extracellular lipid is derived from entry of luminal lipids, and also from degenerating foam cells. Although in early atherosclerotic lesions, macrophages are the predominant lipid-loaded cells, while as the lesion develops, progressively more smooth muscle cells become lipid loaded. In more advanced lesions, and particularly in those with fibrosis, both free and esterifed cholesterol accumulates extracellularly. This cholesterol is thought to be derived from plasma lipoproteins containing apolipoprotein B, such as LDL and very low density lipoproteins (VLDL), while the apolipoprotein A1-containing lipoproteins (HDL) are believed to be important in the removal of cholesterol from the arterial wall [28]. Lipoproteins enter the arterial wall by passing through the endothelial monolayer. It appears that endothelial cells regulate the movement of lipoproteins, possibly by vesicular transport [29]. Hypercholesterolaemia can lead to an increase in endothelial permeability, even in the absence of endothelial loss [30, 31]. The interaction of lipoproteins with endothelial cells can modify the lipoproteins [32], and these modifications may affect subsequent interactions of the lipoproteins with other components of the arterial wall [33].

It is now agreed that macrophages, derived from blood monocytes, are a significant feature of human atherosclerotic lesions [34, 35] (Figure 1.1). These cells can contribute to lipid modifications and accumulation [36], and also secrete platelet-derived growth factor (PDGF)-like mitogens [37]. In view of the rapidly increasing knowledge of how leukocyte adhesion and emigration can be modulated by alterations of endothelial cell properties, it seems highly likely that the endothelium plays an active role in recruiting monocytes. Once present, macrophage-derived interleukin-1 (IL-1) could serve to maintain and amplify such alterations in endothelial cell function [8]. Macrophages also produce fibroblast growth factors and transforming growth factor a and b. The latter may stimulate the synthesis of proteoglycans by arterial smooth muscle cells.

Arterial smooth muscle cells within the intima (see below) also play an important role in the development of atherosclerotic lesions. A common feature of atherosclerosis is proliferation of intimal smooth muscle cells [38, 39]. Growth factors which may stimulate smooth muscle cells may be derived from platelets [40], macrophages [36] or endothelial cells [41]. While there is no doubt that growth factors may be released within the vessel wall, there has been some controversy concerning the role of circulating growth factors. Platelets secrete PDGF, epidermal growth factor, transforming growth factor b, and other less well-characterised mitogens. In a model of endothelial injury induced by homocystinaemia, sulphinpyrazone, an inhibitor of the platelet release reaction, has been shown to suppress the smooth muscle mitogenic response [42]. Insulin has been shown to stimulate the growth of many tissues [43], and there appears to be an association between hyperinsulinaemia and the development of atherosclerosis [44], and hyperinsulinaemia may be an independent risk factor for atherosclerosis. Insulin may have atherogenic effects on serum and arterial wall lipids [45], while chickens that are made hyperinsulinaemic by injecting insulin develop arterial lipid-containing lesions [46].

Inappropriate proliferation and migration of vascular smooth muscle cells is an important part of the pathogenesis of the lesion [33]. In most situations the intima contains few if any smooth muscle cells until the stimuli responsible for atherogenesis begin to induce smooth muscle cell migration from the media, and the consequent change to the synthetic phenotype. It is likely that smooth muscle cells migrate into the intima from the media in response to a variety of stimuli, and some growth factors have been shown to induce smooth muscle cell migration. Once in the intima, some smooth muscle cells accumulate cholesteryl ester, and so develop into foam cells,

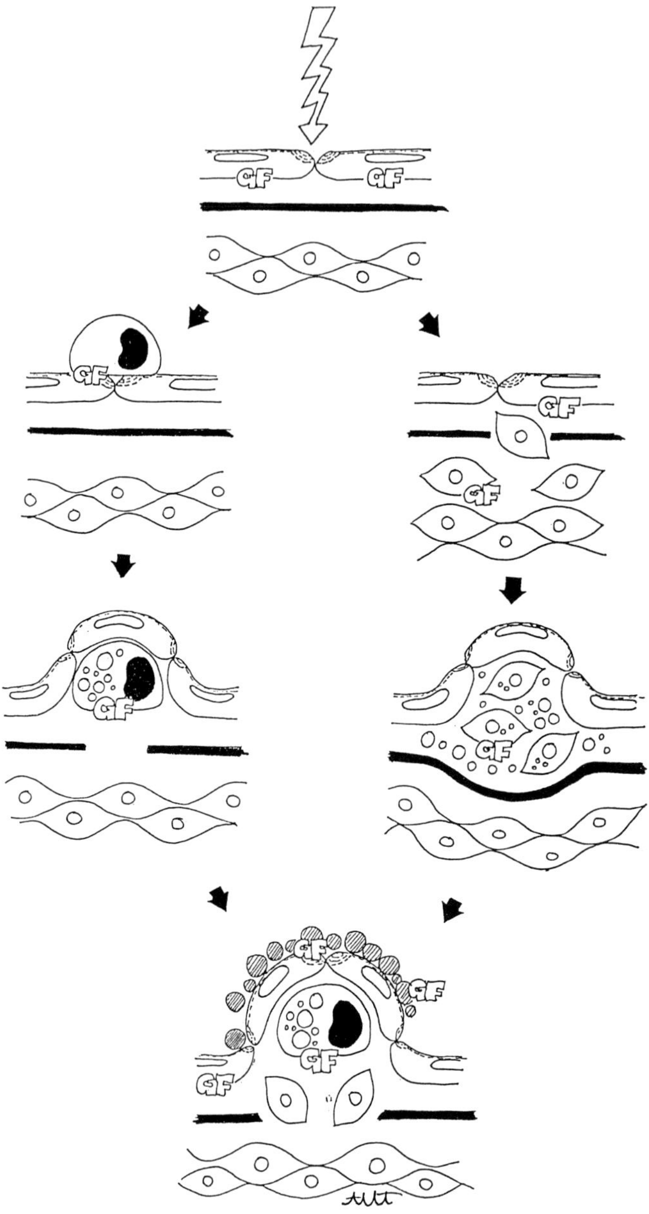
GF
GF
GF
GF
GF
GF
GF
GF
GF
GF
GF

while others accumulate little cholesteryl ester, and instead synthesis large amounts of connective tissue components. These ultimately form the fibromuscular cap which is common in advanced lesions [21].

Cell death and necrosis is an important aspect of the development of the advanced atherosclerotic plaque. *In vitro* studies [47] and studies of the developing atherosclerotic plaque in the hyperlipidaemic swine model of atherosclerosis [48], have indicated cell death is an invariable feature of plaque development. A number of toxic substances may lead to smooth muscle cell necrosis, including oxidized forms of cholesterol [49], peroxides of polyunsaturated fatty acids, and free radical generation within the plaque [50, 51]. Furthermore, there is some evidence that the action of monocytes and neutrophils may oxidize LDL to render it cytotoxic [52]. Local angiogenesis, with endothelial cell profileration is frequently found near these necrotic areas, and may reflect local release of growth factors which act on endothelial cells, for instance fibroblast growth factor [53].

Endothelial cells in culture produce a vascular smooth muscle cell mitogen indistinguishable from PDGF [41], as well as a separate factor which supports the growth of other endothelial cells [54]. It appears that once smooth muscle cell profileration has been set in motion, it is difficult to stop it. Smooth muscle cells from human atheroma have been shown to transcribe the genes for PDGF, and to produce PDGF-like molecules [55]. However, *in vivo* observations that intact endothelium inhibits intimal smooth muscle cell proliferation have led to the demonstration that heparin-like oligosccharides secreted by endothelial cells powerfully inhibit smooth muscle cell growth [56]. These effects are dose-dependent and specific to smooth muscle cells. Heparin, either the anticoagulant or non-anticoagulant species, has been shown to be the most effective glycosaminoglycan at preventing smooth muscle cell growth, raising the possibility that it may have therapeutic potential. Similar anti-proliferative effects have been shown with heparan

Figure 1.1. The revised response to injury hypothesis of atherogenesis [Based on Ross 1986 (Ref 34)]. Intimal proliferation may occur by at least two separate pathways. Injury to endothelium is the primary event, and this injury may lead to the release of smooth muscle cell mitogens (GF) by endothelial cells. On the left endothelial damage is followed by monocyte adhesion, and persistent release of growth factor. Subsequently monocytes migrate through the endothelial monolayer, and lead to the formation of the fatty streak. Further growth factor release leads to the formation of fibrous plaque. Monocytes may also injure or stimulate the overlying endothelium, resulting in platelet attachment. Finally endothelial cells, monocytes and platelets continue to secrete factors, as may neo-intimal smooth muscle cells. On the right, injured but intact endothelium increases its turnover and production of smooth muscle cell mitogens. These growth factors lead to smooth muscle cell migrating from the media to the intima. These migrating smooth muscle cells also produce growth factor – probably PDGF. The interaction of endothelial and smooth muscle cell growth factors lead to fibrous plaque formation. (Reproduced from Ref 2, by permission of the Editor, Journal of the Royal College of Physicians.

sulphate. There has been considerable progress in identifying the chemical structures involved in the antiproliferative effect, indicating a minimum polysaccharide length of five monosaccharides, and the necessary presence of a $O\text{-}SO_3^-$ group in heparin [57].

There is an interplay of growth factors within the vessel wall. Under normal conditions smooth muscle cells in the media are surrounded by extracellular matrix, and their position behind the endothelial cell monolayer prevents them being exposed to circulating platelet- and monocyte-derived growth factors. Endothelial cells themselves secrete low amounts of PDGF and thrombospondin, both of which promote smooth muscle cell proliferation and migration. It is postulated that the effects of these compounds are counterbalanced by matrix heparin and heparan sulphate. Smooth muscle cells themselves synthesis and secrete matrix associated macromolecules, including heparan sulphate and thrombospondin. Smooth muscle cell thrombospondin is released only when the cell is stimulated by low levels of PDGF, while heparin prevents thrombospondin synthesis [58]. The control by matrix macromolecules may be over-ridden if the endothelial cell monolayer is perturbed, allowing access of circulating growth factors to the smooth muscle cells. It is also of interest that while chondroitin and dermatan sulphate proteoglycans increase in atherosclerotic lesions, there is little change, or even a decrease in the anti-proliferative heparan sulphate proteoglycan [59].

The atherogenetic process

Atherosclerosis can be seen as a response of the vascular wall to injury, and it has many of the features of the inflammatory response in other tissues [60]. Endothelial cell damage or dysfunction is widely regarded as a critical initiating factor [33, 38] (Figure 1.1). Frank endothelial cell damage may promote at least two atherogenic processes. First, it reduces the significant barrier to lipoprotein accumulation within the vessel wall. Second, it initiates smooth muscle cell migration and proliferation, as suggested above.

An important, and incompletely understood question is why atherosclerosis develops primarily at certain sites in the vasculature. Although it occurs primarily at sites of turbulence where there is shear stress and disturbed flow, this is not the whole explanation. The distribution of lesions is heterogenous both between and within individuals. For example, some patients have disease only in the coronary arteries and not in the cerebral circulation, or vice versa, while others have severe atherosclerosis throughout the aorta, but clear coronaries.

Mechanical damage to endothelium can lead to lipid-rich atherosclerotic lesions in normalipidaemic animals [61]. Homocystinaemia, which causes endothelial cell injury, is associated with aggressive premature atherosclerosis [62, 63], while accelerated peripheral vascular and cerebral occlusive disease occurs even in heterozygotes [64]. Hypertension, a recognized risk factor for ischaemic heart disease, has been shown to disrupt endothelial integrity [65]. Regenerated endothelium has properties, related either to increased permeability to lipoproteins or altered lipoprotein metabolism, that enhance intimal lipid accumulation [66].

Both viral and immunological injury to endothelium have been implicated in atherogenesis. Human endothelial cells can be infected with several viruses, including herpes viruses [67], and this virus has been shown to induce atherosclerosis in animals [68]. The possibility of immunological involvement in accelerated atherosclerosis derives from clinical observations in certain patients with auto-immune diseases including rheumatic fever [69], systemic lupus erythematosus [70, 71], and rheumatoid arthritis [72], and the finding that rapidly progressive atherosclerosis is one of the most important long-term complications of graft rejection [73]. A possible role for immunological injury *in vivo* has been suggested in a number of different experimental models, including one in which endothelial cells were used as immunogen [74–76].

Finally, endothelial cell dysfunction, particularly in relation to the maintenance of thromboresistance or vascular tone, may play a critical role in the precipitating events of myocardial ischaemia: thrombus formation or vasospasm. Arterial thrombosis is usually precipitated by rupture of an atherosclerotic plaque. Until recently there has been no evidence linking thrombosis to the earlier process of plaque formation. However, if now emerges that lipoprotein(a), a variant of LDL, promotes coagulation and is an independent risk factor for atherosclerosis. Lp(a) is a physiological inhibitor of plasminogen activation, and so prevents unopposed plasmin generation [77, 78]. Plasminogen-binding sites are widely distributed on vascular endothelial cells, which also secrete and bind tPA. The close association of binding sites for plasminogen and tPA accelerates tPA-mediated plasmin generation, and it is likely that surface binding protects plasmin and tPA from their inhibitors. Lp(a) competes with plasminogen for the plasminogen binding site but has no effect on the fluid-phase activity of plasmin. There is a marked accumulation of Lp(a) on the endothelium of atherosclerotic coronary arteries, but not in normal blood vessels [78]. Plasminogen is readily detectable in normal vessels, but not in atherosclerotic vessels. Patients with familial hypercholesterolaemia show a three-fold increase in plasma Lp(a), and those with the highest Lp(a) levels are at the greatest risk of developing coronary artery disease. Plasma concentration of Lp(a) is influenced by metabolic factors such as diabetes mellitus and nephrotic syndrome, in which cases it increases, while it is decreased by dietary fish oil [79].

Disturbances in endothelial cell function may lead to vascular spasm. It has recently been shown that atherosclerotic segments of coronary artery fail to dilate *in vivo* during infusion of acetylcholine (a potent stimulus for release of EDRF) and respond with paradoxical vasospasm [80].

Summary

Hyperlipidaemia, or some component of hyperlipidaemic serum as well as other risk factors, such as cigarette smoking, cause endothelial cells injury, resulting in platelet and/or monocyte adhesion and emigration, and release of growth factors, which lead to smooth muscle migration and proliferation. Foam cells derived from both macrophages and smooth muscle cells may already be found in the fatty streak, and always form within the atherosclerotic lesion. We are now close to being able to provide a complete pathophysiological and biochemical description of atherosclerosis, which will inevitably contribute to our ability to treat, and perhaps to prevent, this disease.

References

1. Wight TN. Cell biology of arterial proteoglycans. Arteriosclerosis 1989; 9:1.
2. Petty RG, Pearson JD. Endothelium – the axis of vascular health and disease. J Roy Coll Phys 1989; 23:92.
3. Sage H. Collagen synthesis by endothelial cells in culture. In: Jaffe EA (ed). Biology of Endothelial Cells. Martinus Nijhoff, Boston 1984; 161.
4. Madri JA, Pratt BM, Yannariello-Brown J. Matrix-driven cell size change modulates aortic endothelial cell proliferation and sheet migration. Am J Pathol 1988; 132:18.
5. DeGroot PG, Sixma JJ. Role of von Willebrand factor in the vessel wall. Semin Haemostas Thromb 1987; 13:416.
6. Rodgers GM, Greenberg CS, Shuman MA. Characterisation of the effects of cultured vascular cells on the activation of blood coagulation. Blood 1983; 61:1155.
7. Johnsen ULH, Lyberg T, Galdal KS, Prydz H. Platelets stimulate thromboplastin synthesis in human endothelial cells. Thromb Haemost 1983; 49:69.
8. Mantovani A, Dejana E. Modulation of endothelial function by interleukin-1. A novel target for pharmacological intervention? Biochem Pharmacol 1987; 36:301.
9. Machovich R. Choices among the possible reaction routes catalysed by thrombin. Ann NY Acad Sci 1986; 485:170.
10. Esmon NL. Thrombomodulin. Semin Haemostas Thrombosis 1987; 13:454.
11. Stern DM, Brett J, Harris IC, Nawroth PP. Participation of endothelial cells in the protein C-protein S anticoagulant pathway. J Cell Biol 1986; 102:1971.
12. Hekman CM, Loskutoff DJ. Fibrinolytic pathways and the endothelium. Semin Haemostas Thrombosis 1987; 13:514.
13. Jaffe EA. Cell biology of Endothelial Cells. Hum Pathol 1987; 18:234.
14. Moncada S. Biological importance of prostacyclin. Br J Pharmacol 1982; 76:3.
15. Radomski MW, Palmer RMS, Moncada S. Comparative pharmacology of endothelium-

dependent relaxing factor, nitric oxide and prostacyclin in platelets. B J Pharm 1987; 92:181.
16. Pearson J D, Gordon J L. Nucleotide metabolism by endothelium. Ann Rev Physiol 1985; 47:617.
17. Harlan J M. Leukocyte-endothelial interactions. Blood 1985; 65:513.
18. Gabbiani G, Kocher O, Bloom W S, Vandekerckhove J, Weber K. Actin expression in smooth muscle cells of rat aortic intimal thickening, human atheromatous plaque, and cultured rat aortic media. J Clin Invest 1984; 73:148.
19. Chamley-Campbell J H, Campbell G R, Ross R. The smooth muscle cell in culture. Physiol Rev 1979; 59:1.
20. Campbell G R, Chamley-Campbell J H. The cellular pathobiology of atherosclerosis. Pathology 1981; 13:423.
21. Benditt E P, Benditt J M. Evidence for a monoclonal origin for human atherosclerotic plaques. Proc Natl Acad Sci USA 1973; 70:1753.
22. Stary H C, Malinow M R. Ultrastructure of experimental coronary artery atherosclerosis in Cynomolgus macaques. A comparison with the lesions of other primates. Atherosclerosis 1982; 43:151.
23. Faggioto A, Ross R. Studies of hypercholesterolemia in the nonhuman primate: II. Fatty streak conversion to fibrous plaque. Arteriosclerosis 1984; 4:341.
24. Aquel N M, Ball R Y, Waldman H, Mitchinson M J. Identification of macrophages and smoot muscle cells in human atheroma using monoclonal antibodies. J Pathol 1985; 146:197.
25. Munro J M, van der Walt J D, Munro C S, Chalmers J A C, Cox E L. An immunohistochemical analysis of human aortic fatty streaks. Hum Pathol 1987; 18:375.
26. Fowler S, Shio H, Haley N J. Characterization of lipid-laden aortic cells from cholesterol-fed rabbits. IV. Investigation of macrophage-like properties of aortic cell populations. Lab Invest 1979; 41:372.
27. Ghidoni J J, O'Neal R M. Recent advances in molecular pathology. A review of ultrastructure of human atheroma. Exp Mol Pathol 1967; 7:378.
28. Picardo M, Massey J B, Kuhn D E *et al.* Partially reassembled high density lipoproteins. Effect on cholesterol flux synthesis and esterification in normal skin fibroblasts. Arteriosclerosis 1986; 6:434.
29. Stein O, Stein Y, Eisenberg S. A radiographic study of the transport of 1251-labelled serum lipoproteins in rat aorta. Z Mikr-Anat Forsch 1973; 138:223.
30. Stemerman M B. Effects of moderate hypercholesterolemia on rabbit endothelium. Arteriosclerosis 1981; 1:25.
31. Navab M, Hough G P, Berliner J *et al.* Rabbit beta-migrating very low density lipoprotein increases endothelial macromeolecular transport without altering electrical resistance. J Clin Invest 1986; 78:389.
32. Henricksen T, Mahoney E M, Steinberg D. Enhanced macrophage degradation of biologically modified low density lipoprotein. Arteriosclerosis 1983; 3:149.
33. Thomas W A, Lee K T, Reiner J M, Kim D N, Florentin R A, Scott R F, Schmee J. Population dynamics of arterial cells during atherogenesis. XII. Mitogenic and cytotoxic effects of a hyperlipidemic (HL) diet on cells in advanced lesions in the abdominal aorta of swine fed an HL diet for 270–345 days. Exp Mol Pathol 1983; 39:257.
34. Ross R. The pathogenesis of atherosclerosis – an update. N Engl J Med 1986; 314:488.
35. Mitchinson M J, Ball R Y. Macrophages and atherogenesis. Lancet 1987; II:146.
36. Steinberg D S. Lipoproteins and the pathogenesis of artherosclerosis. Circulation 1987; 76:508.
37. Shimokado K, Raines E W, Madtes D K *et al.* A significant part of macrophage-derived growth factor consists of at least two forms of PDGF. Cell 1985; 43:277.

38. Clarkson T B, Weingard K W, Kaplan J R, Adams M R. Mechanism of atherogenesis. Circulation 1987; 76 (Suppl I): I–20.
39. Davies P F. Vascular cell interactions with special reference to the pathogenesis of atherosclerosis. Lab Invest 1986; 55:5.
40. Ross R, Glomset J, Kariya B, Harker L. A platelet-dependent serum factor that stimulates the proliferation of arterial smooth muscle cells *in vitro*. Proc Natl Acad Sci USA 1974; 71:1207.
41. DiCorletto P E, Bowen-Pope D F. Cultured endothelial cells produce a platelet-derived growth factor-like protein. Proc Natl Acad Sci USA 1983; 80:1919.
42. Harker L A, Marlan J M, Ross R. Effect of sulfinpyrazone on homocstein-induced endothelial injury and arteriosclerosis in baboons. Circ Res 1983; 53:731.
43. Straus D S. Growth-stimulatory actions of insulin *in vitro* and *in vivo*. Endocrine Rev 1985; 5:359.
44. Stern M P, Haffner S M. Body fat distribution and hyperinsulinaemia as risk factors for diabetes and cardiovascular disease. Arteriosclerosis 1986; 6:123.
45. Stout R. Insulin and atheroma – an update. Lancet 1987; I:1077.
46. Stout R W, Buchanan K D, Vallance-Owen J. The relationship of arterial disease and glucagon metabolism in insulin-treated chickens. Atherosclerosis 1973; 18:153.
47. Chen R M, Getz G S, Fisher-Dzoga K, Wissler R W. The role of hyperlipidemic serum on the proliferation and necrosis of aortic medial cells *in vitro*. Exp Mol Pathol 1977; 26:359.
48. Thomas W A, Lee K T, Reiner J M, Kim D N, Florentin R A, Scott R F, Schmee J. Population dynamics of arterial cells during atherogenesis. XII. Mitogenic and cytotoxic effects of a hyperlipidemic (HL) diet on cells in advanced lesions in the abdominal aorta of swine fed an HL diet for 270–345 days. Exp Mol Pathol 1983; 39:257.
49. Peng S K, Taylor C B, Mosbach E H, Huang W Y, Hill J. Mikkelson B. Distribution of 25-hydroxycholesterol in plasma lipoprotein and its role in atherogenesis: A study in squirrel monkeys. Atherosclerosis 1982; 41:395.
50. Belch J J F, Chopra M, Hutchinson S. Free radical pathology in chronic arterial disease. Free Rad Biol Med 1989; 6:375.
51. Stringer M D, Gorog P G, Freeman A, Kakkar V V. Lipid peroxides and atherosclerosis. Br Med J 1989; 298:281.
52. Cathcart M K, Morel D W, Chisholm G M. Monocytes and neutrophils oxidize density lipoprotein making it cytotoxic. J Leukocyte Biol 1985; 38:341.
53. Klagsbrun M, Edelman E R. Biological and biochemical properties of fibroblast growth factors. Implications for the pathogenesis of atherosclerosis. Arteriosclerosis 1989; 9:269.
54. Gajdusek C M, Schwartz S M. Ability of endothelial cells to condition culture medium. J Cell Physiol 1982; 110:35.
55. Libby P, Warner S J C, Salomon R N. Production of platelet-derived growth factor-like mitogen by smooth muscle cells from human atheroma. N Engl J Med 1988; 318:1493.
56. Castellot J, Addonizo M L, Rosenberg R *et al.* Cultured endothelial cell produce a heparin-like inhibitor of smooth muscle cell growth. J Cell Biol 1981; 90:372.
57. Castellot J J, Choay I J, Lormeau J C, Petitou M, Sache E, Karnovsky M J. Structural determinants of the capacity of heparin to inhibit the proliferation of vascular smooth muscle smooth muscle cells. II. Evidence for a pentasaccharide sequence that contains a 3-O-sulfate group. J Cell Biol 1986; 107:1979.
58. Majack R A, Cook S C, Bornstein P. Control of smooth muscle cell growth by components of extracellular matrix. Autocrine role for thrombospondin. Proc Natl Acad Sci USA 1986; 83:9050.
59. Dalfreres E R, Radhakrishnamurthy B, Ruiz H A, Berenson G S. Composition of proteoglycans from human atherosclerotic lesions. Exp Mol Pathol 1987; 47:363.
60. Munro J M, Cotran R S. The pathogenesis of atherosclerosis: atherogenesis and inflammation. Lab Invest 1989; 58:249.

61. Moore S. Thromboatherosclerosis in normolipemic rabbits; a result of continued endothelial damage. Lab Invest 1973; 29:478.
62. Harker L A, Ross R, Schlichter S J, Scott C R. Homocystine-induced arterioclerosis. The role of endothelial injury and platelet response in its genesis. J Clin Invest 1976; 58:731.
63. De Groot P G, Willems C, Boers G H J, Gonsalves M D, Van Aken W G, Van Mourik J A. Endothelial cell dysfunction in homocystinuria. Eur J Clin Invest 1983; 13:405.
64. Boers G, Smals A, Trijbels F *et al.* Heterozygosity for homocystinuria in premature periphery and cerebral occlusive arterial disease. N Engl J Med 1985; 313:709.
65. Reidy MA, Schwartz S M. A technique to investigate surface morphology and endothelial cell replication of small arteries; a study in acute angiotensin-induced hypertension. Microvasc Res 1982; 24:158.
66. Minick C R, Stemmerman M B, Insull W. Effect of regenerated endothelium on lipid accumulation in arterial wall. Proc Natl Acad Sci USA 1977; 74:1724.
67. Bruggeman C A, Debie W H, Muller A D, Schutte B, van-Dam-Mieras M C. Cytomegalovirus alters the von Willebrand factor content in human endothelial cells. Thromb Haemost 1988; 59:264.
68. Fabricant C G. Herpes-induced atherosclerosis. Diabetes 1981; 30 (Suppl. 2):29.
69. Zeek P. Studies in atherosclerosis. II. Atheroma and its sequelae in rheumatic heart disease. Amer I Med Sci 1932; 184:356.
70. Tsakraklides V G, Bleiden L C, Edwards J E. Coronary atherosclerosis and myocardial infarction associated with systemic lupus erythematosus. Am Heart J 1974; 87:634.
71. Bulkley B H, Roberts W C. The heart in systemic lupus erythematosus and the changes induced in it by corticosteroids. Am J Med 1975; 58:243.
72. Bywaters E G L. Peripheral vascular obstruction in rheumatoid arthritis and its relationship to other vascular lesions. Ann Rheum Dis 1957; 16:84.
73. Rider A K, Copeland J C, Hunt S A *et al.* The status of cardiac transplantation. Circulation 1975; 52:531.
74. Klimov A N, Yu N Z, Nagornev V A. Immunochemical aspects of atherosclerosis. Atherosclerosis Rev, Vol. 4, 1979, Ed. Paoletti R. and Gotto A M.:119.
75. Klurfeld D M. Interactions of immune function with lipids and atherosclerosis. C R C Crit Rev Toxicol 1981; 11:333.
76. Klurfeld D M, Weber M M, Levine E M, Mueller S N, Kritchevsky D. Increased atherosclerosis in rabbits immunized with endothelial cells. Atherosclerosis 1985; 55:283.
77. Miles L A, Fless G M, Levin E G, Scance A M, Plow E F. A potential basis for the thrombotic risks associated with lipoprotein (a). Nature 1989; 339:301.
78. Hajjar K A, Gavich D, Breslow J L, Nachman R L. Lipoprotein (a) modulation of endothelial cell surface fibrinolysis and its potential role in atherosclerosis. Nature 1989; 339:303.
79. Rainwater D L, Manis G S, VandeBerg J L. Hereditary and dietary effects on apolipoprotein (a) isoforms and Lp(a) in baboons. J Lipid Res 1989; 30:549.
80. Ludmer P L, Selwyn A P, Shook T L *et al.* Paradoxical vasoconstriction by acetylcholine in atherosclerotic coronary arteries. N Engl J Med 1986; 315:1046.

2. The pathology of atherosclerosis

ASEEL N. FATTAH and ABDUL-KADIR ABDULLA

Atherosclerosis is a disease of large and medium sized muscular arteries (e.g. coronary, carotid and arteries of the lower limbs) and the elastic arteries such as the aorta and iliac vessels. It is a long term process which starts early in life. The process may reflect the haemeostatic imbalance of the vessel wall and its attempt to restore its protective intimal covering [1]. The basic lesion (the atheroma or fibrofatty plaque) consists of a raised focal plaque within the intima, having a core of lipid (mainly cholesterol, usually complexed to proteins and cholesterol esters) and a covering fibrous cap. These atheromata are sparsely distributed at first but as the disease advances they become more numerous and sometimes cover the entire intimal surface of the severely affected arteries.

Epidermiology and incidence

Death from ischaemic heart disease in England and Wales is among the highest in the world [2] although it has been superseded by Finland, Scotland and USA. Conversly the rate is remarkably lower in Asia, Africa and South and Central America. In 1986 statistics, it has been shown that death from ischaemic heart disease increases with age groups. The trend shows an increase in the incidence from the age of 25 onward. From the age of 80 years onward the incidence of the disease is higher in females than in males.

In the age group 25–44 the incidence of the disease is highest in Scotland both in men and women. This is followed by Northern Ireland. The lowest incidence among this age group is in England and Wales.

In the age group 45–64 years, the pattern of the disease changes in that the incidence in Northern Ireland increases in men and women and exceeds that in Scotland, while England and Wales maintain a lower incidence. In

A.-M. Salmasi and A. N. Nicolaides (eds.), Occult Atherosclerotic Disease, 19–31.

the age group 64–84 the pattern changes again in that Scotland becomes highest for men and women followed by Northern Ireland then England and Wales. In the age group 85 and over, however, the incidence in Northern Ireland becomes highest for men and women followed by Scotland then England and Wales.

Pathophysiology of atherosclerosis

There has been great advances during the past two decades in our understanding of the pathogenesis of atherosclerosis. These have been derived mainly from modern epidermiological studies [3–5] and intensified clinico pathological investigations, [6, 7] as well as improved animal model research [8, 9], pioneering cellular pathobiological [10–13] and molecular biochemical studies [14, 15].

The current concept emphasises that the impairment of endothelial function and structure plays a key role in the pathogenesis of atherosclerosis [16]. This concept is illustrated in detail in the Reaction to Injury Theory. This theory, formulated by Ross and Glomset in 1976 and modified in 1986 [17], states that atherosclerotic changes are initiated as a response to some form of injury to the arterial endothelium [18]. The endothelial injuries in experimental animals induced by mechanical denudation, immune complex, deposition, irradiation, and chemical substances lead to desquamation of endothelial cells which result in increase permability to plasma constituents including lipid and permit platelets and monocytes to adhere to subendothelial connective tissue. The initial interaction of platelets with the damaged surface is important in stimulating the smooth muscle cell changes that can occur with the loss of the endothelium and exposure of the subendothelium. Platelet derived growth factor (PDGF) released from the activated platelet stimulates smooth muscle cell proliferation and smooth muscle cell migration from the media to the intima [19]. It has been suggested that only smooth muscle cells in the synthetic states (in contrast to the contractile state) can be stimulated to proliferate [20]. Platelets may also influence smooth muscle proliferation by releasing heparitinase and platelet factor 4. Glycosaminoglycans have been implicated in the regulation of smooth muscle cells proliferation [21]. It has been shown that the normal vessel wall contains heperans and proteoglycans that inhibit smooth muscle cell proliferation. The factors released from the stimulated platelets inactivate these inhibitory substances so that smooth muscle cells are released from growth inhibition [20].

The role of macrophages

It is well known that subendothelial migration and localization of macrophages is the earliest events in fatty streak formation. Macrophages have receptors for both native and modified LDL [22–23]. The capacity of the macrophages to take up these lipoproteins and to de-esterify and re-esterify cholesterol may be important in their ability to accumulate lipid and become foam cells. The sub-endothelial localization of macrophages and the phagocytosis of extracellular material are probably normal functions of the macrophages.

In hypercholesteremia the earliest cellular interactions is the attachment of monocytes to endothelial cells [24–26]. The macrophages/monocytes are preferentially adherent to injured or regenerating endothelial cells in culture.

Bevilaequa *et al.* [27] found that interlukin-1, a product of both macrophages and endothelial cells will enhance adherence of neutorphils and monocytes to arterial endothelium. Also the macrophages produce one of the most potent chemoattractant known leukotriene 30 (product of lipoxygenase system).

This and other lipoxygenase products may be very important in modulating the artery wall during and after atherosclerosis. Macrophages can injure the neighbouring cells by forming toxic substance such as superoxide anion and lysosomal hydrolases and by oxidising lipid. Thus the subendotheial migrating macrophages may injure the overlying endothelium. In this sense development of a fatty streak could be considered to represent an inflammatory response to local changes in the wall of the artery [28].

Activated macrophages secrete growth factors for fibroblasts, smooth muscle cells and endothelium [29]. The fibroblast growth factor secreted by macrophages is a potent mitogen for connective tissue cells and endothelial cells [30].

The role of viruses

The role of the viruses as a causative agent of atherosclerosis has been strongly supported by the experimental atherosclerosis. However the evidence in human from the electron microscopic and immunofluorescent studies was only suggestive and less compelling than the experimental work in animals.

In late 1940 Patterson and Cottal showed that there was a strong association between coronary atherosclerosis and lymphomatosis, known as

Marek's disease in the chicken. A decade later, it was discovered that the causative agent of Marek's disease is Herpes type virus. The virus was then called Marek's virus (MDV) [31].

The same observation was noted by fabricant and associates in 1978 [32] who found that infected chickens with MDV have lymphomatous disease and vascular changes resembling human atherosclerosis. Subsequent work by Melnik *et al.* [33] showed that a macroscopical evidence of atherosclerosis was seen in 14% of the animals infected with MDV. Microscopical changes were also seen in 65%. However none of these changes were seen in the control group.

Experimental work, by using immunofluorescent technique, showed that vascular muscle contained MDV despite the absence of endothelial injury. These findings suggest that viral transformation [33] of vascular smooth muscle might be of critical aetiological significance in atherosclerosis, and that the endothelial cell damage may not be required for the initiation of the disease process.

Fabricant and colleagues in 1981 [34] studied the effect of MDV on the metabolism of lipid by the cultured chicken aortic smooth muscle cell. It was found that the infected cells contained significantly higher amount of cholesterol, cholestrol esters, fatty acids and triglycerides. The total lipid was also higher than those in the uninfected cells.

The degree of athersclerosis of the ascending aorta in patients who died from coxsakie virus myocarditis is out of proportion compared to the age and the definable risk factors in these patients. More recent work has shown that herpes virus can alter the cellular metabolism and the lipid content and composition in human arterial smooth muscle cells, inducing similar changes to those produced by MDV in chickens [35].

The viral infection may prove to be an important factor in the initiation of atherosclerosis. Viruses may act as an injurious agent by altering the cellular lipid metabolism. This is compatible with response to injury hypothesis.

Risk factors

It is important to demonstrate the contribution of the following risk factors in the pathogenosis of atherosclerosis. Their effect compliment the injury theory in the causation of atherosclerosis.

Lipid and atherosclerosis

Long standing elevated levels of plasma lipoprotein particularly LDL and ULDL have been associated with an increased incidence of atherosclerosis. In many epidemiological studies [36, 37] the decrease in cholesterol levels was correlated with a reduction in the incidence of atherosclerosis. The cells contain specific receptors for LDL which control cholesterol metabolism. The number of LDL receptors displayed by a cell varies with the need of the cell for cholesterol. This protects the cell against excess cholesterol. However when the number of LDL receptors decreases this also leads to decrease in removal of LDL from the circulation and increase in plasma LDL [38, 39].

Hypercholesterolaemia may induce a subtle form of injury to endothelium. The endothelium may be injured by chronic exposure to high levels of LDL [40]. Alterations in the cholesterol phospholipid ratio of the plasma membrane of cells may lead to an increase in membrane viscosity. Such changes might decrease the malleability of endothelial cells particularly at anatomical sites such as branches or bifurcations where they are exposed to changes in blood flow. Another explanation of how endothelium may be injured in hypercholestrolaemia is that when LDL exposed to macrophages is oxidized and is toxic to fibroblasts in culture [41]. The oxidised LDL is toxic to endothelium. It could be an important source of endothelial injury which may explain the changes occurred during progression of fatty streaks to more advanced lesion.

Diabetes mellitus

Autopsy study showed that diabetes is associated with high incidence of atherosclerosis. The early development of atherosclerosis in diabetes is due to abnormal metabolic factor e.g. high blood glucose or abnormal and high plasma lipids. Raised plasma Von Will-brand factor is probably associated with vessel wall injury in diabetic patients [42].

This therefore may decrease the vessel wall ability to synthesise prostacyclin. It has been claimed that diabetes increases platelets adhesiveness and responds to aggregating agents [43]. However it has not been established whether the thrombo-embolic complications of atherosclerosis in diabetics is the result of platelets hypersensitivity or the result of vessel wall changes that promote platelet adhesion.

Blood flow and hypertension

The blood flow acts as a mechanical factor which may damage or dislodge endothelial cells. Examples of such factors are the wall shear at areas of tight stenosis in an artery [44–46]. The flow disturbance in narrowed arteries promotes platelets aggregation. [45–47]. The low velocity of blood and flow separation has been implicated in the causation of early atherosclerosis.

Most patients with hypertension have a significant coronary atherosclerosis, so it is regarded as an important predisposing factor. Kannel and Sytkowski [48] emphasised that the haemodynamic process plays important role in the causation of vessel wall injury.

Immunological injury

It has been demonstrated that immunologically induced arterial injury may promote the development of atherosclerosis in human arteries [49]. Also vascular injuries induced by circulating immune complexes especially in areas of blood flow disturbance [50–52]. The antigen antibody complexes causes platelets aggregations which in turn causes local vasculitis [53–55]. The aggregated platelets release their granules contents which may indirectly damage the vessel wall.

Other factors like Bacteria can cause platelet aggregate and release of their granules.

Smoking

Epidemiological studies have shown that there is a clear relationship between smoking and the risk of dying from coronary heart disease [48]. The extent of atherosclerosis was greater in heavy smokers than non smokers [56]. In experimental animals it was found that smoking reduced the production of prostacycline and its inhibitory effect on the platelets [57–59]. In experimental animals smoking enhances platelet aggregation and causes obstruction of flow in stenosed coronary arteries [58].

Smoking has not only been implicated in the pathogenosis of atherosclerosis but also in its thromboembolic complications.

Obesity

There is clear association between obesity and atherosclerosis, although most of the risk is the consequence of the associated hypertension, hyperlipidaemia and diabetes. However a small increased risk can be a ascribed to obesity.

Homocystineamia

Homocystineamia has been found to be associated with endothelial cell injury, early development of atherosclerosis and its thromboembolic complication [61].

Stress and catecholamine

Siltanon [62] has found an association between stress and coronary artery disease. Levin and associates [63] demonstrated that in man, emotional stresses cause the release of platelets granules in the circulation and increase the concentration of epinephrine and norepinephrine in the plasma. However it has been found that the raised catecholamine level in the blood which has been caused by stress is insufficient to cause platelet aggregation, but they may potentiate the effect of other aggregating agent. Gordon *et al.* [64] demonstrated that stressful stimuli induce structural changes in the arterial intima of the experimental animals.

Other theories of atherosclerosis

Although the endothelial injury with the effect of risk factors is the most solid explanation for atherosclerosis, the development of the atheromatous plaque could also be explained if smooth muscle proliferation was the initial event. The endothelial injury may be then a secondary phenomenon. The monotypic nature of the smooth muscle cells in the plaque was interpreted by Benditt and Benditt [65] as evidence that plaques may be equivalent to benign monoclonal neoplastic role such as leiomyoma. These may be initiated by mutation [66]. The mutagenic effect may be from an exogeneous chemical (e.g. hydrocarbons) or endogenous metabolite (e.g. cholesterol or some of its oxidants) or a virus. All this has been given the terminology of a monoclonal hypothesis of atherogenesis.

Morphology

The morphological changes which are seen in the arteries of patients with atherosclerosis are variable. But there are two well-documented lesions: (a) fatty streaks; (b) atheromatous plaque. Arteries of patients with occult atherosclerosis may show different stages of the disease, even the superadded complications.

(a) *Fatty streaks* These lesions appear in the aortae of all children older than one year regardless of the geography, race, sex or the environment. Macroscopically they are yellow, flat spots, less than 1 mm in diameter. They grow in size into elongated streaks 1–2 mm wide and 1 cm in length or even longer. Microscopically the lesion is composed of elongated smooth muscle, lipid laden macrophages, extra cellular lipid and few T lymphocytes. Their distribution is mainly in the abdominal aorta and around the ostia of its major branches. The coronary arteries, the thoracic aorta and the arteries of the circle of willis are also involved.

The significance of fatty streaks is because of the disturbance of blood flow that may result. This may therefore be the precusor of the atheromatous plaques. The lesions increase with age from about 10% in the first decade to 30–50% in the 3rd decade. They subsequently decrease in number as the atheromatous plaques predominate.

(b) *Atheromatous plaque* This is the fundamental lesion of atherosclerosis. Macroscopically they are white to whitish-yellow in appearance. They protrude into the lumen of the artery and vary in size diameter from 0.3 to 1.5 cm. They may coalesce to form a larger mass.

Microscopically the plaque consists of a fibrous cap which is composed of smooth muscle cells, few leucocytes and dense connective tissue. The connective tissue includes collagen, elastic fibre and proteoglycans. Beneath and to the side of the cap there are mixtures of smooth muscle cell, macrophages and T lymphocytes. The necrotic core of the plaque is com-

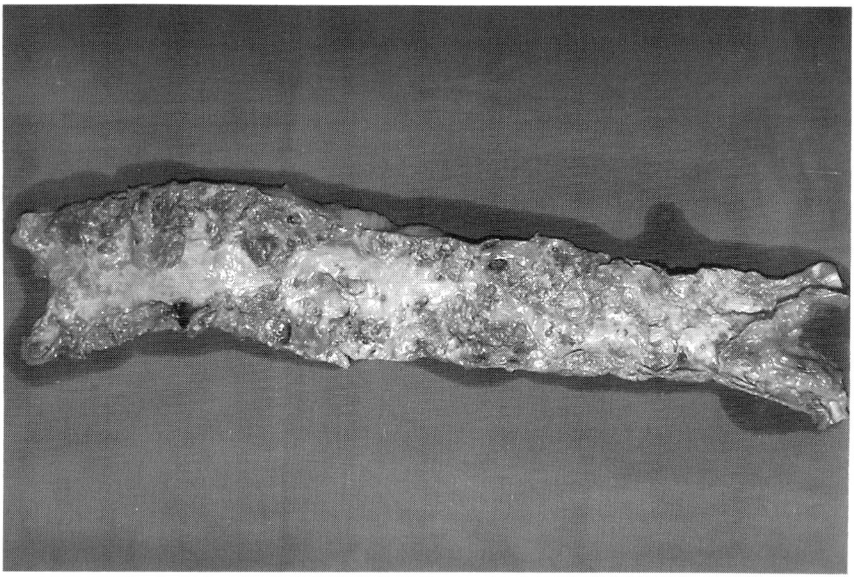

Figure 2.1. Interior surface of thoracic and abdominal aorta from a patient who died suddenly without any previous symptoms or signs of myocardial ischaemia, myocardial infarction or other clinical evidence of atherosclerotic disease. Severe atherosclerosis and ulcerations are seen.

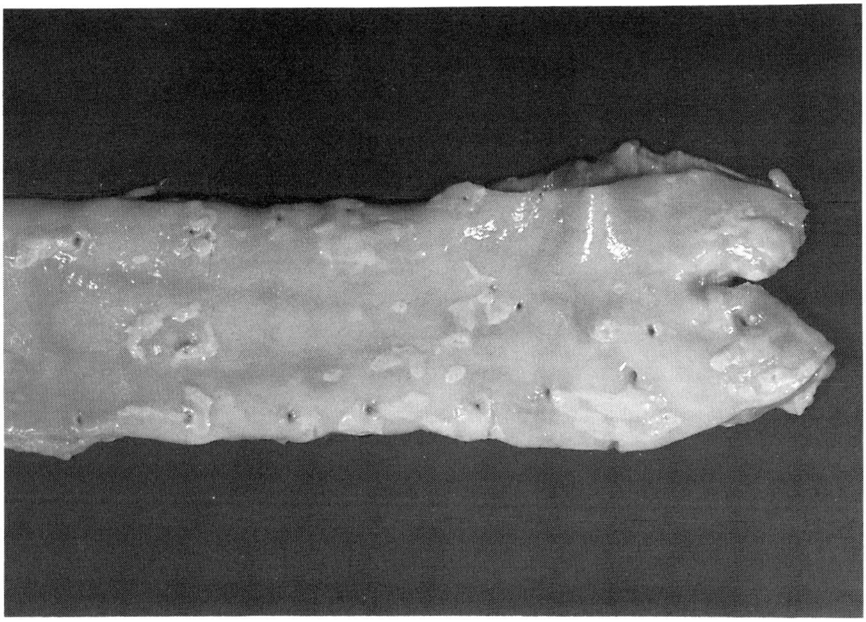

Figure 2.2. The aorta of a totally asymptomatic 29 year-old woman who died in a road traffic accident. Note the atheromatous plaques.

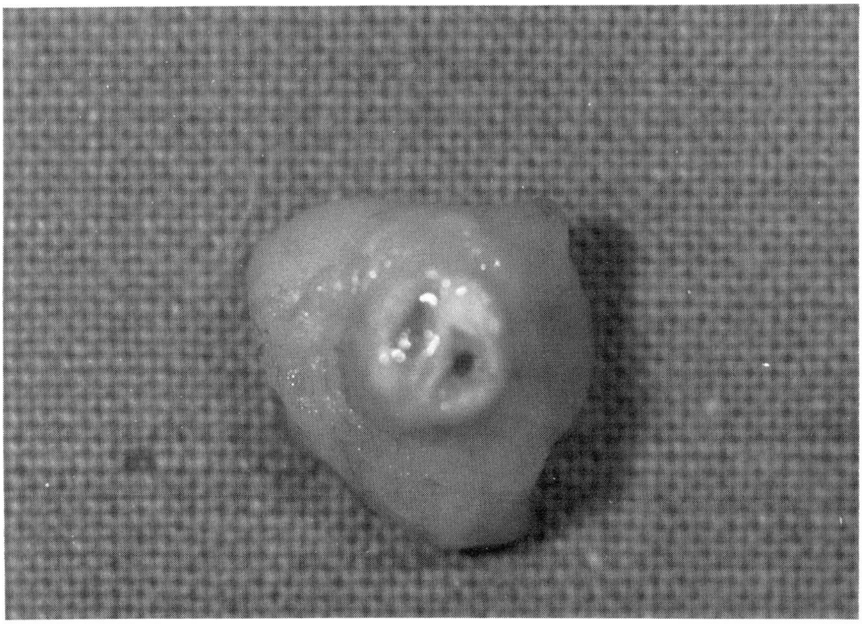

Figure 2.3. Transverse macroscopical section through the right coronary artery of a 43 year-old who died suddenly. The patient was asymptomatic and otherwise normal and without previous history of myocardial infarction. The atherosclerotic process is recanalised.

posed of disorganised lipid material, cholesterol clefts, cellular debris, fibrin and lipid laden macrophages. The lipid is mainly cholesterol and cholesterol esters. Vascular proliferation particularly around the periphery of the plaque may be seen.

The variation in the histological features of the plaque is related to the relative component of smooth muscle cell macrophages and other leucocytes, the extra and intra cellular lipid and other connective tissue. All these variations give rise to the spectrum of lesions seen in atherosclerosis.

In advanced atherosclerosis the progressive fibrosis convert the fatty atheroma into a fibrous plaque. Fully developed atheroma may undergo variable changes such as calcification, ulceration, haemorrhages, rupture and superaded thrombosis (Figs. 2.1, 2.2 and 2.3).

References

1. Gotlieb A I, Wong M K. Atherosclerosis, activation of the injured vessel wall. Cardiovasc Clin 1988; 3:3.
2. Mortality statistics 1978 and 1986 for England and Wales (office of population censuses and surveys).
3. Dawber T R. The Framingham study. The epidemiology of atherosclerotic disease. Harvard Univ. press, Cambridge Massachusettes, 1980.
4. Keys A. Coronary heart disease. The global picture. Atherosclerosis 1975; 22:149.
5. Blackburn H. Conference on the health effects of blood lipids; optimal distributions for populations. Workshop report: Epidemiological section, preventive medicine 1979; 8:612.
6. Roberts W C. The coronary arteries in coronary heart disease morphologic observations. Annu review pathobiol 1975; 5:249.
7. Buja L, Mand J T, Willerson. Clinicopathologic correlates of acute ischaemic heart disease syndromes Am J cardiol 1981; 47:343.
8. Wissler R W, Vesselinovitch. Atherosclerosis in non human primates. In: Advances in veterinary science and comparative medicine, vol 21, Bradley C A, Cornelius C E and Simpson C F (eds). Academic press, New York, 1977; p. 351.
9. Watanabe Y. Serial inbreeding of rabbits with hereditary hyperlipidemia. Atherosclerosis 1980; 36:261.
10. Wissler R W. The emerging cellular pathobiology of atherosclerosis. Artery 1979; 5: 409.
11. Ross R. Atherosclerosis: A problem of the biology of arterial wall cells and their interactions with blood components. Arteriosclerosis 1981; 1:293.
12. Wissler R W. The pathobiology of atherosclerotic plaque in the mid 1980's in regression of atherosclerotic lesions. In: Experimental studies and observations in humans. Melinow M R and Blaton V H (eds). Plenum press NY, 1984; p. 5.
13. Steinberg D. Lipoproteins and atherosclerosis. A look back and a look ahead. Arteriosclerosis 1983; 3:283.
14. Goldstein J L, Brown M S. The low density lipoprotein pathway and its relation to atherosclerosis. Ann Rev Biochem 1977; 46:897.
15. Mahley R W. Atherogenic hyperlipoproteinemia. The cellular and molecular biology of plasma lipoproteins altered by dietary fat and cholesterol. Med Clin North Am 1982; 66:375.
16. Ross R, Horker L. Hyperlipidemia and atherosclerosis. Chronic hyperlipidemia initiates

and maintain lesions by endothelial cell desquamation and lipid accumilation. Science 1976; 193:1094.
17. Ross R. The pathogenesis of atherosclerosis. In E. Braunwald (ed): Heart disease. A text book of cardiovascular medicine. 3rd ed. W. B. Saunders Co Philadelphia 1988; p. 1135.
18. Steinberg D. Current theories of the pathogenesis. In D. Steinberg and J. Olefsky (eds) Hypercholesterolemia and atherosclerosis. Pathogenesis and prevention. Churchill, Livingstone, New York, 1987; p. 5.
19. Ross R. The pathogenesis of atherosclerosis. An update. N Engl J Med 1986; 2:488.
20. Schwartz S M, Campbell G R, Campbell J H. Replication of smooth muscle cells in vascular disease Circ Res 1986; 58:427.
21. Guyton J R, Rosenberg R D, Clowes A W, Karnovsky M J. Inhibition of rat arterial smooth muscle cell proliferation by heparin *in vivo* studies with anticoagulant and non anticoagulant heparin. Cir Res 1980; 46:625.
22. Mazzone T, Jensen M, Chief A. Human arterial wall cells secrete factors that are chemotactic for monocytes. Proc Natl Acad Sci, USA 1983; 80:5094.
23. Brown M S. Goldstein J L. Lipoprotein metabolism in the macrophage implications for cholesterol deposition in atherosclerosis. Annu Rev Biochem 1983; 52:223.
24. Faggiotto A, Ross R, Harker L. Studies of hypercholesterolemia in the non human primate. 1. changes that lead to fatty streak formation. Arteriosclerosis 1984; 4:323.
25. Gerrity R G, Naito H K Richardson M, Schwartz C J. Dietary induced atherogenesis in swine: morphology of the intima in prelesion stages. Am J pathol 1979; 95:775.
26. Rosenfield M E, Faggiotta A, Ross R. The role of the mononuclear phagocyte in primate and rabbit models of atherosclerosis. Proceedings of the fourth Leiden conference on mononuclear phagocytes. The Hague; Martinus Nijhoff. 1965; p. 795.
27. Bevilacqua M P, Pober J S, Cotran R S, Ginabrone M A Jr. Interleukin 1 (JL1) acts upon vascular endothelium to stimulate procoagulant activity and leukocyte adhesion. J cell Biochem 1985 (suppl. 9A); p. 148 (abstract).
28. Martin T R, Altman L C, Albert R K, Henderson W R. Leukotriene B4 production by human alveolar macrophage; a potential mechanism for amplifying inflammation in the lung. Am Rev Resp Dis 1984; 129:106.
29. Bitterman P B, Rennard S I, Hunninghake G W, Crystal R G. Human alveolar macrophages growth factor for fibroblasts; regulation and partial characterization, Clin Invest 1982; 70:806.
30. Baird A, Mormede P, Bohlen P. Immunoreactive fibroblast growth factor in cells of peritoneal exudate suggests its identity with macrophage derived growth factor. Biochem biopsies Res commun 1985; 126:358.
31. Calnek B W. Merek's disease and lymphoma. In: F. Rapp (ed) Oncogenic herpes viruses. Boca Ronton, CRC press Inc. Florida 1980; p. 103.
32. Fabricant C G, Fabricant J, Litrentn M M, Minisk C R. Virus – induced atherosclerosis. J Exp Med 1978; 148:335.
33. Minick C R, Fabricant C G, Fabricant J, Litrentn M M. Atheroarteriosclerosis induced by infection with a herpes virus. Am J pathol 1979; 96:673.
34. Fabricant C G, Hajjar D D, Minick Cr, Fabricant J. Herpes infection enhances cholesterol and cholesterol ester accumulation in cultured arterial smooth muscle cells. Am J pathol 1981; 105:176.
35. Hajjar D D, Grant A J. Human herpes virus induces altered cholesterol metabolism and accumulation in human arterial smooth muscle cell. Circulation 1986; 74 (suppl II): 11.
36. Inkeles S, Eisenberg D. Hyperlipidemia and coronary atherosclerosis a review. Medicine (Baltimore) 1981; 60:110.
37. Lipid research clinics program. The lipid research clinics coronary primary prevention trial results. I. reduction in incidence of coronary heart disease JAMA 1984; 251:351.

38. Goldstein J L, Brown M S. The low density lipoprotein pathway and its relation to atherosclerosis. Annu Rev Biochem 1977; 46:896.
39. Goldstein J L, Kita T, Brown M S. Defective Lipoprotein receptors and atherosclerosis: lessons from an animal counterpart of familial hypercholesterolemia. N Eng J Med 1983; 309:288.
40. Brown M S, Goldstein J L. How LDL receptors influence cholesterol and atherosclerosis. Sci Am 1984; 251 (5):58.
41. Cathcart M K Morel D, Chisolm G M III. Monocytes and neutrophils oxidize low density lipoprotein making it cytotoxic. J Leuk Biol 1985; 38:341.
42. Colwell J A, Winocour P D, Lopes virella M, Halushka P. New concepts about the pathogenosis of atherosclerosis in diabetes mellitus. Am J Med 1983; 75:67.
43. Mustard J F, Packham M A. Editorial retrospective: platelets and diabetes mellitus. N Engl J Med 1984; 311:665.
44. Fry D L. Hemodynamic forces in atherogenesis. In: P Sheinberg (ed). Cerebrovascular disease: Tenth princeton conference; Raven Press New York p. 77.
45. Gertz S D, Uretsky G, Wajnberg R S, Navot N, Gotsman M S. Endothelial cell damage and thrombus formation after partial arterial constriction: Relevance to the role of coronary artery spasm in the pathogenesis of myocardial infarction. Circulation 1981; 63:476.
46. Joris I, Majno G. Hydrodynamic injury of the endothelium in acute aortic stenosis. Am J Pathol 1982; 108:394.
47. Folts J D, Crowell E B Jr, Rowe G G. Platelet aggregation in partially obstructed vessels and its elimination with aspirin. Circulation 1976; 54:365.
48. Kannel W B, Sytkowski P A. Atherosclerosis risk factors. Pharmac Ther 1987; 32:207.
49. Minick C R. Synergy of arterial injurial injury and hypercholesterolemia. In: Moore S (ed): 'Vascular injury and atherosclerosis' New York: Marcel Dekker 1981; p. 149.
50. Cochrane C G. Initiating events in immune complex injury in B Amoe (ed): 'Progress in immunology'. Academic press; Orlando 1971; p. 143.
51. Minick C R, Alonso D R, Rankin L. Role of immunologic arterial injury in atherogenesis. Thromb Haemost 1978; 39:304.
52. Stills H F, Bullock B C, Clarkson T B. Increased atherosclerosis and glomerulonephritis in cynamolgus monkeys (macaca fascicularis) given injections of BSA over an extended period of time Am J pathol 1983; 113:222.
53. Hughes A, Tonks R S. The role of micro emboli in the production of carditis in hypersensitivity experiments. J Pathol Bacteriol 1959; 77:207.
54. Orgensen L, Hovig T, Rowsell H C, Mustard J F. Adenosine diphosphate – induced platelet aggregation and vascular injury in swine and rabbits. Am J pathol 1970; 61:161.
55. Fujimato T, Suzuki H, Tanoue K, Fukushima Y, Yama Zaki H. Cerebrovascular injuries induced by activiation of platelets *in vitro*. Stroke 1985; 16:245.
56. Strong J P, Richards M L. Cigarette smoking and atherosclerosis in autopsied men. Atherosclerosis 1976; 23:451.
57. Pittilo R M, Mackie I J, Rowles P M, Machin, Woolf N. Effects of cigarette smoking on the ultrastructure of rats thoracic aorta and its ability to produce prostacyclin. Thromb Haemost 1982; 48:173.
58. SinZinger H, Kefalides A. Passive smoking severely decreases platelet sensitivity to anti aggregatory prostaglandins. Lancet 1982; 2:392.
59. Lubawy W G, Valentovic M A, Atkinson J E, Gairda G C. Chronic cigarette exposure adversely alters c-arachidonic acid metabolism in rat lungs, aorta and platelets. Life Sci 1983; 33:577.
60. Felts J, Bonebrake F C. The effects of cigarette smoke and nicotine on platelet plugging in stenosed dog coronary arteries. Inhibition with phentolamine: Circulation 1982; 65:465.

61. McCully K G. Homocysteine theory of a therosclerosis: development and current status. Atheroscler. Rev 1983; 11:157.
62. Siltanon P. Stress, coronary disease and coronary death. Ann Clin Res 1987; 19:96.
63. Packham M A, Mustard J F. Normal and abnormal platlet activity. In A lasslo (ed) 'Blood platelet function and medicinal chemistry' Elsevier Biomedical New York 1984; p. 61.
64. Gordon D, Guyton G R, Karnovsky M J. Intimal a Herations in rat aorta induced by stressful stimuli, Lab Invest 1981; 45:14.
65. Benditt E P, and Benditt J M. Evidence for amonoclonal origin of human atherosclerotic plaque proc. Natl Acad Sci USA 1973; 70:1753.
66. Benditt E P. Origins of human atherosclerotic plaque. The role of altered gene expression. Arch. Pathol. Lab Med 1988; 112:997.

PART TWO

Occult carotid and cerebrovascular disease

3. The natural history of asymptomatic carotid artery disease

THOMAS S. HATSUKAMI and D. EUGENE STRANDNESS, JR.

The goal in the management of patients with carotid artery disease is the prevention of cerebral infarction. The means by which this goal should be attained has been the subject of debate for many years. Decisions regarding appropriate management of these patients must be predicated on knowledge of the natural history of the disease.

The increased risk of stroke after the development of ischaemic neurologic symptoms has been well documented by numerous investigators [1, 2]. However, reports on the incidence of stroke in asymptomatic patients with carotid artery disease have differed widely [3–14]. Many of the earlier studies were performed using the presence or absence of asymptomatic cervical bruits as the criteria for inclusion [15]. However, Kartchner and McRae found that only 21% of 1,287 patients with asymptomatic cervical bruits had significant internal carotid stenosis by oculoplethysmography [16] and Moore found that among patients with significant carotid stenosis only 58% had an audible bruit [17]. Similar results were reported in patients studied with angiography [18]. These studies demonstrate that cervical bruits alone are a poor indicator of the severity of carotid artery disease.

Results from series correlating neurologic events with the actual degree of carotid stenosis are difficult to compare, owing to differences in the duration of follow-up, the categorization of symptoms, and the methods of reporting occurrences. Furthermore, in many studies, serial examination of the asymptomatic carotid artery is not performed. Whether occult progression has occurred is not known, and the degree of carotid stenosis at the time of the neurologic event is unspecified.

The advent of duplex ultrasonography facilitated the detection and follow-up of patients with asymptomatic carotid artery disease. The accuracy of duplex ultrasonography has been documented by several investigators [19–24]. Sensitivity, or the ability to detect disease, is 99%, and specificity is 84%. Compared to contrast angiography, the accuracy of carotid duplex

A.-M. Salmasi and A. N. Nicolaides (eds.), Occult Atherosclerotic Disease, 35–44.

scanning for haemodynamically significant, 50–99% diameter-reducing lesions is 91%, and 97% for occlusions [23, 24].

This chapter reviews the natural history of asymptomatic, extracranial carotid artery disease, focusing on results from data acquired over the past decade in our long-term carotid duplex follow-up study.

Disease progression

Reports on internal carotid artery disease progression are few in number. In 1970, Javid and his co-workers [25] performed repeat angiograms on 93 patients with < 60% internal carotid stenosis at intervals of one to nine years (mean of three years). Significant progression was noted in 22% of the non-operated patients.

In 1984, Roederer and associates reviewed the outcome of 167 patients referred to our carotid duplex laboratory for asymptomatic mid-cervical bruits [26]. Patients were examined with duplex ultrasonography at six month intervals for the first year, and annually thereafter for up to 36 months. Disease at the carotid bifurcation was classified into six categories: normal; 1–15%, 16–49%, 50–79%, and 80–99% diameter reduction; and occlusion (Table 3.1).

Table 3.1. Criteria for classification of internal carotid artery disease by spectral analysis of duplex doppler signals, center stream sample volume, with doppler beam angle 60 degrees to vessel axis.

Arteriographic Lesion		Spectral Criteria
A	normal (0% diameter reduction)	Peak systolic frequency up to 4kHz; no spectral broadening
B	1–15% diameter reduction	Peak systolic frequency up to 4kHz; spectral broadening in deceleration phase of systole
C	16–49% diameter reduction	Peak systolic frequency up to 4kHz; spectral broadening throughout systole
D	50–79% diameter reduction	Peak systolic frequency > 4kHz; end diastolic frequency < 4.5 kHz
D+	80–99% diameter reduction	End diastolic frequency > 4.5 kHz
E	total occlusion	No internal carotid flow signal; flow to zero in common carotid artery

At the time of entry into the study, the distribution of internal carotid disease was as follows: normal 2%; 1–15% stenosis 29%; 16–49% stenosis 33%; 50–79% stenosis 29%; 80–99% stenosis 3%; and occlusion 4% (Fig 3.1). Disease progression was observed in 60% of the internal carotid arteries during follow-up. By life-table analysis, the mean annual rate of progression from < 50% to 50–99% stenosis was 8% per year.

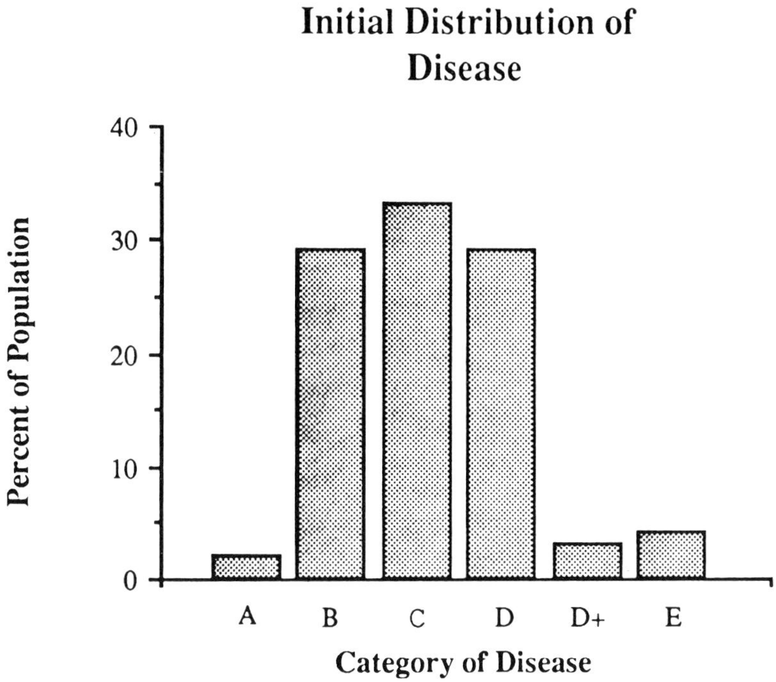

Figure 3.1. Initial distribution of disease in 167 patients referred for asymptomatic mid-cervical bruits, studied with carotid duplex scanning.

A total of ten carotid arteries occluded during the course of follow-up. Disease progression to ⩾ 80% stenosis was observed in all patients before occlusion, when serial studies were available.

Major risk factors associated with disease progression were age, cigarette smoking, and diabetes. In patients older than 65 years at the time of entry into the study, the proportion of those who progresed was lower than in patients less than 65 years old (29% versus 45%; p=0.02). Among cigarette smokers, 42% exhibited disease progression, compared to 24% of the non-smokers (p=0.03). Fifty-eight percent of patients with diabetes were found to have internal carotid disease progression as opposed to 35% of the non-diabetic group (p=0.04).

Neurologic events

Correlation with high-grade stenosis

Roederer found a significant correlation between the presence of 80–99% carotid stenosis and the subsequent development of transient ischaemic attacks (TIAs), strokes, or carotid occlusion. The risk of developing ischaemic symptoms or ipsilateral occlusion was 35% within six months of progression to 80–99% stenosis, and 46% within 12 months. Patients with < 80% stenosis had a significantly lower incidence of these complications (1.5%; $p < 0.00001$). If only TIAs and strokes were considered, the incidence of complications was 33% in patients with 80–99% stenosis, and 0.4% in those with < 80% disease ($p < 0.00001$). All of the strokes occurred in patients with > 80% diameter-reducing lesions, and 75% of the strokes occurred without antecedent TIAs.

Other investigators have similarly documented an increased risk of stroke in patients with high-grade stenosis of the carotid bifurcation. Chambers and Norris followed 500 patients referred for asymptomatic cervical bruits with serial Doppler examination for up to four years [27]. At one year, the incidence of TIAs and strokes was 6% overall. However, in patients with > 75% carotid stenosis, the incidence of these events was significantly higher (18% at one year; $p < 0.001$). When only hemispheric strokes were considered, the overall incidence was 1.7% at one year, compared to 5.5% in patients with > 75% stenosis.

In 1987, Moneta *et al.* reported on 115 patients with 80–99% carotid stenosis followed with serial duplex examination [28]. By life-table analysis, the incidence of hemispheric stroke was 19% at two years, for a calculated annual stroke rate of 9.5%.

Correlation with carotid occlusion

As noted above, Roederer documented an increased risk of carotid occlusion in patients with 80–99% carotid stenosis. The prevention of total occlusion is relevant, since several studies have documented an increased rate of stroke in the distribution of previously asymptomatic occluded carotid arteries [29, 30]. Nichols reviewed the natural history of 212 patients with total carotid occlusion who were referred to our carotid duplex laboratory [29]. During a mean follow-up period of 24.9 months, 31 strokes occurred. By life-table analysis, cumulative stroke-free survival was 75% at five years, for an estimated mean annual rate of 5% per year. (Fig. 3.2)

Correlation with ulcerative lesions

A few investigators have reported an increased risk of stroke in patients with ulcerated lesions of the carotid bifurcation. Moore *et al.* categorized ulceration by measurement of length and depth on angiography [31, 32]. Three categories were described: 'A' for ulcerative lesions with an area measurement of < 10 mm^3; 'B' for ulcers measuring between 10 to 40 mm^3; and 'C' for ulcers > 40 mm^3 or those with a complex, cavernous appear-

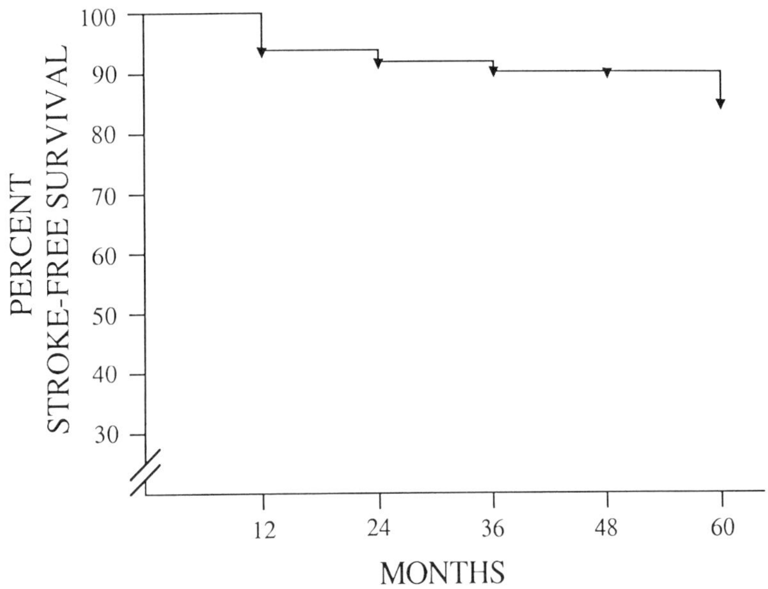

Figure 3.2. Cumulative five-year stroke-free survival by life-table analysis in patients with total carotid occlusion.

ance. Type 'A' ulcers carried a benign prognosis, with only 3% subsequently having strokes, whereas type 'B' and 'C' ulcerations were associated with a stroke incidence of 21% and 19% respectively. The calculated stroke risk was 4.5% per year for 'B' ulcerations and 7.5% per year for 'C' ulcerations. None of these strokes were preceded by TIAs.

Kroener *et al.* reviewed the outcome of 76 patients with 87 nonstenotic, ulcerative internal carotid lesions and confirmed the benign prognosis in patients with 'A' type ulcerations [33]. However, in patients with 'B' ulcerations, a significantly increased stroke risk could not be documented. No data were available for type 'C' lesions as these patients had surgery. Further studies will be needed, particularly in those patients with moderate ulcerations of the carotid bifurcation.

Carotid disease in perioperative patients

In 1984, Ivey reviewed the outcome of 1,433 consecutive patients referred to our institution for cardiac surgery [34]. Ninety-four of these patients were found to have a mid-cervical bruit and were evaluated by duplex scanning. Nine patients developed transient neurologic symptoms and underwent carotid endarterectomy prior to or simultaneously with cardiac surgery. One neurologic complication occurred in this group of patients. Among 82 patients who had asymptomatic neck bruits, 16 had internal carotid stenoses of > 50%, and 66 had less severe lesions. None of these patients underwent carotid endarterectomy, and none developed focal neurologic complications after cardiac surgery.

Other studies have similarly failed to demonstrate a relationship between perioperative neurologic complications and asymptomatic carotid stenosis [35–38]. Of these studies, only Kartchner and McRae were able to show an increased risk of stroke [35]. Using oculoplethysmographic (OPG) criteria, patients with positive OPGs had a 17% risk of stroke, compared to a 1% risk in those with negative OPGs. However, this study did not document the site of symptoms that occurred during follow-up.

Based upon the findings from these studies, prophylactic carotid endarterectomy cannot be recommended in asymptomatic patients. The exception may be those individuals with pre-occlusive, > 90% lesions, since many of the above mentioned investigators performed carotid endarterectomy on these patients, and thus excluded this subgroup of patients.

Carotid disease contralateral to endarterectomy

There are relatively few studies examining the natural history of asymptomatic carotid disease contralateral to a carotid endarterectomy [39–44]. Most studies have shown a low incidence of stroke during follow-up.

Roederer *et al.* reviewed the outcome of 134 patients with patent contralateral carotid arteries after unilateral carotid endarterectomy [41]. Patients were followed with serial duplex scanning for up to four years. A strong relationship was noted between the presence of a high-grade, 80–99% contralateral carotid stenosis and the subsequent development of ischaemic neurologic symptoms. The risk of developing symptoms was 50% in patients with 80–99% stenoses, compared to only 7% in those with < 80% disease ($p=0.003$). A conservative approach was recommended, reserving contralateral carotid endarterectomy until the patient exhibits ischaemic neurologic symptoms or a high-grade, 80–99% stenosis.

Prophylactic surgical intervention on asymptomatic patients with moderate degrees of carotid stenosis (50–70%) is generally not recommended by most investigators. At our institution, we have adopted a management approach by which patients are followed with serial duplex examinations after unilateral carotid endarterectomy. Contralateral carotid endarterectomy is recommended for symptomatic patients and those with 80–99% stenoses. Patients with < 80% contralateral carotid stenoses who remain asymptomatic are followed nonoperatively.

In 1989, the authors reviewed the outcome of 200 patients following

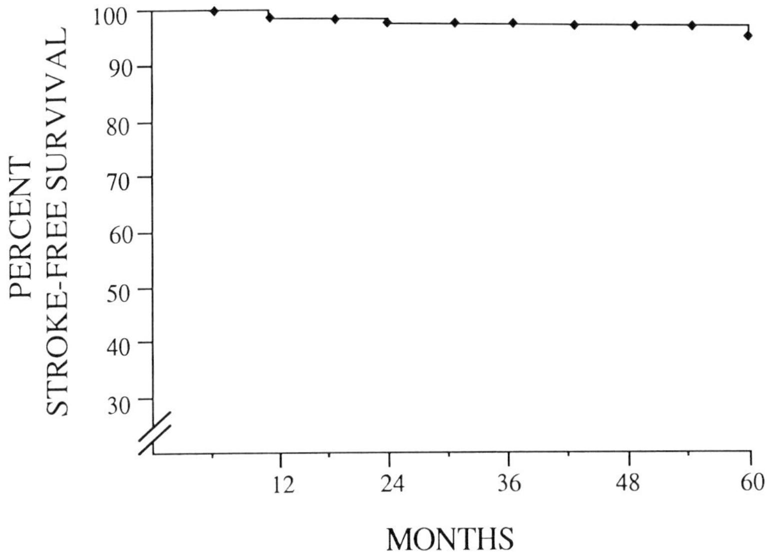

Figure 3.3. Cumulative five-year stroke-free survival on the side opposite a carotid endarterectomy.

unilateral carotid endarterectomy, given this management strategy [45]. Patients were followed for up to ten years (mean of 54 months). The mean annual rate of progression to ⩾ 50% stenosis was 3.9% per year and 1.2% per year for progression to ⩾ 80% stenosis. Cumulative stroke-free survival was 96.1% at five years, and the estimated mean annual rate was < 0.8% per year (Fig. 3.3). Case history review of those patients who had strokes failed to reveal additional subgroups of patients who would have benefited from carotid endarterectomy. We concluded that patients with < 80% contralateral carotid stenosis who remain asymptomatic can safely be followed with serial examination and duplex scanning.

Summary

Patients with asymptomatic, high-grade (80–99%) internal carotid stenoses appear to be at increased risk for subsequent stroke or carotid occlusion. Stroke risk in this subgroup of patients has generally been reported to range from 3–6% per year. Furthermore, patients with 80–99% stenoses have been shown to have a higher risk for subsequent total carotid occlusion, which in turn carries an increased risk for stroke.

Several reports suggest that complex, ulcerative lesions predispose patients to ischaemic neurologic events, with stroke risk ranging from 5 to 7% per year. However, further studies will be needed to validate our diagnostic capabilities to identify these types of lesions.

Studies on patients with asymptomatic carotid artery disease found prior to major surgery have generally failed to demonstrate an increased risk of neurologic complications perioperatively. However, the natural history of patients with > 90% stenoses in unknown, since these patients have been excluded in most of these studies.

In patients with carotid artery disease contralateral to an endarterectomy, operative intervention is recommended for patients exhibiting ischaemic neurologic symptoms or 80–99% diameter-reducing stenoses. Asymptomatic patients with < 80% stenoses appear to follow a benign course.

References

1. Bogousslavsky J, Despland P, Regli F. Asymptomatic tight stenosis of the internal carotid artery: Long-term prognosis. Neurology 1986; 36:861.
2. Committee on Health Care Issues, ANA. Does carotid endarterectomy decrease stroke and death in patients with transient ischaemic attacks? Ann Neurol 1987; 22:72.
3. Moore W L, Beren G, Malone J A, Goldstone J. Asymptomatic carotid stenosis: Immediate and long-term results after prophylactic endarterectomy. Am J Surg 1979; 138:228.
4. Roederer G O, Langlois Y E, Jager K A *et al.* The natural history of carotid arterial disease in asymptomatic patients with cervical bruits. Stroke 1984; 15:605.
5. Hertzer N R, Flanagan R A, O'Hara P J, Beven E G. Surgical versus nonoperative treatment of asymptomatic carotid stenosis. Ann Surg 1986; 204:163.
6. Moneta G L, Taylor D C, Nicholls S C *et al.* Operative versus nonoperative management of asymptomatic high-grade internal carotid artery stenosis: Improved results with endarterectomy. Stroke 1987; 18:1005.
7. Caracci B F, Zukowski A J, Hurley J J, Naunheim K S, Auer A I. Asymptomatic severe carotid stenosis. J Vasc Surg 1989; 9:361.
8. Humphries A W, Young J R, Santilli P H, Beven E G, deWolfe V F. Unoperated, asymptomatic significant internal carotid artery stenosis: A review of 182 instances. Surgery 1976; 80:695.
9. Durward Q J, Ferguson G G, Barr H W K. The natural history of asymptomatic carotid bifurcation plaques. Stroke 1982; 13:459.
10. Yatsu F M, Fields W S. Asymptomatic carotid bruit. Arch Neurol 1985; 42:383.
11. Bogousslavsky J, Despland P, Regli F. Asymptomatic tight stenosis of the internal carotid artery: Long-term prognosis. Neurology 1986; 36:861.
12. Chambers B R, Norris J W. The case against surgery for asymptomatic carotid stenosis. Stroke 1984; 15:964.
13. Chambers B R, Norris J W. Outcome in patients with asymptomatic neck bruits. N Engl J Med 1986; 315:860.
14. Ford C S, Frye J L, Toole J F, Lefkowitz D. Asymptomatic carotid bruit and stenosis. Arch Neurol 1986; 43:219.
15. Heyman A, Wiolkinson W E, Hayden S *et al.* Risk of stroke in asymptomatic persons with

cervical arterial bruits: A population study in Evans County, Georgia. N Engl J Med 1980; 302:838.
16. Kartchner M M, McRae L P. Non-invasive evaluation and management of the asymptomatic carotid bruit. Surgery 1977; 82:840.
17. Moore W S, Bean B, Burton R *et al.* The use of opthalmosonometry in the diagnosis of carotid artery disease. Surgery 1977; 82:107.
18. David T E, Humphries A W, Young J R *et al.* A correlation of neck bruits and atherosclerosclerotic carotid arteries. Arch Surg 1973; 107:729.
19. Blackshear W M, Phillips, D J, Thiele B L *et al.* Detection of carotid occlusive disease by ultrasonic imaging and pulsed Doppler spectrum analysis. Surgery 1979; 86:698.
20. Fell G, Phillips D J, Chikos P M, Harley J D, Thiele B L, Strandness Jr D E. Ultrasonic duplex scanning for disease of the carotid artery. Circulation 1981; 64:1191.
21. Breslau P J, Knox R A, Phillips D J *et al.* The accuracy of ultrasonic duplex scanning as compared with contrast arteriography. Vasc Diag Ther 1982; 3:17.
22. Flanigan D P, Schuler J J, Vogel M *et al.* The role of carotid duplex scanning in surgical decision making. J Vasc Surg 1985; 2:15.
23. Roederer G O, Langlois Y E, Chan A W *et al.* Ultrasonic duplex scanning of extracranial carotid arteries: Improved accuracy using new features from the common carotid artery. J Cardiovasc Ultrasonogr 1982; 1:373.
24. Roederer G O, Langlois Y E, Jager K A *et al.* A simple spectral parameter for accurate classification of severe carotid disease. Bruit 1984; 8:174.
25. Javid H, Ostermiller W E Jr, Hengesh J W *et al.* Natural history of carotid bifurcation atheroma. Surgery 1970; 67:80.
26. Roederer G O, Langlois Y E, Jager K A *et al.* The natural history of carotid arterial disease in asymptomatic patients with cervical bruits. Stroke 1984; 15:605.
27. Chambers B R, Norris J W. Outcome in patients with asymptomatic neck bruits. N Engl J Med 1986; 315:860.
28. Moneta G L, Taylor D C, Nicholls S C *et al.* Operative versus nonoperative management of asymptomatic high-grade internal carotid artery stenosis: Improved results with endarterectomy. Stroke 1987; 18:1005.
29. Nicholls S C, Kohler T R, Bergelin R O, Primozich J F, Lawrence R L, Strandness D E. Carotid artery occlusion: Natural history. J Vasc Surg 1986; 4:479.
30. Cote R, Barnett H J M, Taylor D W. Internal carotid occlusion: A prospective study. Stroke 1983; 14:898.
31. Moore W S, Boren C, Malone J M *et al.* Natural history of nonstenotic asymptomatic ulcerative lesions of the carotid artery. Arch Surg 1978; 113:1352.
32. Dixon S, Pais S O, Raviola C *et al.* Natural history of nonstenotic asymptomatic lesions of the carotid artery. Arch Surg 1982; 117:1493.
33. Kroener J M, Dorn P L, Shoor P M *et al.* Prognosis of asymptomatic ulcerating carotid lesions. Arch Surg 1980; 115:1387.
34. Ivey T D, Strandness D E Jr, Williams D B *et al.* Management of patients with carotid bruit undergoing cardiopulmonary bypass. J Thorac Cardiovasc Surg 1984; 87:183.
35. Kartchner M M, McRae L P Carotid occlusive disease as a risk factor in major cardiovascular surgery. Arch Surg 1982; 117:1086.
36. Barnes R W, Liebman P R, Marszalek P B *et al.* Natural history of asymptomatic carotid disease in patients undergoing cardiovascular surgery. Surgery 1981; 90:1075.
37. Turnipseed W D, Berkoff H A, Belzer F O. Postoperative stroke in cardiac and peripheral vascular disease. Ann Surg 1980; 192:365.
38. Evans W E, Cooperman M. The significance of asymptomatic unilateral carotid bruits in perioperative patients. Surgery 1978; 873:521.
39. Podore P C, DeWeese J A, May A G, Rob C G. Asymptomatic contralateral carotid artery

stenosis: A five-year follow-up study following carotid endarterectomy. Surgery 1980; 88:748.
40. Riles TS, Imparato AM, Mintzer R, Baumann FG. Comparison of results of bilateral and unilateral carotid endarterectomy five years after surgery. Surgery 1982; 91:258.
41. Roederer GO, Langlois YE, Lusiani J *et al.* Natural history of carotid artery disease on the side contralateral to endarterectomy. J Vasc Surg 1984; 1:62.
42. Sterpetti AV, Schultz RD, Feldhaus RJ. Asymptomatic carotid artery stenosis on the side contralateral to endarterectomy: A comparison between patients with and those without operation. J Vasc Surg 1989; 8:453.
43. Sobel M, Imparato AM, Riles TS, Mintzer R. Contralateral neurologic symptoms after carotid surgery: A nine-year follow-up. J Vasc Surg 1986; 3:623.
44. Schroeder T, Helgstrand UJV, Egeblad MR, Engell HC. Asymptomatic carotid lesions after endarterectomy of contralateral carotid artery. Arch Surg 1987; 122:795.

4. Techniques of screening, diagnosis and assessment of occult carotid and cerebrovascular disease

SOPHIE C. RENTON and ANDREW N. NICOLAIDES

The requirement of any screening technique used in the diagnosis and assessment of asymptomatic disease is that the test should be sensitive, specific, reproducible and cheap. It should also cause the patient as little inconvenience or discomfort as possible, and be quick to perform. This is a tall order, but in occult disease of the extracerebral vessels, these needs can be met.

Screening for carotid bruits

Auscultation of the neck for carotid bruits is an unreliable method of detecting the presence and assessing the severity of occult cerebrovascular disease. A bruit usually appears when there is a diameter reduction of 50% or more. If a mid-cervical bruit is audible, the likelihood of a stenosis being present is 64–85% [1, 2]. However, only 60% of patients with a significant stenosis (>50% in diameter) of the internal carotid artery will have a bruit, and, in the presence of a bruit, 31% will have silent disease on the contralateral side [1]. This is because in the presence of severe stenosis (>80%), there is not enough blood flowing through the lesion to produce a bruit. The early natural history studies which relied on the presence of a bruit to indicate asymptomatic disease [3, 4] demonstrated that the risk of stroke in the presence of a carotid bifurcation bruit was 1–2% per annum, and many of the events were related to the contralateral carotid artery [4]. These studies also indicated that the mortality rate due to cardiac events was four times higher than the incidence of stroke in patients with carotid bruits, confirming the global nature of the disease.

A.-M. Salmasi and A. N. Nicolaides (eds.), Occult Atherosclerotic Disease, 45–57.

Noninvasive investigations

Prior to the 1970's, the only method of accurately diagnosing atherosclerotic changes in the extracerebral vasculature was arteriography utilising the intra-arterial injection of radio-opaque contrast. This method was not only invasive, time consuming, and expensive, but it also had an estimated risk of stroke of 2.4% (range 0–11%) [5]. The introduction of digital subtraction angiography has lessened the risk associated with the procedure but it is still invasive and is, therefore, unsuitable as a screening method for the detection of asymptomatic disease. During the 1970's, a number of non-invasive techniques were developed. These measured cerebrovascular disease by direct and indirect methods. The direct methods included carotid phonangiography, the analysis of carotid bruits amplified by an electronic stethoscope [6, 7], and the assessment of the carotid arteries by Doppler ultrasound. These direct methods of assessment have now been superseded by the development of duplex ultrasonography [8, 9].

Indirect methods of assessment exploited the unique anatomy of the ophthalmic artery to measure the haemodynamic effect of a lesion proximal to its origin from the internal carotid artery. They included periorbital Doppler and oculoplethysmographic techniques [10, 11]. However, these indirect methods of assessment had several drawbacks. Firstly, they could only detect lesions producing a stenosis of greater than 50% of the diameter of the internal carotid artery, and the predictive value was reduced in the presence of bilateral disease. Secondly, they could not differentiate between a very tight stenosis and an occluded internal carotid artery. Oculoplethysmography and periorbital Doppler studies have largely been replaced by transcranial Doppler studies [8, 9].

Ultrasound imaging techniques

Ultrasound imaging was developed in the 1970's with two basic types of ultrasonic imaging being available: B-mode imaging and Doppler ultrasound imaging.

B-mode imaging

The principle underlying real time B-mode ultrasonography is that ultrasound transmitted through tissues is absorbed, attenuated and reflected from interfaces depending on the density of the tissue and the transmitted frequency of the sound waves. The return signal is processed to produce a two dimensional image, differences in tissue densities being depicted by the grey scale display. Using an oscillating head and recording the reflected image on an oscilloscope, a two dimensional image is projected continuously and in real time. B-mode imaging was initially developed as an imaging procedure for obstetrics but soon became the method of choice for assessing the size and enlargement of the abdominal aorta in aneurysmal disease [12]. B-mode imaging allows the anatomy to be clearly defined, arteries can be identified by their pulsatility and wall thickness, while veins can be seen to collapse under pressure. Subsequent improvement in resolution and the provision of real time imaging have made it applicable for use in the examination of several vessels. Early B-mode images suffered from a poor resolution, and assessment of the vessel lumen let alone the wall was limited. Furthermore, calcification produced acoustic shadows and fresh thrombus could not be differentiated from flowing blood. Agreement with arteriography could be demonstrated in only 67–86% [13–16].

Doppler imaging

The technique of Doppler imaging was first introduced by Hokanson et al [17] in 1971. Doppler ultrasound uses the principle of the Doppler effect to detect movement of blood within blood vessels. An ultrasonic signal is transmitted through the tissues, and movement of red cells in the vessels produces a Doppler shift frequency which is proportional to the flow velocity, the higher the flow, the higher the frequency. By transmitting the ultrasound in intermittent short bursts (the time gate principle), the depth of the returning signal can be distinguished. By adjusting the time between transmission and the activation of the gate, one can select the depth at which the flow signals will be detected. Unlike the B-mode image, Doppler arteriography gives an image of the flow within the artery.

Frequency spectral analysis

Continous wave Doppler ultrasound may be used to assess the pattern of flow within the artery. In any sample volume, blood cells will be moving a several different velocities, this will be reflected in the Doppler shifted frequency. Furthermore, the amplitude of each frequency corresponds to the number of blood cells travelling at that frequency. Frequency spectral analysis is the interpretation of the Doppler shifted signal by measurement of the frequency and amplitude of each component. Using a fast Fourier transform, this can be displayed graphically. The carotid arteries have characteristic flow patterns which permit their identification. The internal carotid artery has little distal resistance and thus high flow in diastole. The external carotid system has a prominent dicrotic notch with very low flow velocity in diastole. The common carotid artery is a mixture of the two.

When a vessel narrows, the blood velocity must increase if a constant flow is to be maintained. Therefore, on passing through a stenosis the frequency shift of the reflected signal increases. Also turbulence develops in relation to arterial wall irregularities causing a widening of the frequency band of the reflected signal. These two features, spectral broadening and an increase in frequency, form the basis of criteria for classification of carotid artery stenosis with spectral broadening being the most sensitive indicator of early disease and an increase in frequency being the most sensitive parameter in very tight stenoses. There are two main drawbacks to Doppler ultrasonography. Firstly, it insonates all tissues in its path, and therefore provides simultaneous superimposed signals from all the vessels it encounters. Secondly, the angle between probe and vessel cannot be determined thus preventing the conversion of Doppler shift signals into absolute velocity units (ml/sec). The first of these problems was largely overcome by the development of gated Doppler. The second drawback was overcome by the development of the duplex scanner.

Duplex scanning

In 1974, the duplex scanner was created by the combination of real time ultrasonic imaging and gated Doppler ultrasound [18]. Anatomic localisation of the vessel with the B-mode image allowed the accurate positioning of a sample volume in the centre of the lumen, therefore allowing the operator to obtain flow velocities at the area of most rapid flow. A further advantage of the duplex scanner was that it permitted the measurement of the angle of insonation in relation to the axis of the imaged vessel, therefore, the velocity could be calculated (cm/sec) [19]. This allowed carotid artery stenoses to be differentiated into broad categories (under 15%, 15–49%, 50–79%, 80–99% and total occlusion) [21–24].

The accuracy of Duplex ultrasound in detecting stenoses is reported to be between 75% and 96% [23–25]. The greatest inaccuracies lie at the extremes of disease, in particular early disease. Technological improvements have resulted in a superior image quality and greater versatility. Initially developed for use in the detection and grading of carotid bifurcation disease [19], the duplex scanner has become widely used in the non-invasive investigation of all vascular disease. Clinical trials have demonstrated that duplex scanning has a high specificity and sensitivity in the evaluation of carotid occlusive disease. One of the advantages of duplex scanning, over simple ultrasonic imaging, is the ability to detect fresh thrombus and plaques with the same echogenicity as blood. These may be detected by recording the haemodynamic disturbance produced by such a thrombus, stenosis or wall irregularity. Duplex scanning is the only non-invasive method of examining the extracranial carotid arteries from which both functional and anatomical information can be achieved in the one study.

Colour flow imaging

The most recent addition to the range of duplex scanners are instruments which provide real time colour flow imaging superimposed on the real time grey scale imaging. The use of linear array transducers and microchip technology provides a means of testing every pixel on the screen for Doppler shift. Thus, any movement is depicted as colour; red for flow in one direction, blue for the reverse; and the higher the frequency of the Doppler shift, the paler the colour depicted. Absence of colour indicates absence of flow. The colour flow map is superimposed on the real time grey scale image. Thus an artery can be seen as a pulsating red lumen, a thrombus or atherosclerotic plaque as a black area protruding into the lumen and a tight stenosis as a white jet [26]. Localisation of the problem area allows the sample volume to be quickly positioned at the tightest point; velocity and diameter can be measured, and flow will be calculated automatically (ml/min). As yet, the reproducibility and clinical usefulness of the flow measurements have not been fully evaluated. A colour duplex scanner, although approximately twice as expensive as earlier scanners, is three to four times quicker to use. Because more patients can be studied per session, the machine has been shown to be more cost effective.

Assessment in occult carotid disease

At present, Duplex scanning is the method of choice for the routine screening for suspected extracranial cerebrovascular disease [21, 22]. Duplex scanning, either in black and white or using colour flow imaging allows follow up studies to be performed safely and quickly, at regular intervals. This holds the promise of providing a better understanding of the pathophysiological changes that occur in arterial disease (eg. flow patterns in relation to atherogenesis, and progression or regression of disease in response to therapy). Identification of individuals at risk of developing symptomatic disease is the main objective in the assessment of the extracranial carotid arteries. Duplex scanning allows the detection and grading of stenoses of the carotid arteries by spectrum analysis. Natural history studies have shown that stenoses of less than 80% have a 1–3% per annum risk of producing a stroke, whereas in the presence of a stenosis greater than 80%, the risk is 4–12% per annum [23, 24, 27, 28]. The risk is greater still if the end-diastolic flow at the stenosis is greater than 200 cm/s. [25].

The role of plaque morphology in the development of symptoms is recognised and attempts have been made to identify plaques ultrasonographically which are associated with a high risk. Reilly *et al.* [29] identified two distinct ultrasound echo patterns, homogeneous and heterogeneous. These findings correlated well with the presence of intraplaque haemorrhage and ulceration and 78% of the symptomatic patients had heterogeneous plaques. Johnson *et al.* [30] found that 93% of patients with 'soft' lesions and >75% stenosis became symptomatic over 5 years. Gray-Weale *et al.* [31] expanded the classification according to the B-mode appearance and described four ultrasound types [1,2] 97.2% of type 1 lesions contained intraplaque haemorrhage or were ulcerated [32]. The improved resolution achieved with modern day linear transducers allows plaques to be characterised and intraplaque haemorrhage detected, with a sensitivity of 91% and specificity of 65% [33]. Duplex scanning is the most appropriate method available for the noninvasive study of patients with asymptomatic carotid disease, it has allowed us to identify a high risk groups according to haemodynamic stenosis and plaque morphology. Furthermore, to complete the examination of the extracerebral vasculature, duplex scanning may also be used for the examination of the subclavian and innominate arteries as well as the origin of the vertebral artery [34]. These vessels can be identified during their course through the supraclavicular fossa and a stenosis of greater than 50% can be identified with a sensitivity of 88% and a specificity of 98% [35]. Colour flow facilitates the identification of the vertebral arteries at their origin and enables them to be followed along their course between the transverse processes to the base of the skull. With colour flow imaging, the diagnosis of subclavian steal is greatly facilitated as retrograde flow in the vertebral artery will be blue if the flow in the carotid is red, and when the peripheral resistance of the arm is reduced e.g. by releasing a clenched fist, the steal is increased, hence the velocity of the Doppler shift is increased.

High resolution ultrasonography

Recently, the resolution of the ultrasound probes has improved considerably, allowing the identification of ultrasonographic features of the arterial wall. These are best seen in the longitudinal view. Pignoli [38] has shown that these layers correlate with histological layers, the first echogenic and echolucent lines being made up of intima and media, and the second echogenic line, the adventitia. Poli et al [37] have shown changes in the intima-media thickness occur in hypercholesterolaemia, and Salonen and Salonen [40] have followed a population of middle-aged men and shown that it was possible to monitor the progression of atherosclerosis by measuring the intima-media thickness, and that the strongest predictors of progression were age, smoking habit, LDL cholesterol, leucocyte count and platelet aggregability. Epidemiological studies have begun to use this measurement in long term studies. One such study, the atherosclerosis risk in the community study [39] found that cases with an increased arterial wall intima-media thickness at entry, had significantly increased levels of total serum cholesterol, LDL cholesterol, triglycerides, and systolic blood pressures as compared to controls [40]. Intima-media thickness measurement can be made validly and reproducibly within the common carotid, bifurcation and internal carotid arteries and this measurement is now being used to monitor the development of atherosclerosis in a large multicentre studies in the United States [39] and Italy [41]. Identification of arterial wall abnormalities by ultrasound has already been shown to correlate with the presence of cardiovascular risk factors [42].

High resolution ultrasound as described above, is at present, limited to the superficial arteries, in particular the carotid and femoral arteries but, as a screening test for the presence of atherosclerotic disease, the latter seem to be sufficient.

Angiography

The increasing availability of a duplex scanning service has altered the role of angiography in the assessment of occult carotid disease. Whereas previously, angiography was the only anatomical method of assessment of the carotid artery, this role has largely been superseded by duplex ultrasonography. In our hospital, only 18% of asymptomatic and 34% of symptomatic patients will proceed to angiography after duplex scanning. Angiography still has a role in the preoperative assessment of disease and as a confirmation of duplex findings. Conventional angiography may provoke a stroke in 2.4% of patients [5] therefore angiographic techniques have been developed which have a lower risk of producing stroke.

Intravenous digital subtraction angiography (IVDSA)

Using computerised subtraction techniques, large arteries can be examined following the intravenous injection of a contrast medium. This can be performed on an out-patient basis. The technique is suitable for examination of the extracranial and intracranial arteries, with the added advantage that it allows visualisation of the aortic arch and the origin of the great vessels. However the method is not without its disadvantages. It is susceptible to motion artifact and, as the contrast medium fills all the vessels simultaneously, vessel overlap may occur. Furthermore, poor arterial opacification may occur in the presence of cardiac disease and the spatial resolution may be poor in comparison to direct arteriography, this is because a low concentration of contrast reaches the arteries after intravenous injection, therefore the final image has to be amplified and considerable noise develops during the process. Two studies [43, 44] have looked at the complication rates of IVDSA. The overall risk of stroke and TIA was low (0.3% and 0.5% respectively), however the risk of systemic complications was 6–23%. Prospective studies [45–51] comparing the results of IVDSA with conventional angiography or operative specimens report an overall accuracy of between 50–96% with a mean of 64% [52]. Furthermore, the negative predictive value of a normal IVDSA is low, therefore a significant stenosis may be overlooked [53].

In our hospital, it has become routine practice to perform a duplex scan on all patients with suspected carotid disease undergoing an IVDSA examination. This combination is a powerful and yet safe investigative tool while IVDSA on its own leaves a lot to be desired. A study of the relative safety and clinical utility of intravenous carotid DSA has been performed as part of a multicentre survey [54]. This study compared the experience of IVDSA with intra-arterial studies, both conventional and DSA. No neurological complications were reported in 3710 IVDSA studies. Adverse reactions included local extravasation of contrast (0.2%) and transient chest pain (0.2%), but no angina occurred in patients with known ischaemic heart disease who were being examined prior to elective coronary by-pass surgery. Out of 510 IADSA's and 780 conventional cerebral angiograms, severe, sudden neurological deficits occurred in four and six examinations respectively (0.7% and 0.8%). In an assessment of the clinical utility of IVDSA, it was found that in only 6% was an intra-arterial study requested after an initial IVDSA, the reasons for the request being poor quality of the original study in half, the rest were requested to confirm an occluded internal carotid artery. Furthermore, during the study period, IVDSA was the only form of contrast angiography performed prior to carotid endarterectomy in 75.2%, although most also had duplex ultrasonography. This study confirms the safety of IVDSA compared with other invasive vascular imaging techniques. In our centre, we advocate duplex ultrasonography as the first line investigation for occult cerebrovascular disease, supplemented where necessary by IVDSA. A small number (6%) may require an intraarterial DSA as well.

Computerised tomographic (CT) scanning

The main role of CT scanning in occult carotid artery disease is to demonstrate intraparenchymal changes and silent infarcts. In early studies, the yield was small due to the poor resolution of the CT scanners. However silent infarcts on CT are common; their incidence increases with increasing degrees of carotid stenosis and their presence in patients with ipsilateral carotid plaques suggests plaque ulceration [54–56]. In our own study of asymptomatic patients undergoing carotid endarterectomy for tight stenoses, the incidence of cerebral infarction is 31%. CT scanning has also been used in the evaluation of carotid plaques [57, 58].

Magnetic resonance imaging

Magnetic resonance imaging is a new imaging technique that offers particular promise in the examination of the vascular system since vessels can be delineated without the need for contrast material. Furthermore, magnetic resonance imaging has better soft tissue contrast than radiography, ultrasound or CT and has the unique potential for tissue characterisation and analysis of blood flow. It is therefore ideally suited for the examination of the cerebral circulation. Magnetic resonance imaging uses radiofrequency pulses to generate echoes. In vascular imaging, as well as conventional spin echo imaging, three further imaging techniques can be used: flow-void, flow enhanced and flow-only imaging. Spin echo imaging has been used to diagnose carotid artery stenosis and dissection [59–61]. MR angiography can be used to examine the intracerebral [62] and extracerebral circulations [62–65] with excellent results; it has the potential to replace conventional and digital subtraction angiography. Furthermore, MR has been shown to be the most sensitive method of diagnosing a cerebral infarct [66–72]. Should an MR scan of the brain be performed at the same time as an examination of the carotid arteries, it would eliminate the need for two separate studies (angiography and CT) with potentially a greater yield, the examination could then become cost effective.

No data exists at the present on the incidence of silent infarction in the population or in patients with asymptomatic carotid artery disease.

Positron emission tomography (PET)

This scanning technique provides pathophysiological information of cerebral blood flow, cerebral metabolism and other physiological variables, as a function of the site of injury, the time course of the injury and the aetiology of the ischaemia. Studies using PET scanning in cerebral ischaemia have provided important into the interrelationship between cerebral blood flow and metabolism [73]. However in the screening diagnosis and treatment of occult cerebrovascular disease, its role is restricted to a research tool.

Conclusion

The detection of asymptomatic disease of the carotid artery can be achieved with the minimum of intervention. Duplex scanning and high resolution ultrasonography are currently being used in a number of long-term follow-up studies [38, 39, 41]. These will permit the accurate documentation of disease progression and allow a greater understanding of the pathology of atherosclerosis, its risk factors and the role of therapy, whether surgical or medical, in bringing about a cessation of disease progression or frank regression. A greater understanding of the natural history of asymptomatic disease of the carotid artery will provide the answer to the vexing question of when to perform a carotid endarterectomy for asymptomatic disease.

Furthermore, high resolution ultrasonography can be used as a quick and easy method of screening for evidence of atherosclerosis, with a greater predictive power than any of the non-invasive methods used in current practice. In the future, we may see this test replacing the ECG in the screening of healthy people.

References

1. Chambers B R and Norris J W. Clinical significance of asymptomatic neck bruits. Neurology 1985; 37:742.
2. Fields W S, Lemak N A, Frankowski R F *et al.* Controlled trial of aspirin in cerebral ischaemia. Stroke 1977; 8:301.
3. Wolf P A, Kannel W B, Sorlie P *et al.* Asymptomatic carotid bruit land the risk of stroke, the Framingham study. JAMA 1981; 245:1442.
4. Heyman A, Wilkinson W E, Heyden S *et al.* Risk of stroke in asymptomatic persons with cervical arterial bruits: a population study in Evans County, Geogia. N Eng J Med 1980; 302:838.
5. Leow K, Murie J A. Cerebral angiography for cerebrovascular disease: the risks. Br J Surg 1988; 75:428.
6. Kistler J P, Lees R S, Miller A *et al.* Correlation of spectral phonangiography and carotid angiography with gross pathology in carotid stenosis. New Eng J Med 1981; 305:417.
7. Duncan G W, Gruber J O, Dewet C F *et al.* Evaluation of carotid stenosis by phonangiography. New Eng J Med 293:1124.
8. Thiele B L. Standards in noninvasive cerebrovascular testing. In: Recent advances in noninvasive diagnostic techniques in vascular disease (ed) Eugene Bernstein. The CV Mosby Co. 1990.
9. Neath Folger W. Noninvasive studies. In: Occlusive cerebrovascular disease. Diagnosis and surgical management Sundt T M (Ed) WB Saunders Co. 1987.
10. Blackshear W M, Thiele B L, Harley J D *et al.* A prospective evaluation of oculoplethysmography and carotid phonoangiography. Surg Gynecol Obstet 1979; 148:201.
11. Neath Folger W. Non-invasive studies in Occlusive Cerebrovascular disease, Diagnosis and surgical management Sundt T M (Ed) WB Saunders Co. 1987.
12. Bernstein E F, Dilley R B, Goldberger L E, Gosink B B, Leopold G R. Growth rates of small aortic aneurysms. Surgery 1976; 8:765.
13. Barnes R W, Bone G E, Reinertson J *et al.* Non-invasive ultrasonic prospective carotid angiography: prospective validation by contrast arteriography. Surgery 1976; 80:328.
14. Hokanson D E, Mozersky D J, Sumner D S *et al.* Ultrasonic arteriography: a noninvasive method of arterial visualization. Radiology 1972; 102:435.
15. Mozersky D J, Hokanson D E, Baker D W *et al.* Ultrasonic arteriography. Arch Surg 1971; 103:663.
16. Lusby R J, Ferrell L D, Ehrenfeld W K *et al.* Carotid plaque haemorrhage. Its role in the production of cerebral ischaemia. Arch Surg 1982; 117:1479.
17. Hokanson D E, Mozersky D J, Sumner D S *et al.* Ultrasonic arteriography: A new approach to arterial visualization. Biomed Eng 1971; 6:420.

18. Barber F, Baker D, Nation A *et al.* Ultrasonic duplex echo-Doppler scanner. IEEE Trans Biomed Eng 1974; 21:109.
19. Breslau PJ, Fell G, Phillips DJ, Thiele BL, Strandness DE Jr. Evaluation of carotid bifurcation disease: the role of common carotid artery velocity patterns. Arch Surg 1982; 117:58.
20. Roederer GO, Strandness DE Jr. A simple spectral parameter for the classification of severe carotid disease. Bruit 1984; 8:174.
21. Kohler TR, Zierler RE, Strandness DE, Duplex scanning and spectral analysis. In: Surgery for cerebrovascular disease S Wesley Moore (ed) Churchill Livingstone, 1987.
22. Williams MA, Deacon DFS, Szendro G, Belcaro G, Nicolaides AN. Duplex scanning in the detection and grading of internal carotid artery stenosis: improved criteria. In: Cardiovascular applications of Doppler ultrasound. AM Salmasi, AN Nicolaides (eds) Churchill Livingstone. Edinburgh 1989.
23. Roederer GO, Langois YE, Lusiani L *et al.* Natural history of carotid artery disease on the side contralateral to endarterectomy. J Vasc Surg 1984; 1:62.
24. Boggousslavsky J, Despland P-A, Regli F, Asymptomatic tight stenosis of the internal carotid artery: long term prognosis. Neurology 1986; 36:861.
25. Moneta GL, Taylor DC, Zieler RE, Kazmers A, Beach K, and Strandness DE Jr. Asymptomatic high-grade internal carotid stenosis: Is stratification according to risk factors or duplex spectral analysis possible.? J Vasc Surg 1989; 10:475.
26. Persson AV. Use of ultrasonic colour imaging in the evaluation of the venous system. In: Cardiovascular applications of Doppler ultrasound. AM Salmasi, AN Nicolaides (Ed) Churchill Livingstone Edinburgh, 1989.
27. Moneta GL, Taylor DC, Nicholls SC *et al.* Operative versus non-operative ámanagement of asymptomatic high-grade internal carotid artery stenosis: Improved results with endarterectomy. Stroke 1987; 18:1005.
28. Caracci BF, Zuckowski AJ, Hurley JJ, *et al.* Asymptomatic severe carotid stenosi J Vasc Surg 1989; 9:361.
29. Reilly LM, Lusby RJ, Hughes L, Ferrell LD, Stoney RJ, Ehrenìeld WK. Carotid plaque histology using real time ultrasonography. Clinical and Therapeutic Implications. Am J Surg 1983; 146:188.
30. Johnson TJ, Kenelly MM, Decasare D *et al.* Natural history of asymptomatic carotid plaque. Arch Surg 1985; 120:1010.
31. Gray-Weale AC, Graham J, Burnett JR, Byrne K, Lusby RJ. Carotid artery atheroma. Comparison of preoperative B-mode ultrasound appearance with carotid endarterectomy specimen pathology. J Cardiovasc Surg 1988; 29(6):676.
32. Langsfield M, Gray-Weale AC, Lusby RJ. The role of plaque morphology and diameter reduction in the development of new symptoms in asymptomatic carotid arteries. J Vasc Surg 1989; 9:548.
33. Bluth EI, Kay D, Merritt CRB *et al.* Sonographic characterisation of carotid plaque: detection of haemorrhage. Am J Radiol 1986; 1061.
34. Visona A, Lusiani L, Castellani V *et al.* The echo-Doppler (duplex) system for the detection of vertebral occlusive disease: comparison with angiography. J Ultrasound Med 1986; 5:247.
35. Ackerstaff RGA, Eikleboom BC, Hoeneveld H, Moll FL, Vries AR, Ultrasonic duplex scanning in atherosclerotic disease of the innominate, subclavian and vetebral arteries. A comparitive study with angiography. Ultrasound Med Biol 1984; 10:409.
36. Pignoli P. Ultrasound B-mode imaging for arterial wall thickness measurement. Atherosclerosis Rev 1984; 12:177.
37. Poli A, Tremoli E, Colombo A *et al.* Ultrasonographic measureìment of the common carotid wall thickness in hypercholesterolaemìic patients. Atherosclerosis 1988; 70:233.

38. Salonen R and Salonen J T. Progression of carotid atherosclerosis and its determinants: a population based ultrasonography study. Atherosclerosis 1990; 81:33.
39. The ARIC Investigators, The atherosclerosis risk in communities (ARIC study) design and objectives. Am J Epid 1989; 129:687.
40. Heiss G, Risk factors for carotid atherosclerosis. Proceedings of the Milan International Workshop on ultrasound methods for atherosclerosis and research and prevention. Milan, 1990.
41. Ventura A. The carotid artery Italian ultrasound study (CAIUS). Proceedings of the International Workshop on ultrasound methods for atherosclerosis and research and prevention. Milan, 1990.
42. Scheinberg P. Controversies in the management of cerebrovascular disease. Neurology 1988; 38:1609.
43. Aaron J O, Hesselink J R, Oot R *et al.* Complications of intravenous DSA performed for carotid artery disease: a prospective study. Radiology 1984; 153:675.
44. Ball J B, Lukin R R, Tomsick T A, Chambers A A, Complications of intravenous digital subtraction angiography. Arch Neurol 1985; 41:969.
45. Chilcote W A, Modie M T, Pavlicek W A *et al.* Digital subtraction angiography of the carotid arteries: a comparative study in 100 patients. Radiology 1981; 139:287.
46. Russell J B, Watson T M, Modi J R *et al.* Digital subtraction angiography for evaluation of extracranial carotid occlusive disease: comparison with conventional angiography. Surgery 1983; 94:604.
47. Wood G W, Lukin R R, Tomsick T A, Chambers A A. Digital subtraction angiography with intravenous injection: assessment of 1000 carotid bifurcations. Am J Radiol 1983; 140:855.
48. Reilly L M, Ehrenfild W K, Stoney R J. Carotid digital subtraction angiography: the comparative roles of intraarterial and intravenous imaging. Surgery 1984; 96:909.
49. Mendel H J, Olbert F, Schlegl A, Nebosis M. Duplex ultrasonography, intravenous digital subtraction angiography, intraarterial digital subtraction angiography and conventional angiography in assessing carotid atherosclerosis. Ann Radiol 1987; 30:115.
50. Glover J L, Bendick P J, Jackson V P *et al.* Duplex ultrasonography, digital subtraction angiography and conventional angiograìphy in assessing carotid atherosclerosis. Arch Surg 1984; 119:664.
51. Turnispeed W D, Sackett J F, Strother C M, Crummy A B, Mistretta C A. A comparison of standard cerebral arteriography with noninvasive Doppler imaging and intravenous angiography. Arch Surg 1982; 117:419.
52. Turner W H, and Murie J A. Intravenous digital subtraction angiography for extracranial carotid artery disease. Br J Surg 1989; 76:1247.
53. Eikelboom B A, Ackerstaff R G A, Ludwig J W *et al.* Digital video ìsubtraction angiography and duplex scanning in the assessment of ìcarotid artery disease: comparison with conventional angiography. Surgery 1983; 94:821.
54. Grigg M J, Papadekis K, Nicolaides A N *et al.* The significance of cerebral infarction and atrophy in patients with amaurosis fugax and transient ischaemic attacks in relation to internal carotid artery stenosis. J Vasc Surg 1988; 7:215.
55. Norris J W and Chambers B R. Stroke risk and critical carotid stenosis. J. Neurol. Neurosurg and Psych 1990; 53:235.
56. Zukowski A J, Nicolaides A N, Lewis R T *et al.* The correlation between carotid plaque ulceration and cerebral infarction seen on CT scan. J Vasc Surg 1984; 1:782.
57. Frisen L *et al.* Detection of extracranial carotid stenosis by computed tomography. Lancet 1979; 1:1319.
58. Culebras A, Leeson M D, Cacayorin E D *et al.* Computed tomographic evaluation of cervical carotid plaque complications. Stroke 1985; 16:425.

59. Heinz E R, Yeates A E, Djang W T. Significant extracranial carotid stenosis: detection on routine cerebral MR images. Radiology 1989; 170:843.
60. Hinshaw D B, Holshouser B, Hasso A N. Magnetic resonance áimagìing of the normal carotid bifurcation. Neuroradiology 1987; 29:7.
61. Asbury A K, Bilanuik L T, Zimmerman R A. Cervical internal carotid artery dissecting haemorrhage: diagnosis using MR. Radiology 1986; 158:157.
62. Masaryk T J, Modic M T, Ross J S *et al.* Intracranial circulation: preliminary clinical results with three dimensional (volume) MR Angiography. Radiology 1989; 171:793.
63. Nitz W R, Mawad M E, Wendt R E. MR angiography of the extracranial cerebral circulation Magn Reson Imag 1989; 7(s1):38.
64. Masaryk T J, Ross J S, Modic M T, Lenz G W, Haacke E M. Carotid bifurcation: MR imaging. Radiology 1988; 166:461.
65. Ruszkowski J T, Damadian R, Giambalvo A. MRI angiography of the carotid artery. Magn Reson Imag 1986; 4:497.
66. Sipponen J T, Kaste M, Ketonen L. Serial nuclear magnetic resonance (NMR) imaging in patients with cerebral infarction. áJ Comput Assist Tmomgr 1983; 7:575.
67. Bradley W G, Waluch V, Yadley R A, Wycoff R R. Comparison of CT and MR in 400 patients with suspected disease of the brain and cervical spinal cord. Radiology 1984; 152:695.
68. Kricheff I I. Arteriosclerotic ischaemic cerebrovascular disease. Radiology. 1987; 162:101.
69. Brandt-Zawadzki M N, Weinstein P, Bartkowski H. MR imaging and spectroscopy áin clinical and experimental cerebral ischaemia: áa review. Am J Neuroradiol 1987; 8:39.
70. Brandt-Zawadzki M N. MR imaging of the brain. Radiology 1988; 166:1.
71. Brown J J, Hesselink J R, Rothrock J F. MR and CT of lacunar infarcts. Am J Neuroradiol 1988; 9:477.
72. Black S E, Helpern J A, Kertesz A. Nuclear magnetic resonance imaging and spectroscopy in stroke. In: Surgery for Cerebrovascular Disease W S Moore (ed) Churchill Livingstone 1987.
73. Mazziotta J C. Positron Emission Tomography. In: Surgery for Cerebrovascular Disease W S Moore (Ed) Churchill Livingstone 1987.

5. The diagnosis and management of occult atherosclerotic disease of the extra-cranial carotid artery

MICHAEL J. GRIGG and KENNETH A. MYERS

Carotid artery surgery has been employed for more than thirty years to prevent stroke in patients considered to be at risk. In the past, suspicion of increased risk has been prompted by the development of focal hemispheric events such as transient ischaemic attacks (TIA's) or amaurosis fugax, or the clinical finding of a mid-cervical bruit. More recently, the availability of duplex ultrasound technology has enabled risk free and accurate examination of the extra-cranial carotid circulation and the detection of carotid bifurcation atheromatous plaques even in patients without symptoms or signs – that is, with occult disease.

Whilst stroke is a common cause of death and disability in western society, the role of prophylactic carotid endarterectomy in asymptomatic patients remains controversial. Attitudes vary as evidenced by the marked disparity in the prevalence of the operation in different countries ranging from about 20 operations per million in Great Britain to more than 400 per million in the USA [1]. The debate, at times heated, continues to founder in a sea of uncertainty and will continue to do so until the natural history of specific subgroups of patients is known and management options assessed by properly controlled trials. It should be recognized that valid trials may not be possible until a greater understanding of the development and progression of atheromatous plaque has been achieved. At the present time, management recommendations for asymptomatic carotid bifurcation disease range from observation alone to aggressive surgical intervention.

A recent report from Lausanne re-emphasizes that there is a demonstrable relationship between extracranial carotid disease and stroke [2]. One thousand consecutive patients suffering from their first stroke were studied by computerised cerebral tomography (CT) and duplex ultrasound scanning of the carotid bifurcations. Approximately one half of the patients had evidence of extracranial atherosclerosis. In the patients with carotid territory infarcts, one third had internal carotid artery stenosis greater than 50% or

A.-M. Salmasi and A. N. Nicolaides (eds.), Occult Atherosclerotic Disease, 59–73.

occlusion. Stroke had been preceded by premonitory transient ischaemic attacks in only 25% of patients. Thus, the occurrence of warning symptoms cannot be relied upon to indicate carotid bifurcation disease with stroke producing potential – the first manifestation of occult carotid disease is frequently stroke [3, 4].

However the presence of carotid artery disease *per se* confers only a low overall risk of stroke. The challenge of occult atheromatous disease of the carotid artery is to identify the subset of patients who are at sufficiently high risk to justify operative intervention. In the past, the severity of the stenosis produced by the atheromatous plaque has been used as the primary criterion for defining risk. This chapter will review the results of this approach and examine other variables which may assist in defining the risk of stroke, and thus the need for prophylactic surgery.

Methods of identifying asymptomatic carotid disease

Cervical bruit

Certainly the simplest method is auscultation of the neck and the finding of a mid-cervical bruit. However the value of this physical sign has been questioned [5–7] and many clinicians believe its only relevance is as a marker for coronary artery disease rather than significant carotid disease [8]. David and associates [9] investigated 265 patients with cervical bruit and found only a 47% incidence of significant carotid lesions. Of more concern was the 25% of arteries without bruits but which had stenoses greater than 50%. Severe stenoses may not produce a murmur if the flow is low [10]. Kartchner and McRae [11] studied 1,287 patients with asymptomatic cervical bruits using oculoplethysmography and carotid phonoangiography. Only 21% of these patients were shown to have a significant stenosis of the internal carotid artery.

The Framingham [8] and Evans County [12] population studies showed that the risk of subsequent strokes in patients with carotid bruits was low – approximately 2% per annum, although this was two to three times greater than for the general population. Ellis and Greenhalgh [13] followed patients with lower limb ischaemia for a mean period of 5.5 years. The stroke rate was 9% per annum for patients with a bruit and 8% for those without suggesting that the presence or absence of a bruit was of little value in defining risk, but the presence of arterial disease elsewhere may be a risk factor for future stroke. In fact, a greater than 75% stenosis of the internal carotid artery has been reported in 10% of asymptomatic patients with risk factors for arterial disease such as non-insulin dependant diabetes, hypertension or hyperlipidaemia [14–16].

Past reports have used a cervical bruit as a marker for occult carotid disease in natural history studies. Since it is now apparent that 40–60% of asymptomatic patients with bruits do not have haemodynamically significant lesions, such studies are of little or no value. Attempts have been made to increase the clinical relevance of a cervical bruit by subjectively assessing pitch and duration with respect to the cardiac cycle and this approach may be of some benefit to some clinicians. For individual patients found to have a cervical bruit, a reasonable course of action is to non-invasively assess the carotid bifurcation by way of a duplex scan.

Oculoplethysmography (OPG)

This indirect, non-invasive method of assessing the carotid circulation is largely of historical interest and is no longer widely used as an investigative technique. Nevertheless, Kartchner and McRae [17], using OPG, were among the first to demonstrate that haemodynamically significant carotid lesions, i.e. OPG positive, were associated with a higher risk of future stroke than less severe lesions (OPG negative). Similar results were reported by Busuttil and colleagues [18]. The three- to four-fold increased risk of stroke helped focus attention on a high risk subset of patients with occult carotid artery disease. Whether this increased risk is sufficiently high to justify the risks of surgery remains contentious. It is worth noting that not all severe carotid stenoses result in strokes which suggests that there are other factors exerting influence.

Ultrasound and duplex scans

The ability to directly, accurately and non-invasively study the extracranial carotid circulation by way of ultrasound has precipitated enormous interest in occult carotid disease and thus stroke prevention. Criteria for grading stenoses from Doppler ultrasound peak velocities and spectral broadening have already been established [19, 20]. Glover *et al.* [21] compared duplex scans and angiographic results in 494 arteries and found that agreement was 'absolute' in 71%, 'good' in 20% and 'poor' in only 9%. It has been shown that duplex scans diagnosed stenoses of greater than 50% with a 95% sensitivity and an 85% specificity [22].

The advent of a safe, non-invasive method of assessing the carotid bifurcation has enabled some assessment of the natural history of occult atheromatous plaques by way of longitudinal studies. Roederer *et al.* [23] prospectively studied 167 asymptomatic patients with duplex scans at six monthly intervals for the first year and then yearly for three years. There was a 4% annual incidence of neurological symptoms with ten patients becoming symptomatic during follow-up and a further six developing silent occlusion of their internal carotid arteries. One of the most significant findings of this study was that 89% of patients becoming symptomatic (TIA's or stroke) or who silently occluded the internal carotid artery demonstrated disease progression, developing stenoses of 80% or greater. Moreover, patients with a stenosis of the internal carotid artery of 80% or greater had a 35% incidence of TIA, stroke or occlusion at six months. For patients with stenoses of less than 80% the outcome was good with only a 1.5% risk of symptoms.

The importance of severe carotid stenosis as a risk factor for future stroke in asymptomatic patients was also shown by Chambers and Norris [24]. They studied and then followed 500 patients with continuous wave Doppler examinations. Patients who developed severe stenoses (i.e. >75%) had an incidence of neurological symptoms (TIA or stroke) of 22% at two years (annual stroke rate 5.5%).

Two important points emerge from these and other studies [25–28]: i) some occult atheromatous plaques are capable of relatively rapid progression to become severely stenotic lesions, and; ii) severely stenotic plaques are more dangerous in terms of future risk of stroke than milder lesions. Unfortunately the small number of events in such studies makes quantification of the conclusions difficult. As an example, in the report by Roederer and associates [23], only 4 patients developed strokes during follow-up and only 7 patients in the Chamber and Norris study [24]. In addition, the factors which promote progression and increase in size of plaques remain unknown and are a fertile area for future research.

Arteriography

Arteriography has been the most accurate investigation available for assessing the degree of stenosis of the carotid artery. The inherent stroke risk of this invasive investigation makes it inappropriate for screening for severe occult carotid disease. Even intravenous digital subtraction angiography (IV DSA), which reduces the well recognized risks of intra-arterial cannulation and injection, is not without significant morbidity [29, 30]. IV DSA has other limitations as a screening technique for carotid disease. Russell *et al.* [31] found that 26% of lesions producing stenoses greater than 50% had IV DSA studies indicating either lesser degrees of stenosis or were technically inadequate. Moreover, two-dimensional angiography will only display the residual lumen of the vessel and not the 'true' dimensions of the arterial wall. Thus mild to moderate occult plaques may not be recognized, particularly in the region of the carotid bulb [32].

Longitudinal studies employing serial arteriography are not possible. However, Hertzer and colleagues [33] followed 195 patients with asymptomatic carotid stenoses who had angiography. They found that the cumulative stroke rate correlated with the initial degree of stenosis of the internal carotid artery. For patients with stenoses of 50 – 69%, the five-year cumulative incidence of stroke was 20%, for stenoses of 70 – 89% it was 24% and for stenoses of 90% or greater, it was 32% at five years. These risks of stroke contrasted with 106 patients who did not have a demonstrable carotid lesion at angiography, the incidence of stroke during follow-up being only 5%.

Dixon and colleagues [34] performed a similar follow-up study on 153 asymptomatic patients undergoing carotid angiography. However, they were interested not in the degree of stenosis produced by the plaque, but rather the presence of ulceration in the plaque which they classified as small, large or extensive [35]. They found annual stroke rates of 0.9% for small ulcers, 4.5% for large ulcers and 7.5% for extensive ulcers. Kroener *et al.* [36] reported their experience with 87 non-stenotic ulcerative lesions followed conservatively. Their study confirmed a low stroke risk with non-stenotic shallow ulcers and a significant stroke risk with extensive, cavernous, complex ulcers.

With the availability of increasingly sophisticated ultrasound technology, it is apparent that plaque ulceration can be more accurately diagnosed with this modality than with angiography. Indeed Eikelboom and colleagues [37] found that arteriography had only a 73% sensitivity and 62% specificity for diagnosing ulceration as judged by examination of endarterectomy specimens. Goodson *et al.* [38] reported an accuracy for diagnosing plaque ulceration of 54% for arteriography compared to 90% for B-mode ultrasound scans.

Are all stenotic atheromatous plaques similar?

Historically, reliance upon angiography for diagnosis has made it necessary to classify atheromatous plaques at the carotid bifurcation on the basis of the degree of stenosis. From the discussion thus far, it is apparent that this approach does distinguish a subset of patients with occult disease who are at increased risk of stroke, i.e. those with severe stenoses of 75%–80% or more. However the risk is low such that a decision to recommend operation in every case is not possible. Certainly patients require time for statistical benefit to accrue, i.e. they must have a reasonable life expectancy to justify the immediate risks of surgery. Also the risk of 'unheralded' strokes is even lower since a proportion of patients will develop warning symptoms. Although there is debate over the incidence of warning symptoms [3, 23, 24, 39–41] probably one third to one half of strokes attributed to carotid artery disease are the first manifestation of an asymptomatic lesion.

In order to determine the factors at work on or within a severely stenotic plaque which make it a danger, it may first be necessary to ascertain the mechanisms by which extracranial disease produces a stroke. Two theories have been advanced – 'haemodynamic failure' and 'embolism'. The former is supported by the fact that an 80% reduction in luminal diameter will be flow-limiting. However the ultimate flow limiting lesion (carotid occlusion) tends to produce more extensive hemispheric events, both clinically and on CT scan [42]. Occlusion of the carotid artery significantly increases the risk of future stroke [43] and is often preceded by a severe stenosis [23] suggesting that prevention of occlusion may be worthwhile.

The embolic theory is perhaps more attractive to surgeons who have observed the debris associated with atheromatous plaques when performing carotid endarterectomy. In addition, the focal nature of symptomatic events is better explained. The validity of this postulate requires an explanation as to why severely stenotic plaques should be more likely to produce emboli. Consequently, there is interest in the characteristics of carotid plaques other than just the degree of stenosis – more particularly this interest has focused on carotid plaque morphology.

Langsfeld and coworkers [44] used duplex scanning to assess plaque constitution in patients. They classified plaques as heterogeneous if they contained echolucent areas or as homogeneous if they were uniformly echogenic. Four hundred and nineteen carotid arteries were followed by duplex scan for a mean period of 22 months. About one quarter changed from homogeneous to heterogeneous with time. Few patients developed symptoms during follow-up but those that did were mostly from the small group of heterogeneous plaques causing more than 75% stenoses. Johnson *et al.* [45] also used B-mode ultrasound to describe atheromatous plaque morphology as either calcified, dense (echogenic) or soft (echolucent). Over a three year follow-up, only 10% of calcified, severely stenotic plaques developed neurological symptoms in contrast to 92% of patients with soft plaques, irrespective of the degree of stenosis. Verification of this study is urgently required.

Several histological studies suggest that morphological characteristics of the plaque contribute to the risk of neurological symptoms. These include intraplaque haemorrhage, lipid accumulations [15, 46–48] and ulceration [49–51]. It seems the larger the atheromatous plaque the greater the likelihood of these changes developing. It may be possible in the future to classify plaques as 'stable' or 'unstable' on the basis of morphological changes detected by ultrasound [38, 52–54] but quantification of the risk of stroke is not possible at this time.

Should the clinical situation affect management decisions?

An alternative approach is to determine whether specific clinical situations affect the risk of stroke, particularly in asymptomatic patients with significant carotid lesions. Various clinical scenaria are often discussed which utilise 'accessory' information such as:

i) the state of the contralateral carotid artery
ii) the presence of intracranial disease
iii) the cerebral CT scan appearance
iv) planned major surgery, e.g. coronary artery bypass grafts.

Bilateral carotid artery disease

An asymptomatic carotid artery lesion is often detected during investigation of the symptomatic contralateral side. It has been argued that these patients are not strictly asymptomatic but there is little evidence to suggest that they are at greater risk of stroke on the asymptomatic side other than the risk imposed by the severity of the stenosis alone [55–60]. Conversely, they do appear to be at greater risk of developing symptoms [56] i.e. TIA's are reported more frequently than by other asymptomatic patients with comparable degrees of unilateral stenosis suggesting 'sensitisation' to symptoms. Either this subset of patients is over-reacting to minor symptoms or our ability to educate other asymptomatic patients to 'warning' symptoms is inadequate.

Even occlusion contralateral to an asymptomatic stenosis does not appear to increase the risk of future stroke on the stenotic side [61, 62] although surgery for the stenosis is more dangerous [63]. Unfortunately, the comparatively high risk of future stroke ipsilateral to carotid artery occlusion is not reduced by operation on the stenosed contralateral side [64, 65].

The presence of coexisting intracranial disease

The natural history of severe intracranial disease appears to be poor. In one study [66], 43% of patients suffered stroke within a mean follow-up period of 30 months; two thirds were ipsilateral and most were fatal. In another study [67] the ipsilateral stroke rate with significant intracranial disease was about 8% per annum. Tandem intracranial disease is found in about 50% of patients with extracranial disease but most intracranial lesions are mild to moderate with little correlation between the severity of intra- and extracranial disease [68].

Lord *et al.* [69] observed that about 15% of patients treated with carotid endarterectomy had a 50–80% ipsilateral intracranial stenosis but only one quarter had abnormal OPG studies. In addition, the incidence of low stump pressure at operation was not increased and the small number of strokes in the series occurred in patients without coexisting intracranial disease. They concluded that tandem disease does not increase the risk of perioperative stroke. Although some surgeons are prepared to operate on the evidence of duplex scan alone [70], most continue to require arteriography, mainly to demonstrate coexisting intracranial disease. Although longer term prognosis is affected, there is little evidence to suggest that the decision for or against carotid endarterectomy should be influenced by intracranial disease.

Cerebral CT scans

Grigg *et al.* [71] performed cerebral CT scans and duplex ultrasound scans on all patients prior to carotid endarterectomy. The incidence of cerebral infarction seen on preoperative CT scan was 20% for carotid stenoses less than 50%, 40% for stenoses greater than 50% and 58% if the ipsilateral carotid artery was occluded. Interestingly the vast majority of CT infarcts were clinically silent. Even in patients with a history of focal TIA's there was a correlation in the incidence of CT infarction with the severity of carotid stenosis – 25% for stenoses less than 50% and 48% for stenoses greater than 50%.

Preoperative CT scans have also been correlated with the histology of endarterectomy specimens. Zukowski *et al.* [50] reported CT infarction in 8% of patients with non-ulcerated carotid plaques compared to 62% if ulceration was present. Street *et al.* [72] found CT infarcts in 20% of asymptomatic patients, in 33% of patients with TIA's and in 76% of patients with stroke. Similar findings have been reported by others [73–75].

Undoubtedly preoperative CT scans provide interesting information. However, for individual patients with occult carotid artery disease, interpretation of this information to allow better clinical decisions is not yet possible. The significance of 'clinically silent' cerebral infarction requires more knowledge with respect to natural history. Understanding would be enhanced if the cause of infarction could be defined on the basis of the appearance of the infarct. Magnetic resonance imaging appears to be more accurate in detecting cerebral infarction, particularly in patients with stroke, but the same problems of interpretation apply. The answer to the question 'do asymptomatic patients with a severe carotid stenosis (>75%) and evidence of a silent cerebral infarction on CT scan have a higher incidence of future stroke than patients with a normal CT scan?' is not known.

Perioperative patients

There is a lack of evidence that asymptomatic carotid bifurcation disease significantly increases stroke risk during abdominal aortic or aorto-coronary bypass surgery [76]. The immediate stroke risk after aorto-coronary bypass has been reported as 3–10% [77–79] and this appears to be most dependent on the patients age and the time on pump bypass [80]. Brener *et al.* [78]

investigated 4000 patients having coronary revascularisation procedures with non-invasive carotid studies and found an incidence of significant, asymptomatic carotid disease in only 5%. In patients with no carotid disease the incidence of perioperative stroke was 2% compared to 4–5% when uni- or bilateral carotid stenosis was present. In patients with carotid occlusion, the incidence of perioperative stroke was 15.6%. Even if stroke risks of coronary surgery are slightly increased with severe carotid stenosis, the increased risks of combined surgery suggest that surgical management of asymptomatic disease is best deferred until after recovery from coronary revascularisation [81].

Management options for asymptomatic carotid disease

The management of the patient with asymptomatic disease requires a decision to recommend for or against surgery. Recommending against prophylactic surgery must be regarded as a decision and the consequences must be weighed. Proponents of a conservative approach argue, not so much as to the low risk of the carotid lesion, but point to a supposedly high risk of carotid surgery. However, there are numerous studies which attest to the low morbidity and mortality of carotid endarterectomy performed for asymptomatic disease [82–87]. In this regard the best available operative results should be used so that the value of the operation itself can be assessed rather than the ability of the individual surgeon. Certainly, individual surgeons need to be able to perform the operation with a combined perioperative morbidity and mortality of less than 3% before they can consider undertaking prophylactic surgery [88]. If surgery is not undertaken, it is incumbent upon the clinician to educate the patient to recognise warning symptoms such as TIA's and amaurosis fugax.

Objective evidence of a role for anti-platelet therapy is lacking. Much misconception involving a role for aspirin treatment can be traced to the Canadian Co-operative Trial [89] performed 12 years ago and an American trial [90] performed 13 years ago. During a two year follow-up, strokes occurred in 16% of patients in the American trial and in 12% of patients in the Canadian trial whilst taking aspirin compared to 23% and 17% in the respective placebo groups. These differences were not statistically significant. In 1988, the Physician Health Study Report [91] sponsored by the United States Federal Drug Administration (FDA) suggested that a reinterpretation of the data of both the American and Canadian trials was necessary. In the FDA study, 22,000 volunteer physicians were prospectively randomised into two blinded cohorts receiving either aspirin or placebo. During a five year follow-up there was a significant reduction in myocardial infarction in the aspirin group, but no measurable difference in overall stroke rate. This study confirms a lack of evidence of benefit for aspirin as an alternative to surgery in preventing stroke due to occult carotid disease. It is disappointing that as yet there is no study which specifically examines the response of patients with severe carotid stenosis to aspirin.

Conclusion

In western society, stroke is a leading cause of death and disability. It has been estimated that as many as 60% of all strokes are related to disease of the carotid bifurcation [92] and that approximately 50% or more of these events are not preceded by warning symptoms [2]. There are grounds for being concerned about the occult atheromatous plaque of the carotid bifurcation. Attempts to retrospectively determine risk factors by way of follow-up studies have been largely unsuccessful. There is an emerging feeling that there exists a small subset of patients with occult carotid disease who have a high risk of stroke but who are being disguised by a very low risk of stroke in the majority.

Although there are two controlled randomised studies (United States Veterans Administration trial and National Institutes of Health trial) in progress which compare prophylactic carotid endarterectomy and medical management, the results will not be available for some years and even then they may not be able to define indications for surgery for occult carotid disease above and beyond what is known already.

Advances in ultrasound technology (i.e. duplex scanning) have enabled accurate, non-invasive detection and assessment of occult lesions of the carotid artery. Whilst helping to provide some insights into the natural history of the carotid plaque and into the composition of plaques, this technology has in many ways increased the size of the problem by allowing the detection of occult disease in larger numbers of patients. The greater availability of duplex scanners in the United States may be one reason for the substantially greater prevalence of surgery for asymptomatic disease in that country as compared to the United Kingdom, for example.

Despite attempts to define high risk subgroups, the severity of carotid stenosis remains the major identifiable factor in determining risk of future stroke. Patients with a 75% or greater stenosis are at increased risk of stroke and will experience a stroke rate of approximately 5% per annum. It may be that patients with clinical evidence of atheromatous disease in other vascular beds are at even greater risk. Large, complex ulcerated plaques also appear to impose an increased risk of stroke but other factors such as plaque heterogenicity and cerebral CT scan defects have not yet fulfilled early promise in defining high risk groups. There is little evidence to suggest contralateral carotid disease, impending major surgery or co-existing intracranial disease should influence decisions for or against surgical intervention for occult carotid artery disease.

Provided surgeons can perform prophylactic carotid surgery with a combined morbidity and mortality of less than 3% and provided the life expectancy of the patient is 3 years or more, prophylactic operation for severe stenoses (>75%) appears to be justified at this stage of our understanding of occult carotid disease. However, it is certain the debate will continue, and perhaps it is worth remembering the words of Voltaire – 'A long dispute means both parties are wrong!'

References

1. Murie J A, Morris P J. Carotid Endarterectomy in Great Britain and Ireland. Br J Surg 1986; 73:867.
2. Bogousslavsky J, Van Melle G, Regli F. The Lausanne State Registry: analysis of 1,000 patients with first stroke. Stroke 1988; 19:1083.
3. Mohr J B, Kaplan L R, Melski J W *et al.* The Harvard Cooperative Stroke Registry: A prospective registry. Neurology 1978; 28:754.
4. Roderer G O, Langlois Y E, Lusiani L *et al.* Natural history of carotid artery disease on the side contralateral to endarterectomy. J Vasc Surg 1984; 1:62.
5. Murie J A, Sheldon C D, Quin R O. Carotid artery bruit: association with internal carotid stenosis and intraluminal turbulence. Br J Surg 1984; 71:50.
6. Riles T S, Lieberman A, Kopelman I, Imparato A M. Symptoms, stenosis, and bruit. Arch Surg 1981; 116:218.
7. Hennerici M, Aulich A, Sandmann W, Freund H J. Incidence of asymptomatic extracranial arterial disease. Stroke 1981; 12:750.
8. Wolf P A, Kannel W B. Solie P, McNamara P. Asymptomatic carotid bruit and risk of stroke. The Framingham Study. JAMA 1981; 245:1442.
9. David T E, Humphries A W, Young J R *et al.* A correlation of neck bruits and artherosclerotic carotid arteries. Arch Surg 1973; 107:729.
10. Pessin M S, Panis W, Prager R J, Millan V G, Scott R M. Auscultation of cervical and ocular bruits in extracranial carotid occlusive disease: A clinical and angiographic study. Stroke 1983; 14:246.
11. Kartchner M M, McRae L P. Non-invasive evaluation and management of the asymptomatic carotid bruit. Surgery 1977; 82:840.
12. Heyman A, Wilkinson W E, Heyden S *et al.* Risk of stroke in asymptomatic persons with cervical arterial bruits. A population study in Evans County, Georgia. N Engl J Med 1980; 302:838.
13. Ellis M R, Greenhaigh R M, Management of asymptomatic carotid bruit. J Vasc Surg 1987; 5:869.
14. Chan A, Beach K W, Martin D C, Strandness D E. Carotid artery disease in NIDDM diabetes. Diabetes Care 1983; 6:562.
15. Van Merode T, Hick P, Hoeks A P G, Reneman R S. Serum HDL/total cholesterol ratio and blood pressure in asymptomatic artherosclerotic lesions of the cervical carotid arteries in men. Stroke 1985; 16:34.
16. Sutton K C, Wolfson S K, Kuller L H. Carotid and lower extremity arterial disease in elderly adults with isolated systolic hypertension. Stroke 1987; 18:817.

17. Kartchner MM, McRae LP. Guidelines for non-invasive evaluation of asymptomatic carotid bruits. Clin Neurosurg 1981: 28:418.
18. Busuttil RW, Baker JD, Davidson RK *et al.* Carotid artery stenosis – Hemodynamic significance and clinical course. JAMA 1981; 245:1438.
19. Green FM, Beach DE, Strandness DE, Fell G, Phillips DJ. Computer based pattern recognition of carotid arterial disease using pulsed Doppler ultrasound. Ultrasound Med Biol 1982; 8:161.
20. Langlois YE, Greene FM, Roederer GO *et al.* Computer based pattern recognition of carotid artery Doppler signals for disease classification: prospective validation. Ultrasound Med Biol 1984; 10:581.
21. Lord RSA, Graham AT. The validity of internal carotid back pressure measurements during carotid endarterectomy for unilateral carotid stenosis. Aust N Z J Surg 1986; 56:493.
22. Blackshear WM, Lamb SL, Kollipara VSK *et al.* Correlation of hemodynamically significant internal carotid stenosis with pulsed Doppler frequency analysis. Ann Surg 1984; 199:475.
23. Roederer GO, Langlois YE, Jager KA *et al.* The natural history of carotid arterial disease in asymptomatic patients with cervical bruits. Stroke 1984; 15:605.
24. Chambers BP, Norris JW. Outcome in patients with asymptomatic neck bruits. N Engl J Med 1986; 315:860.
25. Kelley RE, Pina I, Lee S. Cerebral ischaemia and mitral valve prolapse: case-control study of associated factors. Stroke 1988; 19:443.
26. Moore DJ, Miles RD, Gooley NA, Summer DS. Non-invasive assessment of stroke risk in asymptomatic and nonhemispheric patients with suspected carotid disease. Ann Surg 1985; 202:491.
27. Hennerici M, Hulsbomer HB, Hefter J, Lammerts D, Rautenberg W. Natural history of asymptomatic extracranial arterial disease. Brain 1987; 110:777.
28. Taylor LM, Loboa L, Porter JM. The clinical course of carotid bifurcation stenosis as determined by duplex scanning. J Vasc Surg 1988; 8:255.
29. Reilly LM, Elvenfeld WK, Stoney RJ. Carotid digital subtraction angiography: the comparative roles of intra-artrial and intravenous imaging. Surgery 1984; 96:909.
30. Aaron JO, Hesselink JR, Got R, Jones RL, Davis KR, Taveras JM. Complications of intravenous DSA performed for carotid artery disease: a prospective study. Radiology 1984; 153:675.
31. Russell JB, Watson TM, Modi JR, Lambeth A, Sumner DS. Digital subtraction angiography for evaluation of extracranial carotid disease. Comparison with conventional angiography. Surgery 1983; 94:604.
32. Williams MA, Nicolaides AN. Predicting the normal dimensions of the internal and external carotid arteries from the diameter of the common carotid. Eur J Vasc Surg 1987; 1:91.
33. Hertzer NR, Flanagan RA, O'Hara PJ, Beven EG. Surgical versus nonoperative treatment of asymptomatic carotid stenosis. 290 patients documented by intravenous angiography. Ann Surg 1986; 204:163.
34. Dixon S, Pais SO, Raviola C *et al.* Natural history of nonstenotic, asymptomatic ulcerative lesions of the carotid artery. Arch Surg 1982; 117:1493.
35. Moore WS, Boren C, Malone JM *et al.* Natural history of nonstenotic asymptomatic ulcerative lesions of the carotid artery. Arch Surg 1978; 113:1352.
36. Kroener JM, Dorn PL, Shoor PM *et al.* Prognosis of asymptomatic ulcerating carotid lesions. Arch Surg 1980; 115:1387.
37. Eikelboom BC, Riles TR, Mintzer R *et al.* Inaccuracy of angiography in the diagnosis of carotid ulceration. Stroke 1983; 14:882.
38. Goodson SF, Flanigan PD, Bishara RA, Schuler JJ, Kikta MJ, Meyer JP. Can carotid

duplex scanning supplant arteriography in patients with focal carotid territory symptoms? J Vasc Surg 1987; 5:551.

39. Bogousslavsky J, Van Melle G, Regli F. The Lausanne stroke registry: analysis of 1,000 consecutive patients with first stroke. Stroke 1988; 19:1083.
40. Humphries AW, Young JR, Santilli PH *et al.* Unoperated, asymptomatic significant internal carotid artery stenosis: A review of 182 instances. Surgery 1976; 80:695.
41. Barnes RW, Liebman PR, Marszalek PB *et al.* Natural history of asymptomatic carotid disease in patients undergoing cardiovascular surgery. Surgery 1981; 90:1075.
42. Tatemichi TK, Mohr JP, Rubinstein LU *et al.* CT Findings and clinical course in acute stroke. Stroke 1985; 16:138.
43. Pierce GE, Keushkerian SM, Hermreck AS, Iliopoulos JI, Thomas JH. The risk of stroke with occlusion of the internal carotid artery. J Vasc Surg 1988; 8:74.
44. Langsfeld M, Gray-Weale AC, Lusby RJ. The role of plaque morphology and diameter reduction in the development of new symptoms in asymptomatic carotid arteries. J Vasc Surg 1989; 9:548.
45. Johnson JM, Kennelly MM, Decesare D *et al.* Natural history of asymptomatic carotid plaque. Arch Surg 1985; 120:1010.
46. Lusby TJ, Ferrell LD, Ehrenfeld WK, Stoney RJ, Wylie EJ. Carotid plaque hemorrhage. Its role in production of cerebral ischaemia. Arch Surg 1982; 117:1479.
47. Persson AV, Intraplaque hemorrhage. Surg Clin N Am 1986; 66:415.
48. Aldoori MI, Baird RN, Al-Sam SZ, Cole SEA, Mera A, Davies JD. Duplex scanning and plaque histology in cerebral ischaemia. Eur J Vasc Surg 1987; 1:159.
49. Nicolaides AN, Zukowski AJ. The place of computerized tomographic brain scanning in the classification of ischaemic cerebral disease. In: Courbier R (ed). Basis for a Classification of Cerebral Arterial Diseases. Amsterdam, Excerpta Medica, Current Clinical Practice Series 1985; 22:59.
50. Zukowski AJ, Nicolaides AN, Lewis RT *et al.* The correlation between carotid plaque ulceration and cerebral infarction seen on CT scan. J Vasc Surg 1984; 1:782.
51. Padayachee TS, Kirkham FJ, Lewis RR, Gillard J, Hutchinson MCE, Gosling RG. Transcranial measurement of blood velocities in the basal cerebral arteries using pulsed Doppler ultrasound: a method of assessing the circle of Willis. Ultrasound Med Biol 1986; 12:5.
52. Reilly LM, Lusby RJ, Hughes L, Ferrell LD, Stoney RJ, Ehrenfeld WK. Carotid plaque histology using real-time ultrasonography. Clinical and therapeutic implications. Amer J Surg 1983; 146:188.
53. Hennerici M, Reifschneider G, Trockel U, Aulich A. Detection of early atherosclerotic lesions by duplex scanning of the carotid artery. J Clin Ultrasound 1984; 12:455.
54. Rubin JR, Bondi JA, Rhodes RS. Duplex scanning versus conventional arteriography for the evaluation of carotid artery plaque morphology. Surgery 1987; 102:749.
55. Humphries AW, Young JR, Santilli PH *et al.* Unoperated, asymptomatic significant internal carotid artery stenosis: A review of 182 instances. Surgery 1976; 80:695.
56. Levin SM, Sondenheimer FK, Levin JM. Contralateral diseased but asymptomatic carotid artery: To operate or not? An update. Am J Surg 1980; 140:203.
57. Roderer GO, Langlois YE, Lusiani L *et al.* Natural history of carotid artery disease on the side contralateral to endarterectomy. J. Vasc Surg 1984; 1:62.
58. Durward QJ, Furgeson GG, Barr HWK. The natural history of asymptomatic carotid bifurcation plaques. Stroke 1982; 13:459.
59. Podore PC, DeWeese JA, May AG *et al.* Asymptomatic contralateral carotid artery stenosis: A five year follow-up study following carotid endarterectomy. Surgery 1980; 88:748.
60. Johnson N, Burnham SJ, Flanigan DP *et al.* Carotid endarterectomy: A follow-up study of

the contralateral non-operated carotid artery. Ann Surg 1978; 188:748.
61. Cote R, Barnett HJM, Taylor DW. Internal carotid occlusion: A prospective study. Stroke 1983; 14:898.
62. Hennerici M, Hulsbomer HB, Rautenberg W, Hefter H. Spontaneous history of asymptomatic internal carotid occlusion. Stroke 1986; 17:718.
63. Sillesen H, Schroeder T, Rasmussen L, Hansen HJB. Carotid endarterectomy in patients with occulusion of the contralateral carotid artery: Pertioperative risk and late results. Eur J Vasc Surg 1987; 1:85.
64. Nicholls SC, Kohler TR, Bergelin RD, Primozich JF, Lawrence RL, Strandness DE. Carotid artery occlusion: natural history. J Vasc Surg 1986; 4:479.
65. Friedman SG, Riles TS, Lamparello PJ, Imparto AM, Sakwa MP. Surgical therapy for the patient with internal carotid artery occlusion and contralateral stenosis. J Vasc Surg 1987; 5:856.
66. Craig DR, Meguro K, Watridge C, Robertson JT, Barnett HJM, Fox AJ. Intracranial internal carotid artery stenosis. Stroke 1982; 13:825.
67. Marzewski DJ, Furlan AJ, St. Louis P, Little JR, Modic MT, Williams G. Intracranial internal carotid artery stenosis: Longterm prognosis. Stroke 1982; 13:821.
68. Keagy BA, Poole MA, Burnham SJ, Johnson G. Frequency, severity, and physiologic importance of carotid syphon lesions. J Vasc Surg 1986; 3:511.
69. Lord RSA, Raj TB, Graham AR. Carotid endarterectomy, siphon stenosis, collateral hemispheric pressure, and perioperative cerebral infarction. J Vasc Surg 1987; 6:391.
70. Thiele BL, Strandness DE. Distribution of intracranial and extracranial arterial lesions in patients with symptomatic cerebrovascular disease. In: Bernstein EF (ed), Noninvasive diagnostic techniques in vascular disease. St. Louis, CV Mosby 1985; 316.
71. Grigg MJ, Papadakis K, Nicolaides AN *et al.* The significance of cerebral infarction and atrophy in patients with amaurosis fugax and transient ischaemic attacks in relation to internal carotid artery stenosis: A preliminary report. J Vasc Surg 1988; 7:215.
72. Street DL, O'Brien MS, Ricotta JJ *et al.* Observations on cerebral computed tomography in patients having carotid endarterectomy. J Vasc Surg 1988; 7:798.
73. Dornhorf W, Hornig C. Partial non-progressing stroke – clinical criteria and computer tomography findings. In: Corbier R (ed), Basis for classification of cerebral arterial disease. Excerpta Medica, Amsterdam, Current Clinical Practice Series 1985; 22:50.
74. Bullock R, Mendelow AD, Bone I, Patterson J, Macleod WN, Allardice G. Cerebral blood flow and CO_2 responsiveness as an indicator of collateral reserve capacity in patients with carotid arterial disease. Br J Surg 1985; 72:348.
75. Calandre L, Gomara S, Bermejo F, Millan JM, Del Pozo G. Clinical-CT correlations in TIA, RIND, and strokes with minimum residuum. Stroke 1984; 15:663.
76. Hart RG, Easton JD. Management of cervical bruits and carotid stenosis in preoperative patients. Stroke 1983; 14:290.
77. Barnes RW. Asymptomatic carotid disease in patients undergoing major cardiovascular operations: can prophylactic endarterectomy be justified? Ann Thorac Surg 1986; 42:S36.
78. Brener BJ, Brief DK, Alpert J, Goldenkranz RJ, Parsonnet V. The risk of stroke in patients with asymptomatic carotid stenosis undergoing cardiac surgery: a follow-up study. J Vasc Surg 1987; 5:269.
79. Furlan AJ, Craciun AR. Risk of stroke during coronary artery bypass graft surgery in patients with internal carotid artery disease documented by angiography. Stroke 1985; 16:797.
80. Gardner TJ, Horneffer PJ, Manolio TA, Hoff SJ, Pearson TA. Major stroke after coronary artery bypass surgery: changing magnitude of the problem. J Vasc Surg 1986; 3: 684.
81. Brener BJ. When should carotid lesions be operated upon in conjunction with aorto-

coronary bypass. In: Current Critical Problems in Vascular Surgery, F. Veith (ed) Published by Quality Medical Publishing, St. Louis 1989; 518.
82. West H, Burton R, Roon A G *et al.* Comparative risk of operation and expectant management for carotid artery disease. Stroke 1979; 10:116.
83. Thompson J E, Padman R D, Talkington C M. Asymptomatic carotid bruit: Long term outcome of patients having endarterectomy compared with unoperated controls. Ann Surg 1978; 188:308.
84. Sergeant P T, Drom F, Berzsenye G *et al.* Carotid endarterectomy for cerebrovascular insufficiency: long term follow-up of 141 patients followed up to sixteen years. Acta Chir Belg 1979; 79:309.
85. Moore W S, Boren C, Malone J M *et al.* Asymptomatic carotid stenosis: Immediate and long term results after prophylactic endarterectomy. Am J Surg 1979; 138:228.
86. Moneta G L, Taylor D C, Nicholls S C *et al.* Operative versus nonoperative management of asymptomatic high grade internal carotid artery stenosis: Improved results with endarterectomy. Stroke 1987; 18:1005.
87. Quinones-Baldwich W J, Asymptomatic carotid stenoses. Seminars in Vascular Surgery 1989; 2:4.
88. Beebe H C, Clagett G P, DeWeese J A *et al.* Assessing Risk Associated with Carotid Endarterectomy. Stroke 1989; 20:314.
89. The Canadian Cooperative Study Group, A randomized trial of aspirin and sulphicpyrazone in threatened stroke. N Eng J Med 1978; 299:53.
90. Fields W S, Lemark N A, Frankowski R F, Hardy R J. Controlled trial of aspirin in cerebral ischaemia. Stroke 1977; 8:301.
91. Young F E, Nightingale S L, Temple R A. The preliminary report of the findings of the aspirin component of the ongoing physicians health study. JAMA 1988; 259:3158.
92. Moore W S. Current, immediate and long-tern results of surgery for asymptomatic lesions of the carotid artery. In: Current Critical Problems in Vascular Surgery, F. Veith (ed) Quality Medical Publishing, St. Louis 1989; 501.

PART THREE

Occult coronary artery disease

6. Risk factors and epidemiology in the pathogenesis and clinical progress of occult coronary artery disease

VASKAR MUKERJI and BRENT M. PARKER

The risk factors and epidemiology of occult atherosclerotic disease vary in different subsets of patients. While coronary artery disease may cause silent ischaemia, it can also remain occult in patients with diabetes mellitus, in elderly patients and in some young individuals manifesting only as sudden death during athletic activity. Additionally, certain patients with angina pectoris are found to have angiographically normal epicardial coronary arteries, and it has been postulated that some of these patients may have atherosclerosis in the intra-mural coronary branches. In this chapter we will review some of the information on these subgroups of patients, particularly relating to risk factors and epidemiology, and present data from our own research in this area.

Silent ischaemia

Coronary atherosclerosis is a disease that often progresses abruptly from an occult state to a lethal outcome with little or no warning. Sudden death is the first and also the last symptom in approximately 20 percent of patients with coronary artery disease [1]. Fifty percent of all deaths from coronary disease occur suddenly and only half of this group have any prior history of angina pectoris [2, 3]. For men in the Framingham Study population myocardial infarctions occurred in 3 per 1,000 under the age of 45 years, in 6 per 1,000 under the age of 65 years and in 13 per 1,000 after that age. Women lagged behind men by about 20 years for symptomatic infarctions, but by only 10 years for silent infarctions. Further, of the myocardial infarctions that developed in the Framingham Study subjects over 30 years, about a third were discovered only by changes on the routine biennial electrocardiogram [4, 5]. The proportion of silent myocardial infarctions was higher in women than in men and tended to increase with age. There was no

A.-M. Salmasi and A. N. Nicolaides (eds.), Occult Atherosclerotic Disease, 77–89.

difference in the location of the infarct whether it was silent or symptomatic. Other surveys of apparently healthy populations who underwent noninvasive screening with exercise testing followed by coronary arteriography indicate that 2.5 to 10 percent of middle-aged men appear to have asymptomatic coronary artery disease [6, 7].

The clinical progress of occult coronary atherosclerosis has been studied by a number of researchers. Giagnoni *et al.* [8] have demonstrated that symptomatic men with a positive exercise test have a 5.55:1 higher risk for cardiac events compared to those with a negative exercise test. In the Lipid Research Clinics Mortality Follow-Up Study [9] a positive exercise test was associated with a cumulative mortality of 11.9 percent over a mean period of 8.1 years as compared to 1.2 percent in 8.6 years for men with a negative stress test result. In the Norwegian study, Erikssen and Thaulow [6] followed 50 asymptomatic men with angiographically proven coronary artery disease. In 8 years, 3 had died, 7 had myocardial infarction, 16 had developed angina, 27 had more severe electrocardiographic abnormalities during exercise stress testing and only 17 remained clinically unchanged. After 12.5 years, 11 had died, 8 of the remaining subjects had developed myocardial infarction, 18 had angina and 24 of the remaining men demonstrated progression of coronary artery disease by angiography [10]. The mortality rate was 35 percent (3% annually) with three-vessel, 22 percent with two-vessel, and 7 percent with single-vessel coronary artery disease.

Data from the Framingham Study suggests that the risk factors which apply to symptomatic coronary disease also apply to occult disease [11]. However, hypertension and diabetes were identified as posing additional risk for asymptomatic myocardial infarction [12, 13]. The incidence of silent as well as the incidence of symptomatic myocardial infarctions are both increased in hypertensive individuals [12]. However, the proportion of silent myocardial infarctions increases with the severity of hypertension. Among hypertensive subjects in the Framingham Study, 38.6 percent of myocardial infarctions in men and 49.3 percent in women were silent. The risk of suffering a silent myocardial infarction was twice as high for a hypertensive person when compared to a normotensive person. The relationship of diabetes mellitus to occult coronary atherosclerosis is discussed later in the chapter.

Occult coronary atherosclerosis in the elderly

The prevalence of coronary artery disease rises progressively with increasing age. This relationship between age and cardiovascular disease has long been appreciated and has been particularly evident in the Framingham data [13, 14]. Although the overall mortality from ischaemic heart disease in the United States of America has declined since 1963, [15, 16] the relative contribution of the elderly to these mortality statistics has actually risen [17]. While this may be partly attributable to the aging of the general population, [18] other factors may also play a role. One obvious consideration is the extent to which coronary atherosclerosis may remain occult in this group of patients and manifest ultimately as acute myocardial infarction or sudden death.

Several investigators have studied myocardial infarction in the elderly [19–22]. Fodor and Tibblin, [23] assessing the incidence of sudden death as a manifestation of myocardial infarction, found that 45% of patients over the age of 65 years suffering an acute myocardial infarction died before reaching the hospital. In comparison only 25% of patients with acute myocardial infarction who were younger than 65 years of age died before arriving at the hospital. Williams and associates [20] studied 104 patients over the age of 70 years admitted to the Coronary Care Unit and reported that a significantly greater proportion of these patients (30%) developed symptoms while sleeping when compared to patients under the age of 70 years. Since coronary atherosclerosis usually develops gradually over many years preceding acute myocardial infarction, these data suggest that the condition may remain occult or present atypically in some elderly patients. In our own study of elderly patients with angiographically proven coronary artery disease we have reported that the description of angina pectoris in these patients differs significantly from that of younger individuals in several respects [24]. In the elderly, chest pain occurs less frequently in the typically substernal location, is of milder intensity and lasts for shorter periods of time compared to younger patients. It is also more frequently nonexertional and unresponsive to sublingual nitroglycerin in the elderly patients. The cause for these differences in the manifestation of coronary artery disease remains unclear but may be related to the inactivity of these patients, the concomitant presence of other medical problems or a subjective variation in the interpretation of symptoms. It is also possible that those with a more typical presentation are identified and started on treatment at a younger age. Thus, it appears that coronary atherosclerosis may remain occult or manifest atypically in elderly patients.

The traditionally recognized risk factors for the development of coronary atherosclerosis are increased age, male sex, cigarette smoking, hyperlipidemia, diabetes mellitus, hypertension, sedentary life-style and a family history of coronary artery disease [13, 14]. Obesity and the presence of a 'type A' personality have also been implicated as risk factors, but opinion is divided about the degree to which they contribute to the development of coronary atherosclerosis. However, most of the patients followed up in the large epidemiologic studies were middle-aged. The impact of the traditional risk factors for the development of coronary atherosclerosis in the elderly remains uncertain.

We have studied the prevalence of the traditional risk factors in elderly patients with and without coronary artery disease [25]. Our results suggest that in the elderly, male sex, cigarette smoking and diabetes mellitus (even when treated) remain major coronary risk factors; however, hypertension (treated), hypercholesterolemia, family history of coronary artery disease and sedentary life-style do not discriminate patients with and without coronary artery disease. In assessing the impact of smoking, computation of total pack years of smoking may be the most effective method of evaluating risk exposure [26, 27]. In our study we identified those individuals with a smoking history of 20 pack years or more. Cessation was not considered, although in an earlier report we have shown that cessation of smoking reduces the risk of coronary artery disease most effectively in the forty to sixty year old age group [28]. The difference did not reach statistical significance in our study for persons below forty years or over sixty years of age. Although multiple studies have conclusively established hypercholesterolemia as a risk factor for the development of coronary artery disease, we have indicated in an earlier report that hypercholesterolemia may actually cease to contribute to cardiovascular risk in elderly patients who have not developed atherosclerosis [29]. Many elderly patients exposed to the traditional coronary risk factors still have angiographically proven normal coronary arteries. Further studies are required to clarify the role of these risk factors in the development of coronary atherosclerosis in the elderly and the mechanism by which the disease remains occult in some patients.

Occult coronary atherosclerosis in patients with diabetes mellitus

Patients with diabetes mellitus represent an important subgroup having occult coronary atherosclerosis [13, 30]. Myocardial infarction is the cause of death in approximately 20 percent of diabetic patients. According to the Framingham Study, diabetic males have a 60 percent and diabetic females have a 100 percent greater incidence of coronary artery disease compared to non-diabetics. Additionally, diabetic men and women have a 50 percent and 150 percent higher incidence of myocardial infarction than do nondiabetic men and women. We have reported a difference in the mean fasting blood sugar levels for patients with and without coronary artery disease and that this disparity was significantly greater for women than for men [31]. Bradley and Schoenfield [32] have compared the symptoms of diabetic and non-diabetic patients presenting with myocardial infarction. They found severe pain to be almost three times more frequent in nondiabetic patients when compared to diabetic patients. Conversely, mild to moderate discomfort was twice as common in the diabetic group. Almost half the diabetic patients presented with non-specific symptoms such as nausea, fatigue, and dyspnea, compared to only 6% of nondiabetic patients. Soler *et al.* [33] have noted that in their series of diabetic patients with myocardial infarction, about a third had no symptoms suggestive of myocardial ischaemia. Many patients in their study had worsening congestive heart failure, symptoms of hyperglycemia or hypoglycemia, gastrointestinal distress, hypotension, confusion and transient cerebral ischaemia. These patients also had a higher mortality rate when compared to a nondiabetic cohort. Data from the Framingham Study [5] indicate that 23% of myocardial infarctions were discovered only on routine biennial electrocardiograms. Diabetic patients tended to experience more of these electrocardiographically diagnosed infarcts. In an autopsy study 43% of diabetic patients dying from acute myocardial infarction showed evidence of at least one old healed infarction that was not evident from the patient's history [34]. Bellet and Roman [35] performed a two-step exercise tolerance test on a series of diabetic patients without any anginal symptoms. In this group 22 percent displayed ischaemic ST-segment changes, whereas only 8 percent of matched controls showed a similar ischaemia response. Nesto *et al.* [36] studied the relationship of angina to ischaemia in 50 consecutive diabetic and 50 consecutive nondiabetic persons using exercise thallium-201 scintigraphy. They noted that angina is frequently absent in the diabetic patient despite evidence of myocardial ischaemia documented on stress thallium-201 scintigraphy. Chiariello *et al.* [37] performed 24 hour ambulatory ECG monitoring on patients with coronary artery disease and reported that the number of episodes of asymptomatic ST-segment depression is greater in diabetic patients than in nondiabetic patients. Thus, coronary atherosclerosis frequently remains occult in patients with diabetes mellitus.

Occult coronary atherosclerosis manifesting as sudden death with athletic activity

Isolated sudden deaths of certain well known athletes have drawn tremendous public attention to this problem [38]. Fortunately, the incidence is quite low [39–45]. For instance about 20 million Americans are involved in jogging [46] but jogging deaths have been estimated to occur in only 0.01% or one death per 396,000 person-hours of jogging [47, 48]. Hawley *et al.* [49] reviewed all deaths in Marion County, Indiana in 1985 and found that among 6492 deaths only four (0.06%) occurred during or immediately after exercise. Waller [50] also reviewed 147 cases of exertion-related sudden deaths from 32 reports of individual cases or series. None of these subjects had prior evidence of cardiovascular disease and all died during or shortly after exercise. The author noted that the cause of sudden death was reflected by the age of the victim. For those under the age of 30 years, the cause of death was linked to anomalous coronary circulation in 35% and to hypertrophic cardiomyopathy in 22%. On the other hand, for victims over the age of 30 years, the cause of sudden death was occult coronary atherosclerosis in 97%.

Several researchers have attempted to determine whether exercise is an independent risk factor for sudden death in the presence of occult coronary atherosclerosis. Since there is a per hour risk of dying from occult coronary artery disease, it has been postulated that the association between athletic activity and sudden death in some individuals is a chance event [51]. Yet, data suggest the contrary. Athletic training may cause hypertrophy of the left and right ventricles of the heart [52–55] but it is uncertain whether this hypertrophy could predispose individuals with coronary atherosclerosis to myocardial infarction. Thompson and associates [56] studied a series of 18 deaths that occurred during jogging and noted that 13 of them were related to coronary artery disease. The sudden death rate in Finland among cross country skiers is approximately four times the rate for individuals at rest [57]. In a study on fatal coronary atherosclerosis in young soldiers, French and Dock [58] noted that more than 50% died during vigorous effort while only 10% died while asleep. In a similar study on sudden death in young soldiers, Moritz and Zamcheck [59] noted that in nearly 30% the event occurred during or immediately after strenuous physical activity. Weaver *et al.* [60] studied survivors of exertional and non-exertional cardiac arrest and concluded that arrest was more likely to occur during vigorous exercise. Thus, there appears to be convincing evidence at this time that vigorous physical activity is an important risk factor for sudden death in individuals with occult coronary atherosclerosis.

Angiographically normal coronary arteries with possible occult atherosclerosis of small branches

Approximately 20–30% of patients referred to coronary angiography for chest pain are found to have normal or near-normal coronary arteries [61–65]. The Registry Committee of the Society of Cardiac Angiography reported that of 41,204 patients referred for coronary arteriography because of presumed coronary artery disease, 20% had normal arteriograms [64]. Similarly, 25% of patients screened for the Coronary Artery Surgery Study (CASS) had normal or slightly abnormal coronary arteriograms [65]. In a smaller series of 706 consecutive patients who underwent cardiac catheterization because of chest pain, Bertrand and Colleagues found the incidence of normal coronary arteriograms to be as high as 89% in patients with atypical pain and 29% in patients with typical angina [66].

The aetiology of symptoms in patients with normal coronary arteriograms remains unclear. Some have obvious noncardiac pain [67]. When the pain is typical angina, the term syndrome X has been used to refer to this condition

[68, 69]. Coronary artery spasm can be demonstrated in less than 10% of these patients [66, 70–72]. Aesophageal disorders may account for the chest discomfort in about a third of this group [73–79]. Another third suffers from panic disorder [80–83] with or without major depression [84]. The hypothesis that some of these patients may have occult atherosclerosis affecting the small coronary branches is intriguing. Cannon and co-workers [85, 86] studied a series of patients with chest pain and normal or near-normal coronary arteries by measuring great cardiac vein flow, coronary resistance and coronary sinus lactate levels at rest and with pacing and subjected the patients to the cold pressor test and to intravenous ergonovine challenge. Their data suggest that some of the patients may have inappropriate coronary arteriolar or small coronary artery constriction with abnormal vasodilator reserve when subjected to atrial pacing. Opherk *et al.* [87] confirmed this finding and postulated that since this phenomenon could not be explained by obstructive lesions of the coronary arteries, the disease may be isolated in the cardiac microvessels that were not visualized by coronary angiography. Accordingly, they obtained left ventricular endomyocardial biopsies on 18 of these patients but failed to demonstrate any microvascular atherosclerosis. More recently, Mosseri *et al.* [88] reported their findings from endomyocardial biopsy of 6 patients with angina pectoris and normal coronary angiograms. They found fibromuscular hyperplasia, hypertrophy of the media, myointimal proliferation and endothelial degeneration involving small coronary arteries. Mosseri *et al.* have suggested that small vessel disease should be suspected when a patient with angina is found to have large patent arteries with slow flow of the angiographic contrast medium. Based on these observations, Cannon and co-workers [86] have proposed a model for microvascular angina or apparent effort angina without any obvious cardiovascular pathology. In microvascular angina, the major epicardial coronary vessels visualized on arteriography are clean. However, there are fixed anatomic or functional defects in intramural pre-arteriolar coronary segments. Because of this blockage the smooth muscle surrounding subendocardial vessels remain widely dilated in the resting phase. However, subepicardial vessels do not dilate as they supply areas of modest metabolic demand. With exercise, the subepicardial vessels dilate but the subendocardial vessels are unable to dilate any further, resulting in myocardial ischaemia. The validity of this mode has yet to be tested and verified by other centers. Additionally, at this time there appears to be no practical and reliable method for identifying patients with this condition prior to performing coronary angiography and other sophisticated tests [89].

Several studies have shown that the syndrome of angina with normal epicardial coronary arteries carries a favorable prognosis for longevity. Kemp and co-workers [62] reviewed the CASS registry and showed a seven-year survival rate of 96% in patients with normal coronary arteriograms. Papanicolaou *et al.* [61] followed 1491 patients for a period of up to 10 years and reported a 98% survival rate. Proudfit and his group [90] followed a series of 357 patients for a period of 10 years and found a survival rate of 98%. They then compared these patients with 101 patients with mild disease (<30% narrowing) and 63 patients with moderate disease (30–50% narrowing). Coronary events occurred in 2.1% of those with normal arteriograms, 13.8% of those with mild narrowing and 33% of those with moderate coronary narrowing. All these figures reflect a highly favorable prognosis for longevity in patients with normal coronary arteriograms. But, despite the excellent prognosis for longevity, these patients are subject to considerable morbidity as a consequence of continuing chest pain. About 60–80% of the patients continue to experience chest pain with up to 10 years of follow-up and about 50% of them remain disabled because of their symptoms [61, 91, 92]. Marchandise *et al.* [93] performed a second coronary arteriography at a mean interval of 42 months on a series of patients with normal epicardial coronary arteries and persistent chest pain and demonstrated no new development of disease.

Occult atherosclerosis of coronary ostia

In evaluating patients with normal coronary angiograms, it is important that isolated ostial stenosis be ruled out since misdiagnosis of this condition may be disastrous. We have reported the occurrence of coronary ostial stenosis in the absence of other coronary disease [94]. These patients have occult coronary disease of a serious nature and their prognosis is poor without proper treatment. Coronary ostial stenosis usually occurs in association with stenosis of one or more of the major coronary arteries [95]. A review of the literature reveals only 34 reported cases of nonsyphilitic isolated coronary ostial stenosis [94, 96–98]. The overwhelming majority of these patients were premenopausal women. This is in striking contrast to the usual 7:1 male to female ratio for atherosclerotic coronary disease at this age. Only three male patients have been reported to have isolated coronary ostial stenosis of which two occurred in the setting of definite or probable estrogen excess [94, 99, 100]. Careful angiographic technique is crucial to making the proper diagnosis. The condition should be considered when a patient with documented evidence of myocardial ischaemia during exertion has an apparently normal coronary angiogram.

Conclusion

Occult coronary atherosclerosis has been reported to occur in several different subgroups of patients. The pathogenesis, clinical presentation and course are varied. On reviewing information relating to the risk factors and epidemiology of the condition we are faced with a number of unanswered questions. Further research in this area is awaited.

References

1. Kannel W B. Epidemiologic insights into atherosclerotic cardiovascular disease from the Framingham Study. In: M L Pollock, D H Schmidt (eds), Heart Disease and Rehabilitation, 2nd, ch 1. John Wiley & Sons, New York 1986, p. 3.
2. Gordon T, Kannel W B. Premature mortality from coronary heart disease: The Framingham Study. JAMA 1971; 215:1617.
3. Kannel W B, Barry P, Dawber T R. Immediate mortality in coronary heart disease: The Framingham Study, in Proceedings of the IV World Congress of Cardiology, Mexico City, 1962. Int Soc Cardiol 1963; 4B:176.
4. Kannel W B, Abbott R D. Incidence and prognosis of unrecognized myocardial infarction: An update on the Framingham Study. N Engl J Med 1984; 311:1144.
5. Morgolis J R, Kannel W B, Feinleib M *et al.* Clinical features of unrecognized myocardial infarction – silent and symptomatic: Eighteen year follow-up: The Framingham Study. Am J Cardiol 1973; 32:1.
6. Erikssen J, Thaulow E. Follow-up of patients with asymptomatic myocardial ischaemia. In: W Rutishauser, H Roskamm (eds), Silent Myocardial Ischaemia. Springer-Verlag, Berlin 1984, p 156.
7. Langou R A, Huang E K, Kelley M J, Cohen L S. Predictive accuracy of coronary artery calcification and abnormal exercise test for coronary artery disease in asymptomatic men. Circulation 1980; 62:1196.
8. Giagnoni E, Secchi M B, Wu S C, Morabito A, Oltrona L, Mancarella S, Volpin N, Flossa L, Bettazzi L, Arangio G, Sachero A, Folli G. Prognostic value of exercise EKG testing in asymptomatic normotensive subjects: A prospective matched study. N Engl J Med 1983; 309:1085.
9. Gordon D J, Elelund L-G, Karon J M, Probstfield J L, Rubenstein C, Sheffield L T, Weissfeld L. Predictive value of the exercise test for mortality in North American men: The Lipid Research Clinics Mortality Follow-Up Study. Circulation 1986; 2:252.
10. Erikssen L, Cohn P F, Thaulow E, Mowinckel P. Silent myocardial ischaemia in middle aged men: Long term clinical course. In: T V Arnim, A Maseri (eds), Silent Ischaemia: Current Concepts and Management. Steinkopff, Darmstadt 1987, p 45.
11. Droste C, Roskamm H. Experimental pain measurement in patients with asymptomatic myocardial ischaemia. J Am Coll Cardiol 1983; 1:940.
12. Kannel W B, Dannenberg A L, Abbott R D. Unrecognized myocardial infarction and hypertension: The Framingham Study. Am Heart J 1985; 109:581.
13. Shurtleff D. Some characteristics related to incidence of cardiovascular disease and death: Framingham Study, 18 year follow-up. Washington, DC, US Government Printing Office, 1974, p. 30.
14. Kannel W B, Gordon T. Evaluation of cardiovascular risk factors in the elderly: The Framingham Study. Bull NY Acad Med 1978; 54:573.
15. Stern M P. The recent decline in ischaemic heart disease mortality. Ann Intern Med 1979; 91:630.
16. Stamer. The marked decline of coronary heart disease mortality rates in the United States, 1968–81; Summary of findings and possible explanations. Cardiology 1985; 72:11.
17. Levy R I. Declining mortality in coronary heart disease. Atherosclerosis 1981; 1:312.

18. Fries J F, Aging. natural death and the compression of morbidity. N Engl J Med 1980; 303:130.
19. Pathy M S. Clinical presentation of myocardial infarction in the elderly. Br Heart J 1967; 19:190.
20. Williams B O, Begg T B, Semple T, McGuinness J B. The elderly in a coronary unit. Br Med J 1976; 2:451.
21. Kincaid D T, Botti R E. Acute myocardial infarction in the elderly, Chest 1973; 64:170.
22. Latting C A, Silverman M E. Acute myocardial infarction in hospitalized patients over age 70. Am Heart J 1980; 100:311.
23. Fodor J, Tibblin G. One year's experience of the ischaemic heart disease registry in Gothenburg in Ischaemic Heart Disease registers. WHO working document. EURO 1970; 4:10.
24. Mukerji V, Holman A J, Alpert M A. The clinical description of angina pectoris in the elderly. Am Heart J 1989; 117(3):705.
25. Mukerji V, Holman A J, Artis A K, Alpert M A, Hewett J E. Risk factors for coronary atherosclerosis in the elderly. Angiology 1989; 40(2):88.
26. Tajick C L, Osfeld A M, Freeman D H A. Smoking and coronary heart disease mortality in the elderly. JAMA 1984; 252:2831.
27. Weintraub W S, Klein L W, Seelans P A *et al.* Importance of total life consumption of cigarettes as a risk factor for coronary artery disease. Am J Cardiol 1985; 55:669.
28. Mukerji V, Alpert M A, Hewett J E. Comparison of the smoking histories of patients with coronary artery disease and those with normal coronary arteries – Effect of cessation of smoking. Clinical Research 1987; 35(3):307A.
29. Mukerji V, Alpert M A, Burns T, Hewett J E. Differences in serum cholesterol levels of patients with and without moderate to severe coronary artery disease – effect of age. Clinical Research 1986; 34(2):328A.
30. Kannel W B, McGee D L. Diabetes and cardiovascular disease: The Framingham Study. JAMA 1979; 241:2035.
31. Mukerji V, Alpert M A, Burns T, Hewett J E. Fasting blood sugar levels of patients with and without moderate to severe coronary artery disease. Diabetes 1986; 35 (Suppl 1):212A.
32. Bradley R F, Schoenfield A. Diminished pain in diabetic patients with acute myocardial infarction. Geriatrics 1962; 17:322.
33. Soler N G, Bennett M A, Pentecost B L, Fitzgerald M G, Malins J N. Myocardial infarction in diabetics. Q J Med 1975; 44:125.
34. Bradley R F, Partamian J O. Coronary heart disease in the diabetic patient. Med Clin North Am 1963; 1093.
35. Bellet S, Roman L. The exercise test in diabetic patients as studied by radioelectrocardiography. Circulation 1967; 36:245.
36. Nesto R W, Phillips R T, Kett K G *et al.* Angina and exertional myocardial ischaemia in diabetic and nondiabetic patients: Assessment by exercise thallium scintigraphy. Ann Int Med 1988; 108:170.
37. Chiariello M, Indolfi C, Cotecchia M R, Sifola C, Romano M, Condorelli M. Asymptomatic transient ST changes during ambulatory ECG monitoring in diabetic patients. Am Heart J 1985; 110:529.
38. Currens J H, White P D. Half a century of running: Clinical, physiologic and autopsy findings in the case of Clarence DeMar ('Mr. Marathon'). N Engl J Med 1961; 265:988.
39. Opie L H. Sudden death and sport. Lancet 1975; 1:263.
40. Virmani R. Jogging, marathon running and death. Prim Cardiol 1982; 4:A-28.
41. Roberts W C, Maron B J. Sudden death while playing professional football. Am Heart J 1981; 102:1061.

42. McManus B M, Waller B F, Grayboys T B *et al.* Exercise and sudden death. Cur Prob Cardiol 1981; 9:1.
43. Maron B J, Roberts W C, McAllister H A Jr *et al.* Sudden death in young athletes. Circulation 1980; 62:218.
44. Jokl E, McClellan J T. Exercise and cardiac death. Med and Sport 1971; 5:1.
45. James T N, Froggatt P, Marshall T K. Sudden death in young athletes. Ann Intern Med 1967; 67:1013.
46. Rennie D, Hollenberg N K. Cardiomythology and marathons. N Engl J Med 1979; 301:103.
47. Fletcher G F. The dangers of exercise. In: The Heart: Update V. J W Hurst (ed), McGraw-Hill, New York 1981; p 161.
48. Waller B F, Csere R S, Baker W P, Roberts W C. Running to death. Chest 1981; 79:346.
49. Hawley D A, Pless J E, Waller B F, Vakili S T. Fatal athletic injuries. Am J Forensic Med Pathol 1987; 8:277.
50. Waller B F. Exercise-related sudden death in young (age ≤ 30 years) and old (age > 30 years) conditioned subjects. Cardiovasc Clin 1985; 15:9.
51. Koplan J P. Cardiovascular deaths while running. JAMA 1979; 242:2578.
52. Mukerji B, Alpert M A, Mukerji V. Cardiovascular changes in athletes. Am Family Physician 1989; 40(3):169.
53. Parker B M, Londeree B R, Cupp G V *et al.* The noninvasive cardiac evaluation of long-distance runners. Chest 1978; 73:376.
54. Mukerji V, Mukerji B, Alpert M A, Brukardt D, Londeree B R, Kelly D L. Electrocardiographic and echocardiographic changes in trained swimmers. Ann Sports Med 1989; 4(3):127.
55. Mukerji V, Mukerji B, Alpert M A, Brukardt D, Londeree B R. Right ventricular alterations in trained swimmers. Medicine and Science in Sports and Exercise 1988; 20(2):52.
56. Thompson P D, Stern M P, Williams P *et al.* Death during jogging or running: A study of 18 cases. JAMA 1979; 242:1265.
57. Vuori I, Makarainen M, Jaaskelainen A. Sudden death and physical activity. Cardiology 1978; 63:287.
58. French A J, Dock W. Fatal coronary atherosclerosis in young soldiers. JAMA 1944; 124:1233.
59. Moritz A R, Zamcheck N. Sudden and unexpected deaths of young soldiers. Arch Pathol 1946; 42:459.
60. Weaver W D, Cobb L A, Helstrom A P. Characteristics of survivors of exertion and non-exertional related cardiac arrest: Value of subsequent exercise testing. Am J Cardiol 1982; 50:989.
61. Papanicolaou M N, Califf R M, Hlatky M A, McKinnis R A, Harrell F E, Mark D B, McCants B, Rosati R A, Lee K L, Pryor D B. Prognostic implications of angiographically normal and insignificantly narrowed coronary arteries. Am J Cardiol 1986; 58:1181.
62. Kemp H G Jr, Vokonas P S, Cohn P F, Gorlin R. The anginal syndrome associated with normal coronary arteriograms: Report of six year experience. Am J Med 1973; 54:735.
63. Proudfit W L, Shirey E K, Sones F M Jr. Selective cine coronary arteriography: Correlation with clinical findings in 1,000 patients. Circulation 1966; 33:901.
64. Registry Committee of the Society for Cardiac Angiography, Complications associated with cardiac catheterization and angiography. Cathet Cardiovasc Diagn 1982; 8:5.
65. Killip T, Fisher L D, Mock M B. The National Heart, Lung, and Blood Institute Coronary Artery Surgery Study. Circulation 1981; 63 (suppl 1):71.
66. Betrand M E, La Blanche J M, Tilmant P Y *et al.* Frequency of provoked coronary artery spasm in 1089 consecutive patients undergoing coronary arteriography. Circulation 1982; 65:1299.

67. Mukerji V. Chest pain in a patient with normal coronary arteries. Primary Cardiology 1989; 15(6):28.
68. Kemp HG. Left ventricular function in patients with anginal syndrome and normal coronary arteriograms. Am J Cardiology 1973; 32(3):375.
69. Arbogast R, Bourassa MG. Myocardial function during atrial pacing in patients with angina pectoris and normal coronary arteriograms. Am J Cardiol 1973; 32(3):257.
70. Heupler FA, Proudfit WL, Razavi M, Shirey EK, Greenstreet R, Sheldon WC. Ergonovine maleate provocative test for coronary arterial spasm. Am J Card 1978; 41(4):631.
71. Curry RC, Pepine CJ, Sabom MB *et al.* Hemodynamic and myocardial metabolic effects of ergonovine in patients with chest pain. Circulation 1978; 58:648.
72. Schroeder JS, Bolen JL, Quint RA *et al.* Provocation of coronary spasm with ergonovine maleate. New test results in 57 patients undergoing coronary arteriography. Am J Cardiol 1977; 40:487.
73. Katz PO, Dalton CB, Richter JE, Wu WC, Castell DO. Esophageal testing of patients with noncardiac chest pain or dysphagia. Ann Intern Med 1987; 106:593.
74. DeMeester TR, O'Sullivan GC, Bermudez G *et al.* Oesophageal function in patients with angina-type chest pain and normal coronary angiograms. Ann Surg 1982; 196:488.
75. Svenson O, Stenport G, Tibbling L *et al.* Oesophageal function and coronary angiograms in patients with disabling chest pain. Acta Med Scand 1978; 204:173.
76. Ferguson CS, Hodges R, Heish I *et al.* Oesophageal manometry in patients with chest pain and normal coronary arteriography. Am J Gastroenterol 1981; 75:124.
77. Kline M, Chesne R, Sturdevant RAL *et al.* Oesophageal disease in patients with angina-like chest pain. Am J Gastroenterol 1981; 75:116.
78. Wu WC, Hackshow BP, Nelson JL *et al.* Esophageal motility disorders in patients with angina-like chest pain and normal coronary arteriogram. Gastroenterology 1982; 82:1214
79. Areskog M, Tibbling L. Oesophageal function and chest pain in male patients with recent acute myocardial infarction. Acta Med Scand 1981; 209:59.
80. Mukerji V, Beitman BD, Alpert MA, Hewett JE, Basha IM. Panic attack symptoms in patients with chest pain and angiographically normal coronary arteries. Journal of Anxiety Disorders 1987; 1:41.
81. Mukerji V, Beitman BD, Alpert MA, Lamberti JW, DeRosear L, Basha IM. Panic disorder: A frequent occurrence in patients with chest pain and normal coronary arteries. Angiology 1987; 38(3):236.
82. Beitman BD, Mukerji V, Flaker G, Basha IM. Panic disorder, cardiology patients and atypical chest pain. Psychiatric Clinics of North America 1988; 11:(2):387.
83. Beitman BD, Mukerji V, Lamberti JW, Schmid L, DeRosear L, Kushner M, Flaker G, Basha I. Panic disorder in patients with chest pain and angiographically normal coronary arteries. Am J Cardiolo 1989; 63:1399.
84. Beitman BD, Basha I, Flaker G, DeRosear L, Mukerji V, Lamberti J. Major depression in cardiology chest pain patients without coronary artery disease and with panic disorder. Journal of Affective Disorders 1987; 13:51.
85. Cannon RO, Watson RM, Rosing DR *et al.* Angina caused by reduced vasodilator reserve of the small coronary arteries. J Am Coll Cardiol 1983; 1:1359–1373.
86. Cannon RO, Schenke WH, Leon MB, Rosing DR, Urqhart J, Epstein S. Limited coronary flow reserve after dipyridamole in patients with ergonovine induced coronary vasoconstriction. Circulation 1987; 75(1):163.
87. Opherk D, Zebe H, Weihe E *et al.* Reduced coronary dilatory capacity and ultrastructural changes of the myocardium in patients with angina pectoris and normal coronary arteriogram. Circulation 1981; 63:817.
88. Mosseri M, Yarom R, Gotsman MS, Hasin Y. Histologic evidence of small vessel

coronary artery disease in patients with angina pectoris and patent large coronary arteries. Circulation 1986; 75(5):964.
89. Mukerji V, Alpert M A, Hewett J E, Parker B M. Can patients with chest pain and normal coronary arteries be discriminated from those with coronary artery disease prior to coronary angiography? Angiology 1989; 40(4–I):276.
90. Proudfit W L, Bruschke A V G, Sones F M Jr. Clinical course of patients with normal or slightly or moderately abnormal coronary arteriograms: 10-year follow-up of 521 patients. Circulation 1980; 62:712.
91. Lavey E B, Winkle R A. Continuing disability of patients with chest pain and normal coronary arteriograms. J Chronic Dis 1979; 32:191.
92. Ockene I S, Shay M J, Alpert J S *et al.* Unexplained chest pain in patients with normal coronary arteriograms. N Engl J Med 1980; 303:1249.
93. Marchandise B, Bourassa M G, Chaitman B R *et al.* Angiographic evaluation of the natural history of normal coronary arteries and mild coronary atherosclerosis. Am J Cardiol 1978; 41:216.
94. Tillman C H, Mukerji V, Alpert M A, Sanfelippo J F. Isolated coronary ostial stenosis in men. Am Heart J 1988; 115(5):1127.
95. Barner H, Cadd J, Mudd V *et al.* Nonsyphilitic coronary ostial stenosis. Arch Surg 1977; 112:462.
96. Thompson K. Isolated coronary ostial stenosis in women. J Am Coll Cardiol 1986; 7:997.
97. Miller G, Honey M, El-Sayed H. Isolated coronary ostial stenosis. Cathet Cardiovasc Diagn 1986; 12:30.
98. Freund T, Missri J, Landry F. Isolated left main coronary ostial stenosis. Cardiovasc Rev Rep 1987; 8:72.
99. Malcolm I, Salerno T. Coronary ostial stenosis [Letter], Can Med Assoc J 1983; 128:371.
100. Rissanen V. Occurrence of coronary ostial stenosis in a necropsy series of myocardial infarction, sudden death and violent death. Br Heart J 1975; 37:182.

7. ECG and stress testing in the diagnosis of occult atherosclerotic disease of the coronary arteries

ABDUL-MAJEED SALMASI

Considerable interest has been gained in the concept of occult atherosclerotic disease of the coronary arteries. Both pathological and arteriographic studies have shown that many patients with asymptomatic coronary artery disease have severe and extensive disease which is indistinguishable from that found in symptomatic subjects [1].

In patients with overt (symptomatic) coronary artery disease most episodes of myocardial ischaemia are asymptomatic and the majority of these episodes are not associated with tachycardia seen in these patients during stress testing [2, 3]. In totally asymptomatic subjects, both with normal and abnormally high blood lipids, the mortality rate for individuals with positive stress ECG tests, as evidenced by S-T segment depression, was considerably higher than the mortality rate for subjects with negative stress tests [4]. However, a relatively higher risk for mortality from coronary artery disease has been reported in individuals with positive ECG stress test [5]. If a small fissure develops in an occult atherosclerotic lesion in a major branch of a coronary artery, it may become acutely occluded by a superimposed thrombus and hence can result in the sudden death of an otherwise asymptomatic individual [6].

Although it is essential, theoretically, to identify patients with occult atherosclerotic coronary lesion, in practical terms this is faced with some difficulty. One of these difficulties would be providing huge resources and trained personnel to identify these subjects with occult atherosclerotic lesion in the population. The other source of hindrance is which technique to be used in order to provide the best, more reliable and the least doubtful answer. Obviously and most practically one would to start with, embark on a reliable noninvasive test in order to screen subjects who are regarded as high risk. If suspicion arose one would then revert to an invasive approach.

A.-M. Salmasi and A. N. Nicolaides (eds.), Occult Atherosclerotic Disease, 91–103.

The resting electrocardiogram

Some changes in the resting ECG are of value when detected accidentally in an otherwise asymptomatic individual. If evidence of an old myocardial infarct is detected it is assumed that an infarct was silent or painless not to warrant concern by the patient or the physician [7].

The presence of S-T segment abnormalities alone may suggest the presence of an underlying coronary artery disease. Such a sign, however, has been detected in a relatively small number of patients, but the predicted value may increase from 8% to 44% when combined with a positive stress ECG test [8].

The presence of left bundle branch block or right bundle branch block may be suggestive of the presence of coronary artery disease. Frolicher and associates [9] found that coronary artery disease was present in 22% of asymptomatic subjects with left bundle branch block and in 18% of subjects with right bundle branch block.

The presence of an inverted U-wave (any discrete negative deflection in the TP segment) on the resting ECG has been reported to be confined to patients with cardiac disease [10, 11]. As an isolated phenomenon on the resting ECG, inverted U-wave has been associated with ischaemic heart disease [11].

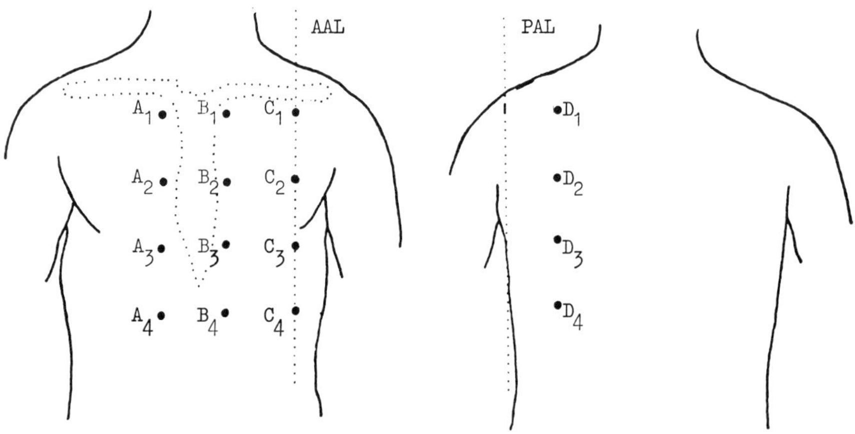

Figure 7.1. Distribution of the 16 leads on the chest wall. Raw D is placed on the back 6 cm medial to the posterior axillary line (PAL). Lead C3 corresponds to lead V5 on the conventional ECG, AAL: anterior axillary line. Raw A projects disease in the right coronary artery territory; Raw B & C project disease in the left anterior descending and/or diagonal coronary artery territory; Raw D projects disease in the circumflex coronary artery territory.

Stress ECG testing

Various techniques have been discussed in this book to identify ischaemic heart disease in asymptomatic subjects. From the theoretical point of view one may assume that combination of these techniques rather than using each one separately may increase the sensitivity to identify occult coronary artery disease. Being inexpensive, totally noninvasive and very commonly used, stress ECG testing has its own value in diagnosing occult coronary artery disease. Our experience dates back to 1981 [12] when we introduced the technique stress ECG testing using 16 chest leads distributed in certain spatial orientation (Figure 7.1) in order to identify disease in individual coronary artery territory [12, 13]. We subsequently used this technique in different groups of high risk subjects and proved the usefulness of this approach to identify individuals with occult coronary artery disease. The usefulness of this approach will be discussed separately in each high risk group.

Hyperlipidaemia

Hypercholesterolaemia is a well known risk factor for the development of atheroma [14]. The inherited metabolic disorder of familial hypercholesterolaemia is commonly associated with premature coronary artery disease [15]. As evidence accumulates for the benefits of intervention with diet and drugs to correct the lipid abnormality the need to identify patients who have advanced asymptomatic disease also increases.

In 1983 a study was carried out at St. Mary's Hospital, London using stress ECG testing and chest wall mapping to identify occult coronary artery disease in asymptomatic patients with hyperlipidaemia [16]. In this study, 100 consecutive totally asymptomatic patients with various forms of hyperlipidaemia were referred to our Laboratory from the metabolic unit in order to identify occult coronary artery disease by stress ECG testing. These patients were originally referred to the metabolic unit because of either 1) being a member of a family with familial (type IIa) hyperlipidaemia or xanthelasmata palpebrarum or 2) referral from their general practitioner because of the high blood lipid concentration. None of the patients had a history of myocardial infarction and all had normal resting ECG. None of the patients developed chest pain during the stress test which was positive in 50% of the patients. Twenty one of the patients with positive stress test (all with type IIa hyperlipidaemia) were persuaded to undergo coronary arteriography. Significant coronary artery disease ($\geq$50% stenosis) was present in 20 of the 21 patients (Table 7.1) and the positive predictive accuracy of the test for individual coronary arterial lesion was 84% (Table 7.2). The cardiac events that subsequently occurred in the 50 patients with positive stress

Table 7.1. Number of coronary arteries with significant stenosis detected by chest wall mapping/ECG stress testing (CWM) in 21 asymptomatic patients with hyperlipidaemia compared to the findings obtained from coronary arteriography.

		No. of coronary arteries with significant stenosis (CWM)			
		0	1	2	3
No. of diseased coronary arteries (>50% stenosis) coronary arteriography	0			1	
	1		1		
	2		1	1	2
	3			2	13

Table 7.2. Sites of lesions as indicated by the stress testing/chest wall mapping (CWM) as compared to results obtained from coronary arteriography in 21 asymptomatic patients with hyperlipidaemia.

		Individual coronary artery territory (CWM)			
		none	LAD	Cx	RCA
Significant (>50%) stenosis (coronary arteriography)	none		1	2	3
	LAD[a]		14		
	Cx[b]	1		13	
	RCA[c]	2			13

[a] LAD: left anterior descending coronary artery
[b] Cx: circumflex coronary artery
[c] RCA: right coronary artery

Table 7.3. Cardiac events in 50 asymptomatic patients with hyperlipidaemia and positive stress ECG test.

event	number of patients
angina pectoris	14
myocardial infarction	2
coronary artery bypass grafting	12

ECG testing are demonstrated in Table 7.3. Similarly in a recent study carried out by Ekelund and associates [17] they studied 3,806 asymptomatic men with hypercholesterolaemia who were included in the lipid research clinics coronary primary prevention trial. Only 8.3% of the patients had positive stress tests. Within the 7 to 10-year follow up period, the authors reported a mortality rate from coronary heart disease of 6.7% in subjects with positive stress tests and 1.3% in subjects with negative stress test [17].

Diabetes mellitus

Although diagnosing occult coronary artery disease in patients with diabetes mellitus is more detailed in chapter 21 the preliminary study which was carried out in our unit at St. Mary's Hospital, using chest wall mapping, is worth referring to. Stress testing using chest wall mapping was carried out on 50 patients with non-insulin dependent diabetes who were totally asymptomatic with normal resting ECG and without history of previous myocardial infarction. The test was positive in 17 patients. Only six patients in whom the chest wall mapping indicated the presence of significant stenosis in three coronary artery territories agreed to undergo coronary arteriography which confirmed the findings of the stress testing. Due to severe disease in the left main stem coronary artery in one patient and the three coronary artery territories in another two, these three patients underwent coronary artery bypass grafting.

Similar to the above results, Hume and associates [18] carried out exercise tests on 60 asymptomatic diabetics, 30 of whom were with demonstrated neuropathy. Stress test was positive in a total of 14 patients equally distributed between those with and without neuropathy.

Intermittent claudication

Patients with peripheral vascular disease are particularly likely to have concomitant coronary artery disease. The incidence of coronary artery disease in patients with intermittent claudication varies between 25% and 90% depending on the patient selection and the diagnostic method used [19–27]. In 1982, Vecht and associates from St. Mary's Hospital [26] carried out stress ECG tests on a series of patients presenting with intermittent claudication. During the exercise, ischaemic ECG changes developed in 20 patients and yet only three of them developed angina pectoris.

More recently the technique of chest wall mapping during exercise was carried out on 100 consecutive patients presenting primarily with intermittent claudication [28]. The stress test was positive in 47 patients indicating disease in three coronary artery territories in 25 patients, in two coronary territories in 16 patients and in one coronary artery territory in 6 patients. On clinical grounds (ECG changes, history of myocardial infarction and/or angina pectoris) coronary artery disease was suspected in 21 patients, thus stress testing indicated occult coronary artery disease in 26 patients. Subsequently coronary arteriography was carried out on 32 patients in whom

Table 7.4. Accuracy of the chest wall mapping (CWM) in detecting number of coronary arteries with significant stenosis in 32 patients presenting with intermittent claudication and who had a positive stress ECG test. Results are compared with these obtained from coronary arteriograms. The predictive accuracy is 82%.

		number of diseased coronary artery territories (CWM)			
		0	1	2	3
number of coronary arteries with significant (>50%) stenosis (coronary arteriography)	0				
	1		2		
	2			6	2
	3			4	20

Table 7.5. Accuracy of the chest wall mapping/stress ECG testing (CWM) in detecting disease in individual coronary artery territory as compared to to coronary arteriography in 32 patients presenting with intermittent claudication. The predictive accuracy is 92%.

		site of the lesion (CWM)			
		0	LAD	Cx	RCA
	0		1		
significant (>50%) stenosis (coronary arteriogram)	LAD[a]		33		
	Cx[b]			28	1
	RCA[c]				24

[a] LAD: left anterior descending coronary artery
[b] Cx: circumflex coronary artery
[c] RCA: right coronary artery

the stress testing raised the suspician of high risk state (25 patients with disease in 3 coronary artery territories and 7 patients with disease in the territories of the left anterior decending and circumflex territories). Coronary arteriography confirmed the findings of the stress testing with high degree of accuracy (Tables 7.4 & 7.5). Amongst the 53 patients with negative stress test the heart rate did not reach a submaximal level in 23 patients during exercise and thus the test was regarded 'inconclusive'. Other methods of diagnosing occult coronary artery disease in this 'inconclusive' group may thus be suggested such as ambulatory ECG monitoring or dipyridamole thallium testing.

Exercise-induced inverted U-wave

Induction of inverted U-waves during exercise in patients with normal resting ECG is highly suggestive of ischaemic heart disease [29–31]. A study from our Laboratory [32] has shown that inverted U-wave during exercise may occur in any lead on the chest wall map indicating disease in the corresponding coronary artery territory. The disappearance of exercise-induced inverted U-wave after coronary artery bypass grafting may confirm its myocardial ischaemic origin [32].

In both the diabetic and the hyperlipidaemic studies (*vide supra*), exercise-induced inverted U-waves contributed to the sensitivity of diagnosing occult coronary artery disease [33]. As a sole ECG criterion of myocardial ischaemia, inverted U-waves during exercise made possible the diagnosis of myocardial ischaemia in 5 coronary artery territories in 5 different patients with hyperlipidaemia and two territories in one patient with diabetes mellitus. The territorial distribution of inverted U-waves on the chest wall map was later confirmed by coronary arteriography.

The nisoldipine study

In a previous study by Salmasi and Besterman [34] it has been shown that the long acting calcium channel blocker, nisoldipine, was useful in patients with angina pectoris. The magnitude of S-T segment depression was significant, and its duration was shorter during the nisoldipine phase of therapy as compared to placebo.

Chest wall mapping was used to study the effect of nisoldipine on silent myocardial ischaemia in totally asymptomatic subjects with known occult coronary artery disease [35]. In a double-blind cross over study and versus placebo, nisoldipine was administered at a dose of 10 mg twice daily to 7 patients with diabetes mellitus and 5 patients with intermittent claudication who were known, by coronary arteriography, to have coronary artery disease and who had positive stress ECG test using chest wall mapping. None of the patients had angina pectoris or history of myocardial infarction and all had normal resting electrocardiogram. The magnitude of S-T segment depression decreased significantly ($p<0.001$) from 6.6 mm during placebo phase of treatment to 1.3 mm during nisoldipine. Similarly the duration of S-T segment depression was significantly longer ($p<0.001$) during placebo (34 minutes) than during nisoldipine (7.1 minutes). This was accompanied by significantly lower episodes of magnitude and duration of S-T segment depression recorded on 24 hour ambulatory ECG monitoring during nisoldipine phase.

Doppler stress testing

The evolution in the use of Doppler ultrasound during physical exercise to assess left ventricular function began in 1982 by the report of Salmasi and associates [36] which was later followed by other reports from the same authors [37–39] and others [40, 41]. Recording aortic blood velocity signals from the suprasternal notch [42] has set up a rather non-expensive and quick outpatient procedure to evaluate noninvasively the changes that occur in the stroke volume and cardiac output during exercise. From these signals the systolic velocity time integral is derived which represent a measure of the stroke volume; hence called the stroke distance. When the stroke distance (Sd) is multiplied by the aortic cross-sectional area a figure equivalent to the stroke volume will therefore result; hence called the minute distance. In previous reports the percentage change, at peak exercise from the resting value in the stroke distance (%$\triangle$ Sd) was found to be correlated to the left ventricular ejection fraction in patients with coronary artery disease [39]. In

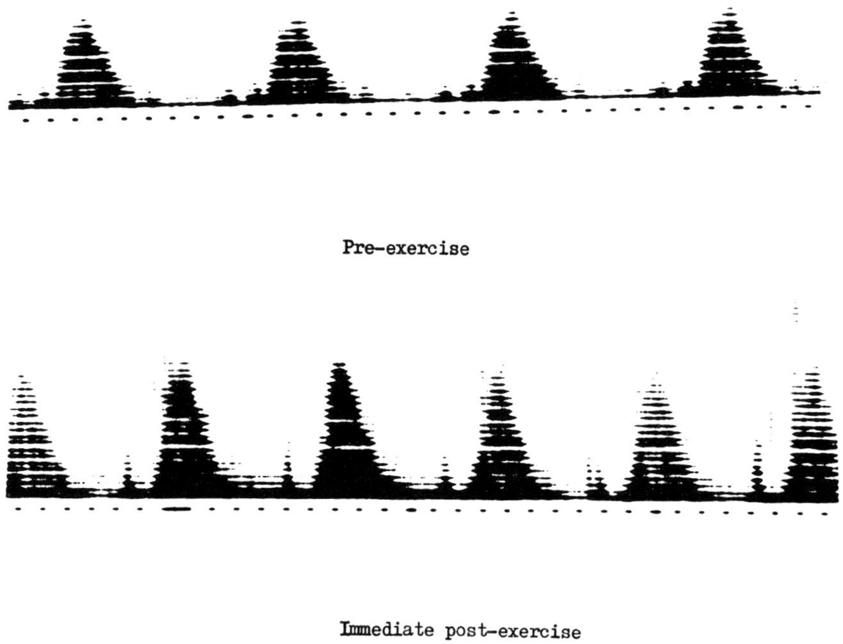

Figure 7.2. Doppler ultrasound signals of the aortic blood velocity in the aortic arch recorded by 2 mHz transducer placed in the suprasternal notch of a normal subject. The top recording is at rest while the bottom one is recorded from the same subject at maximal-tolerated supine exercise which showes an increase in the area under the velocity-time curve, thus indicating increase in the stroke volume with exercise.

normal subjects the stroke distance increased by more than 6% at peak exercise (Figure 7.2) while in patients with coronary artery disease and left ventricular dysfunction the stroke distance decreased at maximal exercise (Figure 7.3). In a subsequent study [43] it has been demonstrated that left ventricular dysfunction the stroke distance decreased at maximal exercise the operation of coronary artery bypass grafting. Such improvement took place irrespective of the presence or absence of history of previous myocardial infarction.

The principle of assessing left ventricular function during exercise by Doppler ultrasound has been used in a fairly recent study to evaluate the relationship between left ventricular dysfunction due to myocardial ischaemia and intermittent claudication in 100 consecutive claudicants. Stress ECG testing (using the technique of chest wall mapping) was positive in 47 patients, in 41 of whom left ventricular dysfunction was indicated by Doppler ultrasound stress testing. With a high degree of predictive accuracy coronary arteriography confirmed the findings on chest wall mapping in the 32 patients who were regarded at high risk on chest wall mapping (see Tables 7.4 & 7.5). Thirteen patients underwent coronary artery bypass graft surgery while 17 patients were treated by transdermal nitrate patches.

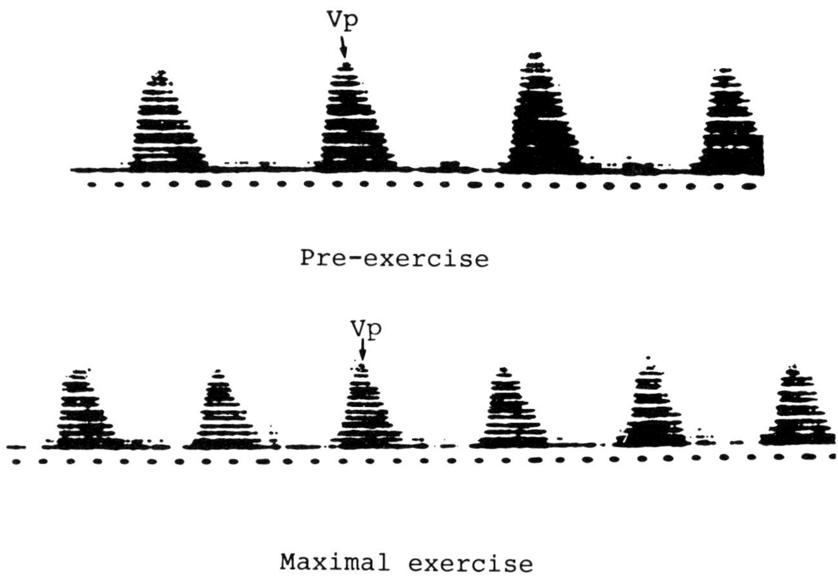

Figure 7.3. Doppler ultrasound velocity signals in a patient with significant stenosis in the three coronary artery territories and poor ejection fraction. The stroke volume (indicated by the systolic velocity-time integral) decreased during exercise (bottom curve) when compared to the resting tracing (top).

Fifteen of the 30 patients who received medical or surgical treatment reported improvement in their walking distance while twelve patients reported that they were able to walk without being limited by claudication. However no change was reported by the remaining 3 patients. The ankle brachial systolic blood pressure index at rest did not change following medical or surgical treatment, while this index, immediately after one minute of standard exercise, increased significantly after treatment. This was accompanied by a significant increase in the %△ Sd following treatment. This study indicated that improving left ventricular function as a result of medical or surgical intervention in patients with intermittent claudication and concomitant coronary artery disease improves or even abolishes the onset of claudication via improving the stroke volume and cardiac output hence regional flow to the lower limbs.

Clinical implications and conclusions

Stress testing is a valuable method for the diagnosis of occult atherosclerotic disease of the coronary arteries as it is of great value for diagnosing symptomatic coronary artery disease. Various centres use different techniques of stress ECG testing but various reports indicated that chest wall mapping gives a high degree of accuracy. Diagnosis of occult coronary artery disease by stress ECG testing was made possible in high risk subjects such as hyperlipidaemia, diabetes mellitus and patients with intermittent claudication. The high degree of accuracy of the chest wall mapping technique in diagnosing coronary artery disease was obtained by combination of both the spatial orientation of the chest electrodes and by using multiple ECG criteria of myocardial ischaemia in addition to S-T segment changes; such as inverted U-waves during exercise. The latter sign contributed also to the diagnosis of occult atherosclerotic disease in patients with hyperlipidaemia and patients with diabetes mellitus.

Stress ECG testing proved a useful tehnique for the evaluation of the effect of the calcium channel blocker, nisoldipine, in occult coronary artery disease and silent myocardial ischaemia. The use may therefore be extended to studying the effect of other calcium channel blocking agents or various anti-anginal therapies.

Doppler ultrasound during exercise has enabled the understanding of the effect of left ventricular dysfunction due to myocardial ischaemia on the onset of claudication in patients who primarily present with intermittent claudication. Left ventricular dysfunction contributed to the onset of claudication; the latter has improved or disappeared after improving left ventricular function following medical or surgical therapy. Accordingly it is established that one of the causes of intermittent claudication is myocardial ischaemia produced left ventricular dysfunction during exercise especially when angiography does not demonstrate an apparent or significant stenosis in the aortoiliac or femoral segments.

Although stress testing has proven of great value in diagnosing occult coronary artery disease, other noninvasive methods of diagnosis and assessment have also proven useful (see other chapters in this book). The usefulness and the predictive power of the combination of these techniques to identify occult coronary artery disease remain to be determined.

References

1. Lindsey HE, Cohn PF. 'Silent' myocardial ischaemia during and after exercise testing in patients with coronary artery disease. Am Heart J 1978; 95:441.
2. Schang SJ, Pepine CJ. Transient asymptomatic ST segment depression during daily activity. Am J Cardiol 1977; 39:396.
3. Deanfield JE, Selwyn AP, Chierchia S *et al.* Myocardial ischaemia during daily life in patients with stable angina: Its relation to symptoms and heart rate changes. Lancet 1983; 1:753.
4. Gordon DJ, Ekelund LG, Karon JM *et al.* Predictive value of the exercise tolerance test for mortality in north american men: The lipid research clinics mortality follow up study. Circulation 1986; 74:252.
5. Giagnoni E, Secchi MB, Wu SC *et al.* Prognostic value of exercise EKG testing in asymptomatic normotensive subjects: a prespective matched study. N Engl J Med 1983; 309:1085.
6. Davies MJ, Thomas A. Thrombosis and acute coronary artery lesions in sudden cardiac ischaemic death. N Eng J Med 1984; 310:1137.
7. Cohn PF. Silent myocardial ischaemia and infarction. Marcel Dekker Inc, New York 1986; p. 100.
8. Joy M, Trump DW. Significance of minor ST segment and T wave changes in the resting electrocardiogram of asymptomatic subjects. Br Heart J 1981; 45:48.
9. Froelicher V, Thompson AJ, Wolthuis R *et al.* Angiographic findings in asymptomatic aircrewmen with electrocardiographic abnormalities. Am J Cardiol 1977; 39:32.
10. Kishida H, Cole JS, Surawicz B. Negative U-wave: clinical significance and possible mechanism. Circulation 1978; 48 (Suppl. II):11.
11. Kishida H, Cole JS, Surawicz B. Negative U-wave: A highly specific but poorly understood sign of heart disease. Am J Cardiol 1982; 49:2030.
12. Nicolaides AN, Salmasi A-M, Vecht RJ et al. ECG chest wall mapping in the diagnosis of individual coronary artery lesion. Europ Heart J 1981; 2(A):35.
13. Salmasi A-M, Nicolaides AN, Vecht RJ et al. Electrocardiographic chest wall mapping during exercise in the diagnosis of coronary artery disease. Brit Heart J 1983; 287:9.
14. Kannel WB, Castelli WP, Gordon T, McNamara PM. Serum cholesterol, lipoproteins and the risk of coronary heart disease. The Framingham study. Ann Int Med 1971; 74:1.
15. Slack J. Risks of ischaemic heart disease in familial hyperlipidaemic states. Lancet 1969; II:1380.
16. Salmasi A-M, Seed M, Salmasi SN et al. Noninvasive detection of coronary artery disease in patients suffering from hyperlipidaemia. Europ Heart J 1983; 4(E):23.
17. Ekelund L-G, Schindran CM, McMahon RP *et al.* Coronary heart disease morbidity and

mortality in hypercholesterolaemic men predicted from an exercise test: The lipid research clinics coronary primary prevention trial. J Am Coll Cardiol 1989; 14:556.

18. Hume L, Oakley G D, Boulton A J M, Hardisty C, Ward J R. Asymptomatic myocardial ischaemia in diabetes and its relationship to diabetic neuropathy: An exercise electrocardiography study in middle-aged diabetic men. Diabetes care 1986; 9:384.
19. O'Donnell T F, Callow A D, Willet C *et al.* The impact of coronary artery disease on carotid endarterectomy. Ann Surg 1983; 198:705.
20. Hertzer N R, Bevan E G, Young J R *et al.* Coronary artery disease in peripheral vascular patients. A classification of 1000 coronary angiograms and results of surgical management. Ann Surg 1984; 199:223.
21. Cutler B S, Wheeler H B, Paraskos J A *et al.* Assessment of operative risk with electrocardiographic exercise testing in patients with peripheral vascular disease. Am J Surg 1979; 137:484.
22. Gage A A, Bhayana J N, Baler V *et al.* Assessment of cardiac risk in surgical patients. Arch Surg 1977; 112:1488.
23. McCabe C J, Reidy N C, Abbott W M *et al.* The value of electrocardiographic monitoring during treadmill testing for peripheral vascular disease. Surgery 1981; 89:183.
24. Kovamees A, Bundin T. Continuous electrocardiographic recording at examination of walking capacity in patients with intermittent claudication. J Cardiovasc Surg 1976; 509:12.
25. Kanazawa M, Rose H, Vyden J K *et al.* The importance of cardiac monitoring in treadmill claudication testing. Prac Cardiol 1981; 7:48.
26. Vecht R J, Nicolaides A N, Brandao E *et al.* Resting and treadmill electrocardiographic findings in patients with intermittent claudication. Int Angiol 1982; 1:119.
27. Carroll R M, Rose H B, Vyden J *et al.* Cardiac arrhythmias associated with treadmill claudication testing. Surgery 1978; 83:284.
28. Salmasi A-M, Nicolaides A N. Noninvasive detection of concomitant coronary artery disease in patients with intermittent claudication. In: A. Strano & S. Novo (eds). Advances in vascular pathology 1989, Excerpta Medica, Amsterdam, 1989; p. 1255.
29. Rogers W R, Hurst W D. Moderate exercise testing in ischaemic heart disease. Northwest Med October 1964:702.
30. Lepeschkin E. The U-wave of the electrocardiogram. Mod Concepts Cardiovasc Dis 1969; 38:39.
31. Faris J V, McHenry P L, Morris S N. Concepts and application of treadmill exercise testing and the exercise electrocardiogram. Am Heart J 1978; 95:102.
32. Salmasi A-M, Salmasi S N, Nicolaides A N *et al.* The value of exercise-induced U-wave inversion on the ECG chest wall mapping in the identification of individual coronary arterial lesion. Europ Heart J 1985; 6:437.
33. Salmasi A-M, Salmasi S N, Nicolaides A N. Is exercise-induced inverted U-wave an indicator of occult ischaemic heart disease in high risk patients? Europ Heart J 1987; 8(2):106.
34. Salmasi A-M, Besterman E M M. Assessment of the antianginal effect of nisoldipine by chest wall mapping during exercise. Proceedings of the cardiovascular pharmacotheraphy 1st international symposium, Geneva, Switzerland, April 1985, p. 123.
35. Salmasi A-M. Effect of nisoldipine on occult ischaemic heart disease. In: R. R. Lichtlen and H. Kreynbuhl (eds). New aspects on Nisoldipine. Schattauer, Stuttgart, New York 1990. p. 29.
36. Salmasi S N, Salmasi A-M, Hendry W G *et al.* Exercise-induced changes in stroke volume measured noninvasively in coronary artery disease. Ultrasound Med Biol 1982; 8(A):170.
37. Salmasi S N A, Salmasi A-M, Hendry W G *et al.* Exercise-induced changes in stroke volume measured noninvasively in coronary artery disease. Acta Cardiol 1983; 6:337.

38. Salmasi A-M, Salmasi S N, Dore C, Nicolaides A N. Noninvasive assessment of changes in aortic blood velocity and its derivatives with exercise in normal subjects by Doppler ultrasound. J Cardiovasc Surg 1987; 28:321.
39. Salmasi A-M, Salmasi S, Nicolaides A N, Dore C, Hendry W G, Kidner P H. Noninvasive assessment of left ventricular function in coronary artery disease by Doppler stress testing. J Cardiovasc Surg 1987; 28:313.
40. Mehta N, Bennett E D. Impaired left ventricular function in acute myocardial infarction assessed by Doppler measurement of ascending aortic blood velocity and maximum acceleration. Am J Cardiol 1986; 57:1052.
41. Bryg R J, Labovitz A J. Doppler treadmill studies in coronary patients: Angiographic correlates. In: Steve Teague (ed). Stress Doppler Echocardiography. Kluwer Academic Publishers, Dordrecht, Holland 1990; p. 107.
42. Light L H. Transcutaneous aortovelography: A new window on the circulation. Br Heart J 1976; 38:433.
43. Salmasi A-M, Salmasi S N, Nicolaides A N, Dore C, Kidner P H. Assessment of the effect of coronary artery bypass grafting on left ventricular performance by Doppler measurement of the aortic blood velocity during exercise. J Cardiovasc Surg 1988; 29:89.

8. Use of Holter monitoring in occult coronary artery disease

SHLOMO STERN and DAN TZIVONI

Our knowledge about coronary artery disease increased rapidly when researchers in the 1920s and 30s started to understand that the ST-T segment of the electrocardiogram provides invaluable information regarding adequate perfusion of the myocardium via the coronary circulation. The electrocardiogram, however, since the early days of Einthoven, was a static test performed while the examinee was sitting or lying in a relaxed and resting state. ST-T abnormalities under such circumstances were interpreted either as an expression of a chronic disturbance in the coronary arterial blood supply and in that case the diagnosis of 'angina pectoris' or chronic coronary artery disease was established, or according to certain patterns acute or healed myocardial infarction could be diagnosed.

The elicitation of ST-T abnormalities in patients in whom the resting electrocardiogram did not show such alterations, by provoking such changes through physical exercise, was pioneered by Goldhammer and Scherf [1] and introduced by Master as a test in the 1940s [2]. However, technical limitations did not allow the recording of the electrocardiogram during the actual exercise of the so-called Master 2-step test, but only immediately after the patient finished climbing the steps. Furthermore, this test or other subsequently developed stress testing methods were limited to the office of the physician, and the classical electrocardiographic recording did not permit one to obtain the information during the usual everyday physical activities of the patient, or stressful conditions of everyday life, etc.

Long-term monitoring of the electrocardiogram

Norman J. Holter in the late 1950s, became interested in recording physiological signals under dynamic conditions. He started to study the electroencephalographic pattern and used radio waves for transmission, while his

A.-M. Salmasi and A. N. Nicolaides (eds.), Occult Atherosclerotic Disease, 105–112.

experimental animals were constantly in motion. He continued with recording the electrocardiogram, using tape recordings of the signals and utilized this method for humans. His first publication in *Science* in 1962 [3] described the use of a system based on continuous tape recording of the electrocardiogram under 'dynamic' conditions, i.e., during daily activities, and offered a technical solution concerning how to interpret a 24-hour recording within a reasonable time.

The medical community promptly realized the ingenuity of Holter's method and its potential to detect abnormalities in the heart rate and rhythm within a 24-hour period, information which the previous classical method of electrocardiographc recording, failed to yield. Hundreds of investigations have been published in the world literature about the use of ambulatory electrocardiographic monitoring for this purpose. Naturally, the ST segment of the electrocardiogram was also recorded during the usual 24-hour Holter monitoring period, but very little attention had been paid to it. In retrospect, this can be explained by the assumption, expressed by Hinkle and his associates in their landmark article on arrhythmia detection through the use of Holter monitoring, that, because of technical limitations, the ST segment was not reliably reproduced by the then available systems [4].

Episodic ST depression without pain ('silent ischaemia')

In a few investigations during the 1970s, our group published proof that if the right equipment is used under meticulous conditions, the ST segment could be reliably recorded with the Holter system [5–7]. In 1974, we published that during a 24-hour monitoring of active subjects suspected of or known to suffer from ischaemic heart disease, during everyday activities episodes of transient ST depression can be observed on the Holter recordings, some of them accompanied by chest pain, but others 'silent'. We expressed the view that ambulatory monitoring of the electrocardiogram during everyday activities can disclose 'silent ischaemic heart disease'. In 1977, Schang and Pepine [8] confirmed our observation concerning asymptomatic ST depression during everyday activities.

Although in the 1960s and 70s ST depression was already an accepted sign of myocardial ischaemia, both when appearing at rest or provoked by exercise, as well as during anginal pain, the idea of 'silent' ST depression being an expression of this disease seemed to be revolutionary. It took a few years of most important investigations by a group of ingenious investigators, led by Maseri, Deanfield, Selwyn and others [9–11], to prove by means of advanced methods of haemodynamic monitoring, radionucleide and other testing that silent changes in the ST segment had a similar significance as the painful ones. This created a breakthrough in our thinking, realizing that 'angina pectoris' is not a *conditio sine qua non* for diagnosing chronic ischaemic heart disease and that patients may suffer from different degrees of coronary artery disease without clinical manifestations.

Reliability of tape-recording systems

There are, today, recommendations to manufacturers and users of specifications for tape recording systems, and the American Heart Association recommended to have a system with a flat amplitude signal for frequency responses between 0.1 and 80 Hz. It has been emphasized that many AM systems may amplify low frequency information normally present in the ST segment, thus overestimating the degree of ST segment depression relative to the height of the R wave. Eight different commercially available Holter systems have been studied by Bragg-Remschel and co-workers [12]. These investigators have demonstrated that although not all systems studied by them were adequate, most of them were valid for ST segment depression documentation, especially if frequency modulated systems were used. Selwyn and co-workers and Pepine and co-workers conducted similar studies [11, 13] and demonstrated accurate reproduction of the ST segment both on AM and FM systems, expressing their view that with faithful reproduction there is no need for extended low frequency range such as found in FM systems. In a recent study, Rotman and co-workers [14] used a precordial and a diaphragmatic lead with semiautomatic and visual analysis; they found that the presence of J point ST depression plus ST depression 80 milliseconds thereafter, of > 0.1mV, predicts the true ischaemic ST depression most accurately. As a practical way of controlling by the individual user his own Holter system, we recommended to record simultaneously during an exercise test both Holter and a 12-lead electrocardiogram, and to expect similar ST shifts on the two systems. We performed such a test on 144 patients, using bipolar V_3 and V_5-like leads [15]. In 138 of the 144 patients (96%), the ST shifts, or lack of shifts, recorded on both systems were concordant. Furthermore, the Holter system identified 6 of the 7 patients whose ischaemic changes were confined to the inferior wall on the 12-lead electrocardiogram, and the addition of the V_5-like lead increased ischaemia detection by 10% over the use of V_3-like lead only. We therefore advocate the use of V_3 and V_5-like leads for detection of ischaemia. Future studies will disclose whether a three-lead system will add further accuracy to Holter recordings.

Characteristics of silent ischaemic episodes as compared with painful episodes

The possibility has been entertained that an ischaemic episode without pain may be an expression of ischaemia of a lesser magnitude than a typical anginal episode. In order to test this hypothesis, we studied 191 patients with transient ST depression on a 24-hour Holter monitoring, all with positive treadmill tests, and 116 with coronary arteriograms [16]. Among the 587 recorded episodes, only 28% were symptomatic. There were no statistically significant differences between the silent and the painful episodes as to the main duration of the episode, the heart rate at onset of the ST depression, the heart rate at time of maximal ST depression and the degree of maximal ST depression. Similar results were published by Selwyn and co-workers [11], using Holter monitoring, and by us, by comparing treadmill tests with >2 mm ST depression in two groups of patients, those who were silent and those who had pain during the stress [17].

It appears thus, that silent and symptomatic ischaemia have similar characteristics and are associated with a similar extent of coronary artery disease. The question that arises is why in some patients, during so many episodes, pain is absent while in others and during some or all the episodes, pain is present. The answer may be in a 'defective warning system', as suggested by Cohn [18] or a higher pain threshold possibly associated with a different apomorphine level in these patients [19].

Prognostic significance of silent ischaemic episodes

The totally silent or 'occult' coronary artery disease cannot be established because these patients go undiagnosed. It should be mentioned, however, that according to various authors, acute myocardial infarction in a patient who previously had no overt coronary artery disease, comprises 20–30% of the total cases of myocardial infarctions. Sudden death, most probably due to acute myocardial infarction as a first manifestation of ischaemic heart disease, occurs in about 20% of the sudden death cases [20]. The prognostic significance of silent ischaemia is based on the observations obtained on a population having dyspnoea, fatigue, or some other manifestations, or those who, by chance, are undergoing ECG, stress testing, Holter monitoring or other diagnostic tests.

In our studies assessing the prognostic significance of ischaemic changes during daily activity, as recorded by ambulatory electrocardiographic monitoring [20, 21, 22] we found that the frequency of future cardiac events (death, reinfarction, hospitalization for unstable angina, percutaneous transluminal angioplasty or coronary artery bypass surgery), was 51% among patients with ischaemic episodes on Holter monitoring as compared with 12% in those without such changes. Patients with ST depression on Holter monitoring had a significantly higher cardiac event rate, compared to those without it. A similar event rate was found in patients with only silent, only symptomatic, or with silent and symptomatic ischaemic episodes. Rocco and co-workers [23] in a prospective follow-up study confirmed the prognostic importance of myocardial ischaemia, silent or painful, detected by ambulatory ECG monitoring in patients with stable coronary artery disease.

Hedblad *et al.* [24] in their study conducted in Malmo, Sweden, on 'Men born in 1914' stated that the occurrence of asymptomatic ST segment depression on Holter monitoring was associated with an increased cardiovascular mortality. Men with ST depression > 0.1mV and no history of coronary artery disease, had a 4.4 times greater relative risk of fatal and non-fatal myocardial infarction, than those without. The increased mortality was independent of a history compatible with angina pectoris or previous myocardial infarction.

Erikson *et al.*, in Norway [25], identified between 1972 and 1975, 60 asymptomatic persons aged 40 to 59 with S-T segment depression. During follow-up, these persons had a worse prognosis than control cases. A similarly high mortality was found in the Duke-Harvard Collaborative Data Bank in totally asymptomatic and partially symptomatic patients. By the end of the four year follow-up in this study, anginal symptoms developed in about 30% of the previously silent patients.

Mody and co-workers [26] found an astonishingly high (90%) frequency of silent episodes in patients with proven coronary artery disease and demonstrated that patients with prolonged duration of myocardial ischaemia (>60 min/24 hours) had several times higher probability for left main, triple, proximal and other forms of advanced coronary disease, than patients without documented ischaemia on Holter monitoring; the specificity of silent symptomatic episodes on Holter monitoring was found to be greater than 90%. This study confirmed what has already been generally accepted by most investigators, that *absence* of S-T segment changes on Holter ECG recording has little predictive value. In other words, for identifying/diagnosing the presence of ischaemic heart disease a test with higher sensitivity, such as exercise ECG testing, should be used.

Long-term electrocardiogram monitoring in unstable angina patients

In a report by Gottlieb *et al.* [27], the frequency and duration of silent ischaemic episodes correlated well with the manifestations of ischaemia induced by stress test: the earlier the exercise test became positive, the longer was the cumulative duration of myocardial ischaemia on the ambulatory 24-hour Holter recordings.

Continuous Holter monitoring in hospitalized patients with ischaemic heart disease indicated that in those unstable, over two-thirds of transient myocardial ischaemic episodes are clinically silent [28]. It is not known, however, whether silent ischaemic episodes are markers of unfavourable outcome in patients with unstable angina, with or without surgical therapy.

Additional data of Nademanee *et al.* [28] suggest that silent myocardial ischaemia documented on Holter recordings in patients with unstable angina is of prognostic significance. Langer and co-workers [29] demonstrated a stratification of unstable patients by Holter monitoring with respect to hospital outcome and coronary anatomy. They found that symptomatic episodes in these patients had a greater magnitude of ST shift and were of longer duration. As their patients had an increase in rate-pressure product, they concluded that myocardial ischaemia may be mediated in part by increased myocardial oxygen demand.

Recent technical developments

The conventional Holter tape playback units use generally visual or semi-automatic interpretation systems, which are inherently time consuming. The printout fully discloses the episodes, which are then confirmed as being ischaemic according to the usual criteria. Recently, more automated trend and custom algorithms are being introduced, which automatically identify not only the isoelectric P-R segment but also the J point and the 60ms or 80ms intervals and provide the slope, upward or downward, of the ST segment. Changes for heart rate are automatically updated by the custom algorithm.

Solid state technology is also available for long-term ambulatory monitoring, although its use is still subject to controversy [30]. Although these microcomputers with solid-state or microcassette storage produced a digitized signal without the probable distortion caused by the tape recording and conventional playback units, but they have the limitation of not having all data stored for review.

Currently, attempts are being made by manufacturers to incorporate into the real-time analysis system 'full disclosure' continuous data storage. So far this has been accomplished for one ECG channel and we may be on the brink of having two-channel continuous storage capabilities. As Kennedy stated recently [31], these methodologies may have a disparity in what they examine and what they provide as evidence to support their decisions. Still, these innovations, together with developments in the conventional Holter tape technologies, promise exciting innovations for even more reliable, less time-consuming methods for recording and demonstrating ischaemic episodes.

Conclusions

Occult ischaemic heart disease can be detected by Holter monitoring. This method, similarly to many other diagnostic methods, is not aimed exclusively at the totally asymptomatic individuals as a screening test, but it seems to be well suited for detecting the silent form of this disease in high-risk individuals and in those who have vague and non-diagnostic symptomatology. The disclosure of silent ischaemic episodes in stable angina pectoris, in the post-infarction patient and in those with unstable angina, seems to carry prognostic value for future cardiac events. Further investigations are required to establish the place of silent ischaemia in the spectrum of coronary artery disease and the position of Holter monitoring in the diagnosis and evaluation of this new clinical entity.

References

1. Goldhammer S, Scherf D. Electrocardiographische Untersuchungen bei Kranker mit Angina Pectoris ('ambulatorischer Typus'). Z Klin Med 1933; 122:134.
2. Master AM, Friedman R, Dack S. The electrocardiogram after standard exercise as functional test of the heart, Am Heart J 1942; 24:777.
3. Holter NJ. New methods for heart studies continuous electrocardiography of active subjects. Science 1961; 134:1214–1220.
4. Hinkle L, Jr, Meyer J, Stevens M, Carver ST. Taperecordings of the ECG of active man. Circulation 1967; 36:752.
5. Stern S, Tzivoni D. The reliability of the Holter-Avionics system in reproducing the ST-T segment. Amer Heart J 1972; 84:427.
6. Stern S, Tzivoni D, Stern Z. Diagnostic accuracy of ambulatory ECG monitoring in ischaemic heart disease. Circulation 1975; 52:1045.
7. Stern S, Tzivoni D. Early detection of silent ischaemic heart disease by 24-hour electrocardiographic monitoring of active subjects. Brit Heart J 1974; 36:481.
8. Schang SJ, Pepine CJ. Transient asymptomatic ST segment depression during daily activity. Amer J Cardiol 1977; 39:396.
9. Biagini A, L'Abbate A, Maseri A. Vasospastic ischemic mechanisms of frequent asymptomatic transient ST-T changes during continuous ECG monitoring. Amer Heart J 1982; 103:13.
10. Deanfield JE, Shea M, Ribiero P *et al.* Transient ST-segment depression as a marker of myocardial ischemia during daily life. Amer J Cardiol 1984; 54:1195.
11. Selwyn AP, Shea M, Deanfield JE, Wilson R, Horlock P, O'Brian HA. Character of transient ischemia in angina pectoris. Amer J Cardiol 1986; 58:21 B.
12. Bragg-Remschell DA, Anderson CM, Winkle RA. Frequency response characteristics of ambulatory ECG monitoring systems and their implications for ST segment analysis. Amer Heart J 1982; 103:30.
13. Pepine CJ. Clinical aspects of silent myocardial ischemia in patients with angina and other forms of coronary heart disease. Amer J Med 1986; 80, Suppl. 40:25.
14. Rotman B, Eber B, Duslag J Fluch N, Weinrauch V. Klein W. Comparison of different methods of ST measurement for evaluation of myocardial ischaemia in Holter monitoring. European Heart Journal 1988; 9 (Suppl. N), 78.
15. Tzivoni D, Benhorin, Gavish A, Stern S. Holter recording during treadmill testing in assessing myocardial ischaemic changes. Amer J Cardiol 1985; 55:1200.
16. Stern S, Gavish A, Weisz G, Benhorin J, Tzivoni D. Characteristics of silent and symptomatic myocardial ischaemia during everyday activity. Amer J Cardiol 1988; 61: 1223–1228.
17. Stern S, Weisz G, Gavish A, Keren A, Tzivoni D. Comparison between silent and

symptomatic ischemia during exercise testing in patients with coronary artery disease. J Cardiopulm Rehab 1988; 12:507.

18. Cohn PF. Silent myocardial ischemia in patients with a defective anginal warning system. Am J Cardiol 1980; 45:697.
19. Droste E, Roskamm H. Experimental pain measurements in patients with asymptomatic myocardial ischemia. JACC 1983; 1:940.
20. Kannel WB, Abbott RD. Incidence and prognosis of unrecognized myocardial infarction. N Engl J Med 1984; 311:1144.
21. Tzivoni D, Gavish A, Zin D *et al.* Prognostic significance of ischemic episodes in patients with previous myocardial infarction. Am J Cardiol 1988; 62:661–664.
22. Tzivoni D, Weisz G, Gavish A, Zin D, Keren A, Stern S. Comparison of mortality and myocardial infarction rates in stable angina pectoris with and without ischemic episodes during daily activities. Am J Cardiol 1989; 63:273.
23. Rocco MB, Nabel EG, Campbells *et al.* Prognostic importance of myocardial ischemia detected by ambulatory monitoring in patients with coronary disease Circulation 1988; 78:877.
24. Headblad B, Juul-Moller S, Hanson BS *et al.* Increased mortality in men with ST segment depression during 24h ambulatory long-term ECG recording. Eur Heart J 1989; 10:149.
25. Erikssen J, Thaulow E. Follow-up of patients with asymptomatic myocardial ischemia. In: W. Rutishauser, H. Roskamm (eds): Silent myocardial ischemia. Springer, Berlin 1984; p. 156.
26. Mody FV, Nademanee K, Intarachot V, Josephson M, Robertson HA, Singh B. Severity of silent myocardial ischemia on ambulatory electrocardiographic monitoring in patients with stable angina pectoris: Relation to prognostic determinants during exercise stress testing and coronary angiography. JACC 1988; 12:1169.
27. Gottlieb SO, Weisfeldt M, Quyang P, Mellits DE, Gerstenblith G. Silent ischemia as marker of unfavorable outcomes in patients with unstable angina. New Engl J Med 1986; 314:1214.
28. Nadamanee K, Intarachot BN, Singh MA, Josephson RW Singh. Characteristics and clinical significance of silent myocardial ischemia in unstable angina. Amer J Cardiol 1986; 58:26 B.
29. Langer A, Freeman MR, Armstrong P. ST segment shift in unstable angina: Pathophysiology and association with coronary anatomy and hospital outcome. JACC 1989; 13 No.7:1495.
30. Kennedy HL, Wiens, RD. Ambulatory (Holter) electrocardiography using real-time analysis. Am J Cardiol 1987 59:1190.
31. Kennedy HL. Ambulatory electrocardiography strategies used in assessing silent myocardial ischaemia. Europ Heart J 1988; 9 (Suppl. N):70.

9. Radionuclide techniques in the diagnosis and assessment of occult coronary artery disease

ABDULMASSIH S. ISKANDRIAN and JAEKYEONG HEO[1]

The diagnosis of coronary artery disease in the absence of symptoms is not an easy task. It is possible that the lack of symptoms is due to the presence of haemodynamically significant coronary artery disease that is entirely silent, yet it is possible that the lack of symptoms is due to the mild and hence, haemodynamically insignificant nature of the coronary stenosis. Such patients are therefore, not expected to produce abnormalities in any of the traditional forms of screening tests, such as exercise electrocardiography, thallium-201 imaging, and radionuclide angiography. These patients are, nevertheless, prone to sudden total occlusion of a coronary artery by a thrombus with the catastrophic results of massive myocardial infarction or sudden death. An argument can be made that patients with severe stenosis which results in a pressure drop across the lesion are protected by well functioning collaterals that are likely to develop and thus, protect the left ventricle in the event of thrombus occlusion of the diseased vessel. Therefore, paradoxically it appears that patients with less severe stenosis who may not be diagnosed by non-invasive testing are at higher risk for sudden death or large infarctions than patients with more severe stenosis who are likely to be detected by exercise studies. Parenthetically, even coronary arteriography will not alter therapy in the former patients because angioplasty or bypass surgery are not recommended for mild stenosis. The role of anti-platelet therapy remains to be determined, but theoretically, it is worth the effort.

During the last two decades, considerable advances have been made in radiopharmaceuticals, gamma cameras and computer systems that have resulted in increasing use of radionuclide techniques in the assessment of patients with coronary artery disease. In this chapter, some of these techniques will be described as they pertain to patients with stable symptoms or

1. The authors wish to thank Phyllis Hartsfield for secretarial assistance.

A.-M. Salmasi and A. N. Nicolaides (eds.), Occult Atherosclerotic Disease, 113–137.

patients with no symptoms; hence, techniques in patients with acute myocardial infarction or unstable angina will not be discussed. The use of nonimaging noninvasive techniques such as exercise electrocardiography, Holter monitoring, two-dimensional echocardiography and electrocardiographic signal averaging are beyond the scope of this chapter.

Myocardial perfusion imaging

Since thallium-201 was introduced into clinical use in 1973, stress thallium imaging has been widely used in the diagnosis, management and risk stratification of patients with known or suspected coronary artery disease. Thallium-201 is a potassium analogue with a physical half-life of 73 hours. Thallium is produced by cyclotron and most of its energy is in the range of 69 to 83 kev and to a much lesser extent, in the range of 167 kev. Studies in animals and man show that the myocardial distribution is proportionate to the regional blood flow over a fairly wide range (from below normal to several folds above normal) [1]. The extraction ratio is high, approximating 85%, during the first-pass at normal flow rates, but diminishes slightly at higher flow rates. It has been demonstrated that with non-recirculating indicators, the fractional uptake of the injected tracer by any organ equals the fraction of the cardiac output perfusing that organ during the measurement. This principle can apply to recirculating indicators, as long as organ extraction and total cardiac extraction of the indicator are the same. This assumption has been proven in animals with potassium-43 and rubidium-86. Studies have shown that myocardial extraction of thallium is significantly higher than the whole body extraction fraction in the control conditions. These results therefore confirm that despite similarities, thallium does not have identical properties to potassium, rubidium or caesium. Further, it has been shown that the myocardial extraction fraction for thallium appears to be higher than that of potassium and its analogues. In addition, the washout of thallium from the myocardium after the initial uptake appears to be slower for thallium than for potassium. Possible reasons for differences between myocardial extraction and total body extraction for thallium include the inclusion of a large high flow compartment such as the renal circulation in the total body extraction. It can be shown for example that the renal extraction of thallium is lower than that of the myocardium. Alternatively, the lower average whole body extraction could be due to the lack of uptake of thallium by the brain because of the inability of the thallium to cross the blood brain barrier. The difference between myocardial and total body extraction of thallium may explain why in the control condition, the myocardial uptake exceeded the fractional myocardial blood flow. However, despite this over-estimation, a linear relation between thallium uptake and myocardial blood flow has been shown. Furthermore, extraction of thallium does not appear to be dependent on sodium potassium pump. When the coronary blood flow was increased by dipyridamole, there was a progressive decrease in the thallium myocardial extraction due to a marked rise in capillary and venous velocity. The decrease in myocardial extraction resulted in an equality between myocardial and systemic extraction fractions. At larger increases in coronary artery flow, myocardial extraction will probably drop even more drastically and therefore cause an underestimation of flow by thallium. Therefore, the correlation between thallium uptake and myocardial blood flow depends on the range of the coronary blood flow in which the experiments are conducted. Increases in flow in the range of 100–200% are comparable to the increases in man during exercise stress testing and suggest that simultaneous measurement of cardiac output and accurate quantification of thallium uptake and correction for background and attenuation could be used to measure absolute coronary blood flow.

Pathophysiology

The basic concept in using thallium-201 in the evaluation of regional coronary blood flow stems from the fact that diseased coronary arteries have limited ability to augment the coronary blood flow in response to exercise or to pharmacologic coronary vasodilatation compared to normal vessels or vessels with less severe stenosis. The disparity in coronary blood flow results in differential thallium concentration, such that the area receiving less coronary blood flow will have less thallium concentration as well, and this area appears to have a perfusion defect detected on the scintigrams. On the other hand, perfusion defects may also reflect the presence of myocardial necrosis. The distinction between ischaemia and scar is based upon comparison of the initial images with 3–4 hour delayed images. In general, ischaemic defects will show redistribution in the delayed images, while fixed defects due to scar will show no change in the perfusion pattern in the delayed images. The lack of redistribution, contrary to earlier predictions, however is not always due to scar. Thus, some fixed defects have been shown to improve after coronary arterial bypass grafting, or percutaneous transluminal angioplasty and have also been shown to maintain metabolic activity detected by positron emission tomography using FDG as a metabolic marker. Some fixed defects have been observed to show redistribution when delayed images were obtained 8–24 hours after exercise but not after 4 hours. The precise mechanism for the lack of redistribution or the 'slow redistribution' is not clear but a very severe coronary stenosis which compromises the coronary flow even at rest has been implicated. Thallium washout depends on the concentration gradient between myocardial cells and blood. Slow washout has been noted in patients with submaximal exercise and when blood thallium is decreased, such as after a meal. We routinely ask our patients to have a light meal between the initial and redistribution images. It is therefore important to remember that fixed defects should be considered as markers of coronary artery disease.

More recently, the re-injection technique has been used to differentiate between fixed and ischaemic defects. With this method, smaller dose of thallium, generally 1 mCi is injected 3–4 hours after exercise and images are obtained 20 minutes after this injection. This technique is a modification of the originally described exercise/rest imaging which were done on separate days. This method has been found to increase the ability to differentiate ischaemia from fixed defects.

Protocol and interpretation

Most clinical studies with thallium-201 have been performed during exercise studies, although similar studies can be performed during coronary vasodilatation with pharmacologic agents and atrial pacing; thallium-201 can be injected directly into the coronary artery, or intravenously during such interventions as balloon occlusion of the coronary artery during angioplasty. During exercise, thallium-201 is injected at peak exercise and the patient is requested to continue exercising for an additional minute to ensure thallium uptake and distribution during the hyperaemic response to exercise.

Planar imaging is done in at least three projections, using usually low energy, all purpose collimator (LEAP) (Figure 9.1) [2]. Images are acquired either for a preset count or time and images contain approximately 250–500 K-counts. The imaging time is approximately 6 to 10 minutes per view. The images are subjected to smoothing and background subtraction; the interpolative background subtraction technique is often used with quantitative

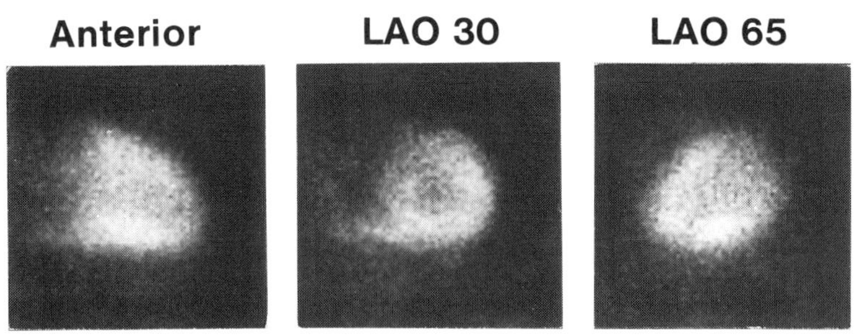

Figure 9.1. Normal planar thallium images in 3 projections; anterior, 30° left anterior oblique and 65° left anterior oblique projections. Images show homogeneous distribution of thallium in all segments of the myocardium.

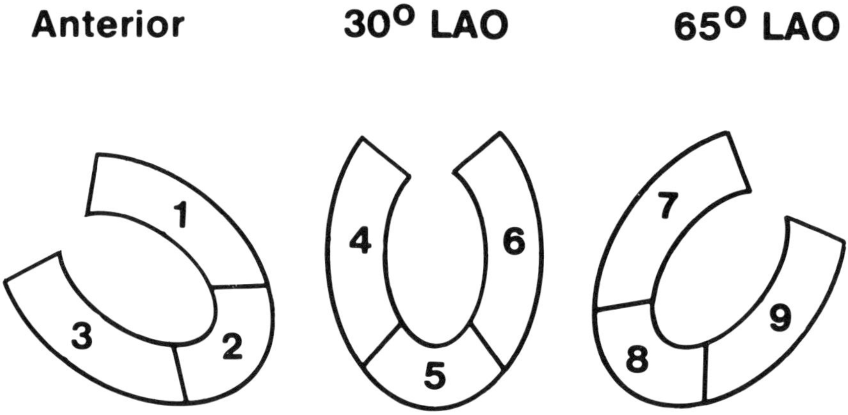

Figure 9.2. Anatomic segments of planar images in 3 projections; segments 1 and 7 represent anterior; 3, inferior wall; 4, septum; 6, posterolateral wall; 9, inferoposterior wall; 2, 5 and 8 represent the apex.

analysis. Images are interpreted either subjectively or quantitatively as to the presence, severity, site and nature of the perfusion abnormality. Perfusion defects involving the anterior wall and septum represent disease of the left anterior descending artery; defects in the inferior wall represent disease in the right coronary artery, and defects in the posterolateral wall represent left circumflex disease (Figure 9.2). It should however be noted that there is considerable overlap in the vascular territories especially between the left circumflex and the right coronary arteries.

A commonly used method for quantitative analysis is referred to as circumferential profile analysis in which the edge of the image is defined and radii are drawn from the centre of the image to the perimeter and counts are measured along each radius, and a plot of the counts versus the angular location is derived. Initial and delayed images are treated in a similar fashion, and the curves are superimposed. Washout curves can be computer derived by subtracting the delayed from the initial curves. These curves can also be compared to a profile. One of the major advantages of this technique has been the improvement in detecting individual diseased vessels by demonstrating washout abnormalities.

Thallium kinetics in relation to coronary stenosis

We studied the relative, spatial and temporal quantitation of myocardial thallium-201 scintigrams and correlated our findings with quantitative coronary artery stenosis measurement [3]. It has been demonstrated that the minimal diameter stenosis and minimal area stenosis of the coronary artery correlated better with regional myocardial thallium concentration than the percent diameter stenosis. In this study we used the ratio of the thallium-201 counts of the segment perfused by the stenosed coronary vessel to the segment perfused by the normal coronary artery to represent the relation of flow in the ischaemic and normal segment of the heart in a group of patients with angiographic evidence of single-vessel disease. This ratio has been shown in dogs to correlate linearly with the flow ratio determined by microspheres, and in man with the flow ratio determined by the regional clearance of xenon-133. This regional difference in perfusion is underestimated by current scintigraphic methods due to overlap of normal and ischaemic myocardium, nonhomogeneous background, attenuation artifact and cardiac motion.

In the clinical setting, other variables may affect the myocardial thallium concentration activity such as muscle viability, dynamic changes in the stenosis severity, the presence of collateral channels, and the level of exercise. In our study, the estimation of the regional difference in perfusion as represented by the myocardial thallium concentration is limited by the characteristics of the planar thallium-201 images. It has been shown that flow differential between the normal and stenotic coronary artery of 2.4 is required to cause a definite defect in the thallium images. This large differential flow requirement is partly explained by the reduced extraction of thallium-201 with increased flow rates. There is however, evidence from experimental studies that the relationship may indeed be linear if flow changes are secondary to metabolic demands as compared to the non-linear response when hyperaemia is produced in excess of oxygen demand, and there is evidence to suggest that the minimal diameter stenosis may not be the ideal measurement in all patients, but may be superior to percent diameter stenosis because it accounts for both localized and diffused disease. This index is useful in proximal stenosis, but unfortunately, no single value for functionally significant minimal cross-sectional areas is possible for a wide range encountered in proximal and distal disease. In our study, there was a significant correlation between a myocardial thallium concentration ratio and the minimal diameter stenosis in 30 patients with one-vessel disease ($r=0.73$, $p<0.001$).

Comparison with exercise electrocardiography

Planar thallium-201 imaging has considerable advantages compared to exercise electrocardiography. These include higher sensitivity, higher specificity, its ability to localize coronary disease, assess the extent of disease, assess muscle viability, and provide more definite and important prognostic data.

The sensitivity of thallium-201 imaging is 80–90% and the specificity is 90–95%. Sensitivity increases as the extent of coronary artery disease increases, i.e. patients with multi-vessel disease are more likely to have an abnormal scan than patients with single-vessel disease, and it increases as the severity of the disease increases, i.e. patients with more severe stenosis, over 90% are more likely to have perfusion abnormalities than patients with 50–70% diameter stenosis as discussed above.

False positive and false negative studies

Causes of false negative exercise planar thallium-201 images include limited extent of coronary artery disease, generally disease confined to the left circumflex, the right coronary artery or to secondary branches, less severe disease (< 70% stenosis), submaximal exercise, misinterpretation of the images and misinterpretation of the coronary angiogram, undue delay between the injection of thallium and the start of imaging allowing redistribution to occur before the initial images are obtained.

False positive scans include misinterpretation of the coronary angiogram, misinterpretation of the thallium scans, attenuation artifacts, especially breast attenuation in women, and diaphragmatic attenuation in heavy men, poor quality images, non-coronary artery diseases, such as cardiomyopathies, valve diseases, collagen vascular diseases and exercise-induced spasm.

Bayes' theorem

Recent studies suggest a decline in the specificity of the radionuclide studies and this has been attributed to referral bias. The argument is that normal subjects are excluded from the cath population in recent years and therefore the study population is skewed towards higher prevalence of disease by the exclusion of these normals. According to the Bayes' theorem, as the population is skewed towards greater prevalence of disease, the number of true negatives or apparent specificity of that study group falls. The term referral bias can therefore be defined as skewing of the study population towards greater disease prevalence. In support of this argument is the normalcy rate of about 90% in uncatheterized patients having less than 5% probability of coronary artery disease by virtue of age, lack of risk factors, or family history of premature coronary arteriosclerosis. An alternative explanation for recent low specificity is that the study population in early reports were made up of patients who had sufficiently advance coronary artery disease to warrant cardiac catheterization anyway without additional data derived from the exercise thallium imaging. More recently, stress thallium imaging has been used in populations without clear clinical evidence of coronary artery disease, and therefore are likely to have a lower prevalence of disease. Supporters of this hypothesis argue that in populations recently studied with lower prevalence of disease in whom a noninvasive test is most needed, the results obtained with thallium imaging must be disappointing because of the lower specificity and hence, lower diagnostic accuracy.

Finally, it can be argued that patients with low pretest probability of disease cannot be used to derive normalcy rate because of differences in risk factors, age, anatomy, including the greater chest diameter, greater body mass, bone density, and the greater prevalence of diaphragmatic and breast attenuation in the older patients with normal coronary angiogram, which may cause false positive images.

In our experience pretest and post-test bias are important factors in the explanation in the decline in the specificity of some of the radionuclide procedures. Another bias could be added to this discussion and that's a personal bias in which the person interpreting the results of the test is the same person who is taking care of the patient. For example, if the angiographer thought that the patient has coronary artery disease, he (or she) is more likely to overestimate the severity of the angiographic disease to fit the pretest hypothesis; normal thallium images in such a patient will be interpreted as false negative! As more and more cardiologists interpret their own results in freestanding laboratories, this issue may become even more important.

Single photon emission computed tomography (SPECT) imaging

Thallium imaging can also be done with single photon emission computed tomography (SPECT) which may be divided into two forms, longitudinal tomography in which the image plane for the patient is parallel to the long axis of the body and transaxial tomography in which the image plane is transverse to the long axis of the body. Seven pinhole and slant hole tomography belong to the former, and rotational tomography belongs to the latter. Rotational tomography could be divided into circular or elliptical. In the former, the camera, as it moves around the patient, describes a circular arc. In the latter, the camera movement is combined with simultaneous patient movement by means of a specially designed body contoured table. The alleged advantage of elliptical tomography is to maintain as close a distance as possible between camera and patient throughout the arc of rotation. Most of the experience with rotational tomography however has been generated with circular tomography. In fact, elliptical tomography may show more image distortion than circular tomography.

In our laboratory, we use a dose of 3.0 mCi thallium-201 and acquire 32 images in an anterior 180° arc, extending from 45° right anterior oblique to 45° left posterior oblique projections. Each image is acquired for 40 seconds [4]. Thus, the total acquisition time is 24 min. The patient is positioned supine on the imaging table, (a prone position has recently been reported to cause less diaphragmatic attenuation) the left arm is strapped above the head, the right arm is placed alongside the body, and the patient is instructed to avoid any motion during the imaging period. Each of the 32 images is then corrected for non-uniformity of camera field with either technetium-99m or cobalt-57 flood source collecting a minimum of 30 million counts. The mechanical center of rotation is determined from the projection data acquired tomographically around the point source, and this information is stored in the computer to be used for reconstruction of patient image data. Filtered back projection is then performed with a Ramp/Hanning filter with a cut-off frequency of 0.83 cycles/cm to construct the transaxial tomogram, each of 1 pixel thickness (approximately 6 mm). The tomograms are then aligned to the long axis of the heart and oblique angled tomograms parallel to the long and short axis of the ventricle are generated from the original transaxial tomograms using a coordinate transformation with commercially available algorithms. This oblique angled tomograms are referred to as short axis, vertical long axis and horizontal long axis projections (Figures 9.3, 9.4). Strict adherence to quality control is essential in SPECT imaging and this includes camera field uniformity, assurance of adequacy of data collection, determination of center of rotation, and testing for component failure that may prove to be source of artifact, loss of resolution, and increase in noise level. The unprocessed images are also reviewed to determine the level of lung thallium uptake and to detect any motion artifact. The tomographic images can also be presented as polar maps (bull's-eye) from the maximal circumferential count profiles of the short axis tomograms. Each point in these profiles represents the maximum

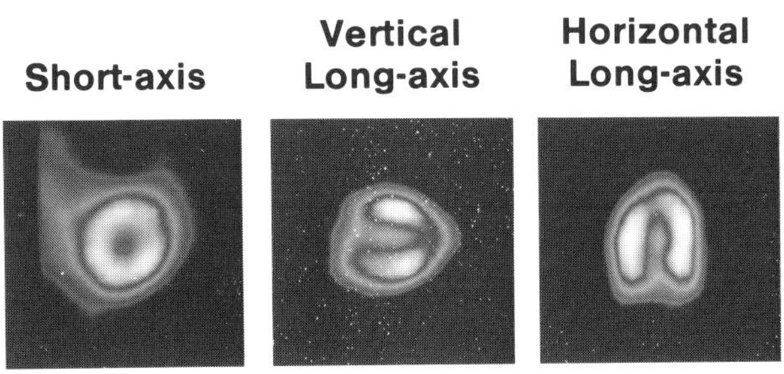

Figure 9.3. Normal SPECT thallium images in oblique-angled tomograms; short-axis, vertical long-axis, and horizontal long-axis planes. There is homogeneous thallium uptake within all segments of myocardium.

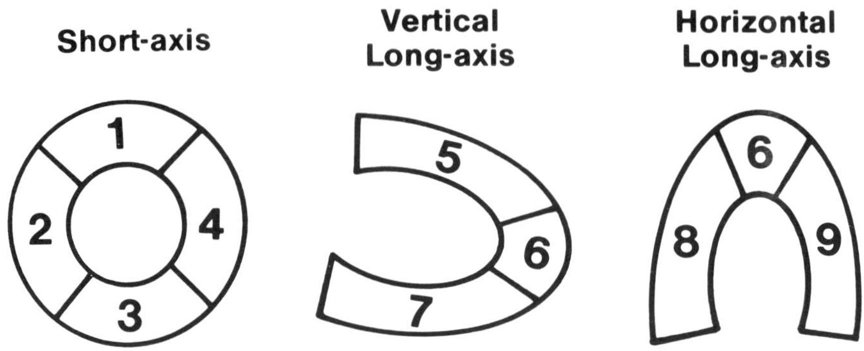

Figure 9.4. Anatomic segments of oblique-angled tomograms in 3 planes. Segment numbers 1 and 5 represent anterior wall; 2 and 8, septum; 3 and 7, inferior wall; 4 and 9, lateral wall; 6 represents apex.

count/pixel along a radius extending from the center of the left ventricle to the limits of the radius. The profiles are constructed by the computer from the values of 40 radii spaced as 9° intervals plotted clockwise. The initial and delayed tomograms are treated similarly and washout profiles are generated for each slice based on the difference between the stress and delayed profiles divided by the stress profile.

The apical position of the left ventricle can be constructed either from the vertical long axis or from the short axis tomograms. Short axis profiles are mapped into two-dimensional polar coordinate presentation. The apex corresponds to the center of the polar presentation and the outermost circle corresponds to the most basal slice that was processed. In this presentation the vascular territories can be defined in terms of quadrants and these profiles can also be compared to normal profiles. A convenient form of presentation is that pixels that have counts 2.5 standard deviation or more below the mean are blackened out; the blackened area hence represents the extent of the perfusion abnormality. In our experience, sole reliance on polar maps results in higher false positive rates, and may also be misleading in some patients with coronary artery disease.

Comparison with planar imaging

Since a slightly higher dose of thallium is used in SPECT than with planar imaging, the cost, and the radiation exposure, especially to the target organ (the bladder) is slightly higher with SPECT than planar imaging. The three-dimensional representation of the images is a clear advantage of SPECT over planar imaging. SPECT imaging provides superb demonstration of the

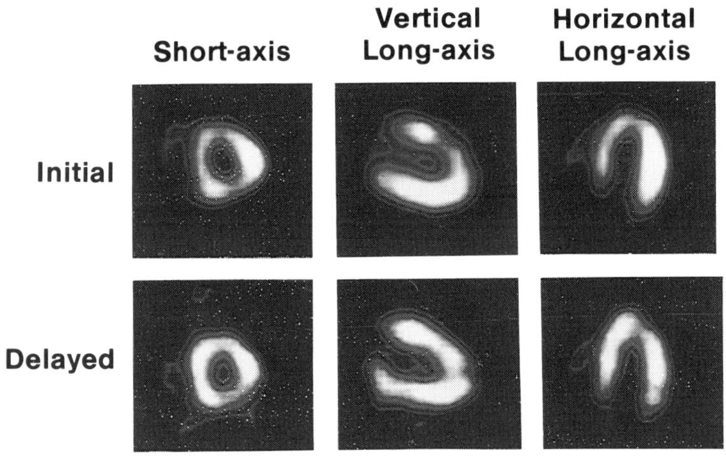

Figure 9.5. Abnormal exercise SPECT thallium images; initial post-stress images reveal extensive perfusion abnormalities involving the anterior wall and septum. Four hour delayed images reveal complete redistribution. This was a 53-year-old man with typical angina. Coronary arteriogram revealed 95% stenosis in the proximal left anterior descending coronary artery.

location of the perfusion abnormality (Figure 9.5). For example, it is possible in a patient with right coronary artery disease to define the extent of the involvement of the inferior wall, and to demonstrate extension of this abnormality to the adjacent septum as well as the posterolateral wall in some patients. SPECT imaging also provides a better contrast for the detection of perfusion abnormality because of a lack of overlap and superimposition. SPECT imaging is better than planar imaging in assessment of the extent of coronary artery disease and recognition of individual diseased vessel, especially left circumflex disease while it is the most difficult with planar imaging. Finally, it is possible, because of the better contrast and higher quality of the images that SPECT imaging is better than planar imaging in detection of moderate or mild coronary artery disease. In fact, the left circumflex distribution is the easiest territory to evaluate by SPECT.

Quantitative analysis of the count distribution in SPECT imaging reveals that the lateral region of the myocardium has slightly higher counts than the septum, both in men and women, and higher counts than the anterior and inferior segments. Furthermore, the anterior and inferior segments have approximately similar counts in women while the anterior segment has slightly higher counts in men than the inferior segment because of the diaphragmatic attenuation. Since SPECT is intuitively three-dimensional, quantitative analysis of the extent of the perfusion abnormality and sizing of the myocardial mass is possible and has been done both in animals and man.

Results

We studied the effect of the level of exercise on the ability of exercise thallium-201 SPECT imaging in the detection of coronary artery disease [5]. These patients were divided into two groups. In group 1, 164 patients achieved adequate exercise end-points defined as positive exercise electrocardiograms or achievement of at least 85% of maximum predicted heart rate. In group 2, 108 patients had submaximal exercise. SPECT thallium-201 images showed perfusion defects in 74% of patients with one-vessel, 88% of patients with two-vessel, and 98% of patients with three-vessel disease in group 1 compared to 52%, 84% and 79% respectively in group 2 ($p < 0.05$ each). Perfusion defects showed partial or complete redistribution consistent with ischaemia in 56% of patients with one-vessel, 80% with two-vessel, and 88% with three-vessel disease in group 1 compared to 35%, 55% and 56%, respectively in group 2 ($p < 0.001$). Thus, in our experience, the level of exercise affects the results of SPECT thallium imaging in the localization of coronary artery disease and the detection of ischaemia.

In a separate group of 131 patients with < 5% pretest probability of coronary artery disease, the specificity of the test was 93%. The sensitivity of exercise SPECT thallium imaging was considerably higher than that of exercise electrocardiography. Patients recruited in this study had stable symptoms and had undergone coronary angiography within 6 months of exercise testing; coronary artery disease was defined as 50% diameter stenosis or greater in any of the major vessels or their branches. It should be noted that contrary to the findings with planar imaging, quantitative analysis using circumferential profile analysis from selected slices in SPECT imaging has not been found to enhance the ability to detect individual disease vessels. This discrepancy between SPECT and planar imaging in the added value of quantitative analysis may be related to the fact that in SPECT imaging no overlap between normal and abnormal segments is present which makes identification of perfusion defects easier and negates the advantage provided by quantitative analysis. We did not expect, neither did we find that all stenoses identified by coronary angiography to be correctly identified by SPECT thallium imaging for several reasons. First, there is sufficient evidence at the present time to indicate that the haemodynamic significance of coronary stenosis cannot be reliably predicted by the percent diameter stenosis. Measurement of the minimal area stenosis as discussed earlier may be more helpful in some patients. However, coronary angiography, which takes into consideration all dimensions stenosis or measurement of the coronary blood flow reserve are more appropriate methods to access the significance of coronary stenosis. Therefore, it is clear that not all vessels with stenosis are necessarily haemodynamically significant and should result in perfusion defects. Second, there is considerable variability in the site, location and anatomic distribution of the major coronary arteries. Hence, it is possible that in some patients with proximal left anterior descending coronary artery stenosis, the perfusion defects may not only be seen in the anteroseptal area, but also involve the inferior wall. Similarly, perfusion defects in patients with a large right coronary artery which supplies multiple posterolateral branches may produce not only inferior perfusion defects, but also posterolateral perfusion abnormality. Third, in patients with multi-vessel coronary artery disease, the most severe regions might be detected whereas the less severe regions might appear normal since thallium imaging deals with relative uptake. Further, some patients with multi-vessel disease might have stopped exercising when ischaemia was achieved in the worst vascular territory which was at the level below which ischaemia will be produced in the territories supplied by a vessel with a less severe stenosis.

Dipyridamole thallium imaging

Several studies have shown that the coronary blood flow in a normal vessel increases by three to five-fold with dipyridamole. This increase is greater than that achieved during exercise testing. The optimum dose of dipyridamole for producing maximum coronary blood flow is 0.56 mg/kg given over 4 min [6]. In some patients however, higher doses are needed to produce maximum coronary vasodilatation. When thallium-201 is injected at the peak hyperemic effect of dipyridamole, variations in the myocardial thallium concentration will correspond to the differences in the regional coronary blood flow. As discussed earlier, at high flow rates, the increased thallium activity in the myocardium is less than the corresponding increase in coronary blood flow because of the decrease in the extraction fraction. In general, the rate of thallium washout is slower in dipyridamole imaging than exercise imaging.

The dipyridamole thallium images have equal to or better quality compared to exercise images. The cardiac activity increases with dipyridamole resulting in an increase in myocardial to background ratio. This ratio is actually higher with dipyridamole than during exercise imaging. These changes can be explained by the relative greater changes in coronary blood flow in relation to the changes in cardiac output. During exercise, the increase in cardiac output is more than the increase in coronary blood flow. Therefore, the fraction of the injected dose of thallium-201 delivered to the myocardium decreases while after dipyridamole infusion, the increase in coronary blood flow is more than the increase in cardiac output, so that the fraction of the dose of thallium delivered to the myocardium increases, and the myocardial thallium activity in consequence increases. The usual protocol involves intravenous injection of 0.142 mg/kg of dipyridamole for 4 minutes while the patient is in the supine position under constant ECG monitoring and with frequent measurement of the blood pressure. Studies have shown that the peak effect of dipyridamole occurs approximately 2–3 minutes after its infusion. Because of this, thallium-201 is injected intravenously approximately 7 minutes from the start of infusion or 3 minutes from the completion of the infusion.

During the early experience, the patients were often asked to stand up and walk in place for 90 seconds before thallium injection. This maneuver was thought to decrease the pulmonary blood volume and the lung thallium uptake, as well as the splanchnic thallium uptake. However, this maneuver is also more likely to produce hypotension, light-headedness and dizziness. In some laboratories, the patient is tilted up to a semierect position before thallium is injected. In other laboratories, the patients perform a handgrip exercise or even submaximal treadmill exercise before thallium is injected in order to increase the double-product. It's important in dipyridamole imaging that all xanthine containing medications and caffeinated beverages be discontinued for 12–24 hours before the test.

The indications for dipyridamole thallium imaging has been the diagnosis of suspected coronary artery disease in patients who are unable to exercise adequate, and also in risk stratification in patients undergoing elective major vascular surgery or patients recovering from acute myocardial infarction. If side effects appear and are severe, they can be treated with slow intravenous injection of aminophylline. In general, a dose of 100 mg is sufficient in most patients. If side effects are unresponsive to aminophylline, nitroglycerin may be used sublingually.

A few fatalities and few instances of life threatening arrhythmias have been reported with dipyridamole thallium imaging and hence, these patients need to be watched carefully. Patients with acute infarction or unstable angina are at higher risk for such complications. The intravenous form of the drug has been recently approved by the FDA in the United States.

The sensitivity of the test has been in the range of 80–90% and the specificity 80–100%.

Oral dipyridamole thallium imaging

We examined the merits of oral dipyridamole SPECT thallium imaging, detecting coronary artery disease in 65 patients who were not candidates for exercise testing [7]. Coronary arteriography revealed no significant coronary artery disease in 17 patients and severe disease in the remaining 48 patients, 12 with one-vessel disease, and 36 with multi-vessel disease.

Thallium-201 was injected intravenously 45 min after an oral dose of

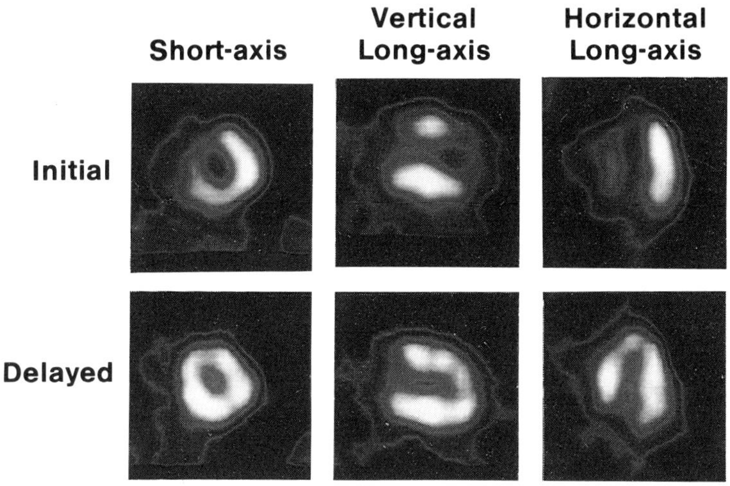

Figure 9.6. Abnormal dipyridamole thallium images showing perfusion defects in the distal anterior wall, apex and the septum. There is complete redistribution on 4 hour delayed images. The coronary angiogram revealed 90% stenosis of the left anterior descending artery after the first septal perforator and diagonal branch.

375 mg of dipyridamole and SPECT imaging was performed within 10 min and 4 hours after injection (Figure 9.6). There were no serious side effects, only 6 patients had ST-segment depression, and 18 patients had chest pains. The heart rate increased slightly from 74 before to 84 at peak effect. The systolic blood pressure did not change significantly. The thallium images were abnormal in 6 of the 17 patients with no coronary artery disease, 7 of 12 patients with one-vessel disease, and 34 of 36 patients with multi-vessel disease (38% vs 58% vs 94%, $p < 0.001$). Twenty-one of 25 patients with perfusion abnormalities in more than one vascular territory had multi-vessel disease by coronary angiography. Thus, oral dipyridamole SPECT thallium imaging is a safe and inexpensive method for detection of coronary artery disease in patients who are otherwise not candidates for exercise testing. Patients with perfusion deficits in more than one vascular territory are likely to have multi-vessel disease by angiography. In our experience, these results are not different from those of patients with submaximal exercise SPECT thallium-201 imaging. All of our patients underwent handgrip exercise before thallium injection. A major problem with oral dipyridamole is that absorption rate is variable, and hence, peak blood levels are unpredictable and cannot be determined by observations in heart rate, blood pressure, electrocardiographic changes or the quality of the thallium images. We have, as well as others, elected to inject the thallium 45 min after the oral dose in the absence of symptoms or electrocardiographic changes.

Other coronary vasodilators

We have recently studied another powerful coronary vasodilator called adenosine which has a very short half-life, (less than 10 seconds). Adenosine is given in a dose of 0.14 mg/kg/min for 6 minutes and thallium-201 is injected intravenously at the third minute and images obtained 5 min after the completion of the injection. Approximately 50 patients have been studied in our laboratories, and the images have proven to be of high quality (Figure 9.7). The sensitivity of adenosine SPECT thallium imaging has been 92%, and the specificity 100%, and the side effects are very few, mild and transient, and the drug is well-tolerated. Most of these perfusion abnormalities are not associated with the corresponding wall motion abnormalities as determined by simultaneous two-dimensional echocardiographic examination, suggesting that the perfusion abnormality is not due to coronary steal but rather due to inability of the diseased coronary vessel to augment the flow as much as the normal vessel.

Newer imaging agents

In 1981 investigations regarding the use of technetium labelled myocardial perfusion labelling agents were started, and since then, a number of these compounds have been tested [8]. The largest experience and the most

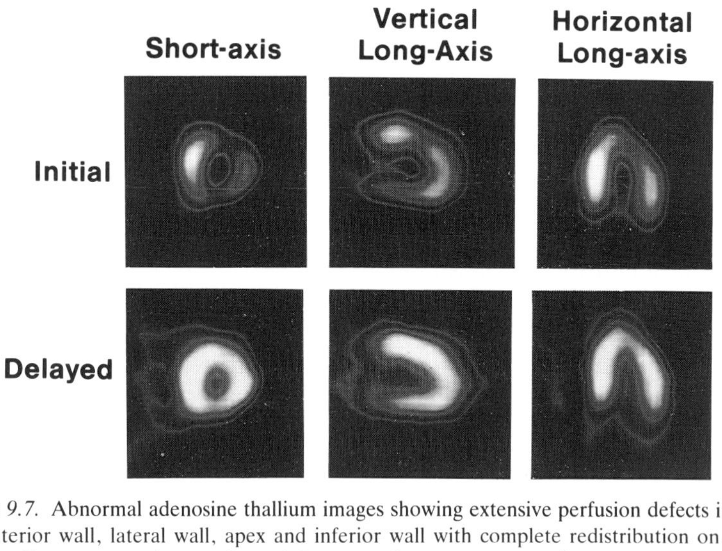

Figure 9.7. Abnormal adenosine thallium images showing extensive perfusion defects involving the anterior wall, lateral wall, apex and inferior wall with complete redistribution on delayed images. Coronary arteriogram showed three-vessel coronary artery disease.

promising agent so far appears to be technetium-99m, hexakis-2-methoxy-2-isobutyl-isonitrile (MIBI, RP-30A, Cardiolite^R, Dupont). The distribution of Cardiolite is according to the regional blood flow. The extraction ratio is lower than that of thallium-201, both at rest and during exercise. After intravenous injection, it is cleared up from the circulation with a half-life time of 1.9 minutes at rest and 1.5 minutes during exercise. Unlike thallium-201, Cardiolite shows no evidence of redistribution, and as a result, images can be obtained 1–2 hours after injection, rather than immediately after injection, as is done with thallium-201.

The lung thallium uptake is generally low, but their is considerable hepatic uptake as the Cardiolite is cleared through the gall bladder into the intestine. In fact, the gall bladder is nicely visualized in all studies at rest and during exercise. Both the dose (20–30 mCi) and the energy level (140 kev) of Cardiolite are considerably higher than those of thallium-201. But the half-life time is shorter (6 hours). Because of the high energy level and the dose, not only image quality is improved, but bolus injection also permits imaging of the transit of the radionuclide in the central circulation, allowing evaluation of right and left ventricular function with first-pass technique.

Recent perfusion studies also have used a gated technique permitting simultaneous evaluation of static perfusion images and wall motion. This dual evaluation may permit assessment of the myocardial viability. Thus, it is possible that segments with perfusion defects which show normal wall motion represent viable myocardium, whereas segments with perfusion defects that show akinesis represents scar. The difference in image qualities is especially apparent in comparing the rest Cardiolite and 4-hour delayed thallium images. Another advantage of Cardiolite, compared to thallium is that it is generator rather than cyclotron produced, being therefore more readily available. Because images are acquired 1–2 hours after injection, this technique may permit assessment of myocardial viability in patients with acute myocardial infarction undergoing emergency thrombolytic therapy or percutaneous angioplasty.

We compared the results of stress and rest SPECT Cardiolite images with stress and redistribution thallium images and results of coronary arteriography in 39 patients, 11 without and 28 with coronary artery disease [9]. Each patient underwent two exercise studies at identical workloads, heart rates and double-products. In a subset of 13 patients, concomitant evaluation of left ventricular function using first-pass radionuclide angiography with a multi-crystal gamma camera was also performed with a bolus injection of the Cardiolite. Cardiolite had similar sensitivity, (82% vs 82%, P:NS) slightly but not significantly higher specificity (100% vs 82%) and similar predictive accuracy (87% vs 82) compared to thallium-201. The tracer uptake was also assessed in 20 segments per study. There was concordance between the Cardiolite and thallium images in 93% of the segments. In

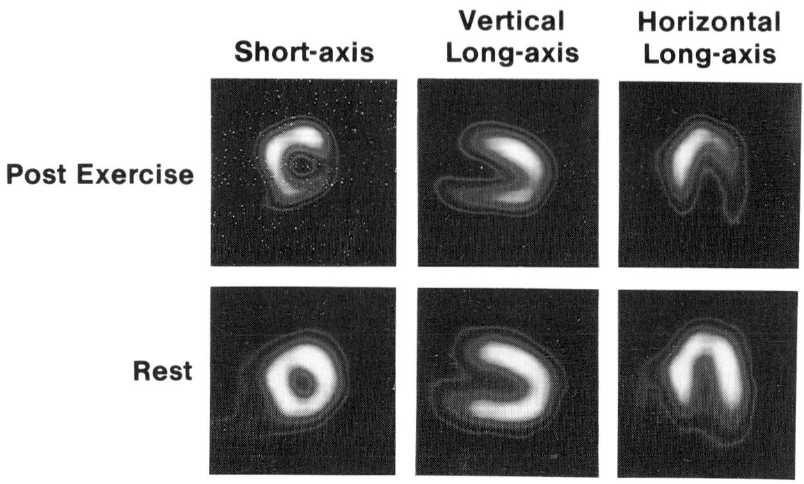

Figure 9.8. Abnormal MIBI images. Post-exercises image show perfusion abnormality involving the lateral wall and inferior wall. These abnormalities are not apparent on rest images performed on a separate date. Note that image quality is excellent and contrast resolution is superb.

general, the Cardiolite images were considered to be of better quality than the thallium images (Figure 9.8). All 10 patients with coronary artery disease who underwent concomitant radionuclide angiography had perfusion abnormalities or abnormal ejection fraction response to exercise.

Radionuclide angiography

In 1927, Blumgart and Weiss measured pulmonary circulation time using radium-C and a small ionization chamber [10]. Twenty years later, Prinzmetal was successful in recording the passage of radiosodium (Na-24) through the cardiac chambers using a Geiger-Mueller counter as a recorder [11]. Since then, there has been major advancement in technology, radiopharmaceuticals, scintillation detectors and computers. In the early 70's, gated and first-pass techniques were introduced and widely accepted as means of evaluating ventricular function and wall motion. The ejection fraction is measured by count changes and hence, is geometrically independent; it is accurate, reproducible and may very well be the 'gold standard' for measuring left ventricular and right ventricular ejection fractions.

Technique

For gated radionuclide angiography, the patient's RBC's are labelled with 20 mCi of Tc-99m. The labelling may be *in vitro*, however the *in vivo* method is most commonly used where a dose of pyrophosphate is injected followed by injection of Tc-99m pertechnetate 20 min later. After equilibration, the computer's acquisition program is synchronized with R-wave of patient's ECG. The R-R cycle is usually divided into 16–48 frames, the first frame representing immediately after R-wave; the study takes 6–10 minutes. Images are filtered and regions of interest drawn and time activity curves created from which various systolic and diastolic parameters are derived.

The first-pass technique uses a different approach. The patient is injected intravenously with a bolus of Tc-99m pertechnetate or other complexes, (sulfur colloid, DTPA, etc.) and time activity is analyzed as it goes through cardiac chambers during the first transit, at a framing rate of 20–40 frames/sec. With proper quality control, these two methods are comparable and produce accurate results. The advantages of gated technique includes ability to analyze wall motion in multiple projections. The first-pass technique however is fast in acquisition (less than 1 minute), thus provides a more accurate determination of events at peak exercise. Shunt calculation and measurement of pulmonary blood volume are also possible with the first-pass technique only. The first-pass technique is the method of choice for right ventricular ejection fraction determination.

Exercise radionuclide angiography

Both gated and first-pass techniques may be used. Using the first-pass technique, the patient is seated in the upright position on a bike. The multicrystal camera, because of its higher count efficiency, is preferred over the single-crystal gamma camera. After a resting study is obtained, the patient is exercised, the workload is increased steadily until the end points of exercise are reached. On the other hand, the gated technique is done usually with the patients in supine position or semi-erect position to avoid any motion artifact and is done with a single-crystal gamma camera. The camera is positioned in LAO projection that best separates left ventricle from right ventricle. The gated technique permits measurements of serial changes in ejection fraction during exercise whereas the first-pass technique provides instantaneous accurate ejection fraction at peak exercise using separate bolus injections.

Normal and abnormal responses to exercise

Studies in normal subjects show a mild increase in end-diastolic volume, (consistent with the utilization of the Starling mechanism) a decrease in end-systolic volume, (consistent with increased inotrophic stimulation) and improvement in ejection fraction (Figure 9.9) [12]. The increase in cardiac output is due to increases in stroke volume and heart rate. The degree of utilization of the Starling mechanism and the improvement in the ejection

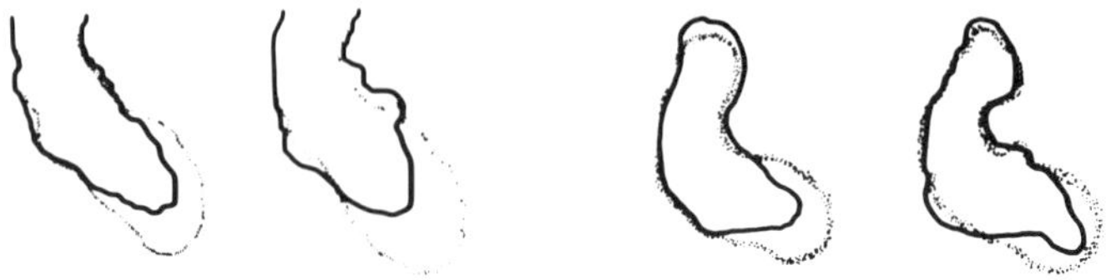

	Normal Response REST	Normal Response EXERCISE	Abnormal Response REST	Abnormal Response EXERCISE
LVEF (%)	64	76	64	58
EDV (ml)	147	185	145	185
ESV (ml)	53	44	52	78
SV (ml)	94	140	93	107
HR (bpm)	86	155	80	136
CO (l/min)	8.1	21.7	7.4	14.6

Figure 9.9. Rest and exercise first-pass radionuclide angiograms; normal response on the left and abnormal response on the right (see rest).

fraction may depend on the level of the exercise, body position during exercise, gender and age; increase in end-diastolic volume is more common at sub-maximal exercise, women, elderly subjects and upright position.

In patients with coronary artery disease, abnormal left ventricular functional response is characterized by regional wall motion abnormalities, an increase in end-systolic volume, a flat response or actual decline in ejection fraction (arbitrarily 5% or greater increase has been defined as a normal response), an abnormal response in the systolic blood pressure/end-systolic volume ratio (so-called the non-invasive index of contractility) (Figure 9.10). This latter index, however is quite different from the E-max.

It is important to remember that conditions other than coronary artery disease could result in abnormalities in left ventricular function during exercise. In a previous study we found that men and women with comparable extent of coronary artery disease demonstrate similar manifestations of myocardial ischaemia and left ventricular dysfunction during exercise [13]; gender did not appear to influence LV function independent of the extent of coronary artery disease. We have also observed that an abnormal ejection fraction response to exercise suggests the presence of reversible ischaemic zones as determined by thallium scintigraphy. We have also examined the changes in ejection fraction and pressure volume relationship in a fairly large number of patients [14]. Normal range for the change in ejection fraction, the absolute ejection fraction during exercise and the relative and absolute pressure volume measurements were established first in 51 subjects with less than 1% probability of coronary artery disease and the results were compared to 53 patients with normal coronary angiograms and 183 patients

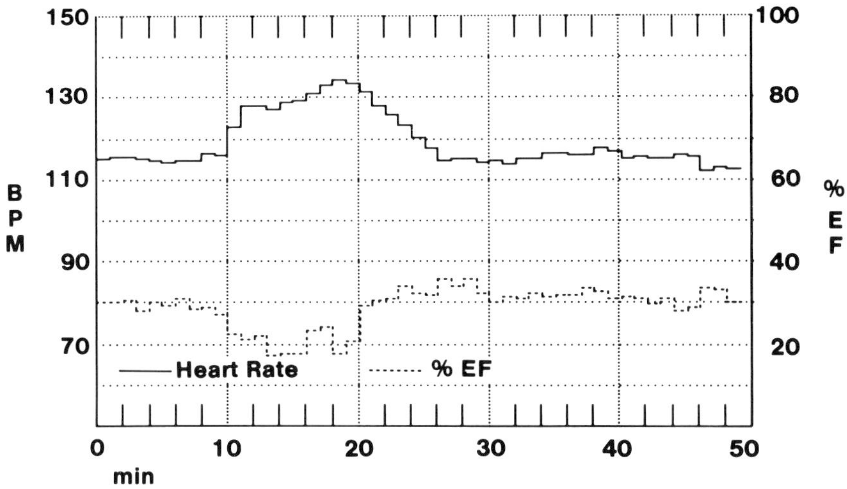

Figure 9.10. A 50 minute recording from the VEST showing EF and heart rate. There is an episode of EF drop of 10% for approximately 10 minutes at which time the heart rate increased from 115 bpm to 134 bpm. The patient had no symptom during this episode and no S-T changes.

with angiographically proven coronary artery disease. We found that abnormality in either the change in ejection fraction or the percent change in the systolic pressure to end-systolic volume ratio were observed in 76% of the patients with one-vessel disease and 91% of the patients with multi-vessel disease. Abnormalities in either the change in ejection fraction or the change in pressure volume ratio were more common than the change in ejection fraction alone in the total coronary artery disease group and in subgroups classified according to the resting ejection fraction, extent of coronary artery disease and adequacy of exercise end-points. Similar results were obtained when absolute exercise ejection fraction or absolute exercise systolic pressure/end-systolic volume ratio were used. In general, patients with more extensive disease have more abnormal response characterized by a greater decrease in ejection fraction with exercise, greater increase in end-diastolic and end-systolic volume and more extensive wall motion abnormality. However, it should be noted that a number of factors beside the extent of coronary artery disease affect the ejection fraction response to exercise [15]; these include age, gender, level of exercise, systolic blood pressure (as a measure of afterloads), end-diastolic volume (as a measure of preload), and medications. In our experience, the exercise ejection fraction correlates better with the extent of coronary artery disease than the ejection fraction response. Furthermore quantitative assessment of the coronary artery disease that takes into consideration severity, site, location and number of stenoses is a better index of the extent of the disease than the simplistic categorization of patients into 1, 2 or 3 vessel disease based on percent diameter stenosis alone.

Silent ischaemia

In our experience, patients with coronary artery disease who experience angina during exercise have a greater increase in end-systolic volume and a greater decrease in ejection fraction and more abnormal response in the systolic blood pressure-to-end-systolic volume ratio than patients with asymptomatic (silent) ischaemia [16, 17]. These results were derived in 108 patients who had angiographically documented coronary artery disease and who had normal resting ejection fraction; 26 patients had angina during exercise (symptomatic ischaemia) and the remaining patients had silent ischaemia. The exercise heart rate, systolic blood pressure and exercise end-diastolic volume were similar in both groups. Of note, however, is that even among the 27 patients with the most severe degree of left ventricular dysfunction during exercise, characterized as a 10% or greater decrease in ejection fraction, only 44% had symptomatic ischaemia.

Since other diseases such as cardiomyopathy, hypertension, diabetes and valvular heart disease may affect the ejection fraction response to exercise, the specificity of the test will depend on the patient population being studied. The newer technetium compounds discussed earlier will permit simultaneous assessment of ventricular function and perfusion and may thus improve the diagnostic accuracy and the information density provided by these procedures.

Diastolic function

In addition to abnormalities in the systolic left ventricular function in coronary artery disease, abnormalities in the diastolic function have also been measured and quantitated by radionuclide angiography [18]. Several indices have been measured such as the peak filling rate (derived from computer manipulation of the time activity curve), the time to peak filling rate, (that is the time from end-systole to peak filling rate), percent filling during one-third of diastole and the percent contribution of atrial systole to ventricular filling. One or more of these parameters is generally abnormal in the vast majority of patients with coronary artery disease, even among those with normal resting ejection fraction. Improvement in these parameters have been observed following revascularization by angioplasty or bypass surgery. Interestingly, in patients with localized coronary artery disease, these abnormalities have been found to be segmental corresponding to the distribution of the diseased vessel. These indices, however, are too sensitive of markers for coronary artery disease and are not specific since they are seen in other forms of heart disease, notably hypertension and diabetes mellitus which are common disorders in association with coronary artery disease. Furthermore, aging also impairs the diastolic function irrespective of associated diseases.

Risk stratification

Both exercise thallium imaging and rest and exercise radionuclide angiography have been found to provide important prognostic data in patients with known or suspected coronary artery disease. For example, patients with normal exercise thallium images have been found to have good prognosis for periods of 5–6 years [19]. Event rate (death or non-fatal myocardial infarction) in these patients is as low as those encountered in patients with normal coronary angiograms. Patients with abnormal thallium images have higher event rates especially in those with evidence of ischaemia (reversible defects), more extensive thallium defects and those with increased lung thallium uptake, suggesting the presence of considerable myocardium at jeopardy during exercise [20]. Similarly, patients with normal exercise ejection fraction or normal ejection fraction response to exercise, have a good prognosis. However, as the exercise ejection fraction decreases or as the change in ejection fraction with exercise becomes greater, the prognosis becomes worse [21]. These techniques may prove useful in patients with occult coronary artery disease; we have found them useful in diabetic patients [22]. Furthermore, since coronary artery disease is a progressive disease, serial studies are necessary to determine the progression of underlying disease in subsets of patients at risk.

Ambulatory nuclear monitor

In recent years we have been working with an ambulatory nuclear detector to measure left ventricular ejection fraction on a beat to beat basis [23]. This device was introduced in 1979 and over the past decade the hardware and the soft-ware have been modified. In principal, it is an improvement over the nuclear probe (or stethoscope) which was introduced in 1968. The ambulatory nuclear detector is composed of a nuclear vest and two detectors; one is a sodium iodide crystal with a parallel-hole collimator approximately 2.5 inches in diameter and is designed to monitor the left ventricular activity and the other is constructed from cadmium telluride and monitors the background activity over the right lung. The left ventricular detector is screwed over a plastic garment which is tightly but comfortably strapped over the chest. In addition to the two detectors there are two leads that constantly monitor the electrical activity of the heart, and both the detectors and the ECG leads are connected by wire to a tape-recorder that may be carried over the shoulder. The entire assembly of detectors and recorder weighs approximately 7.5 lbs. There is an event marker to allow the patient to signal special events during the recording period. The events are recorded on a cassette tape and analyzed by a dedicated IBM computer.

Technetium-99m pertechnetate is used for labelling the red blood cells. The detector is then positioned over the left ventricular region and the recorder system is activated and data are obtained continuously for many hours. The recording period is approximately 2–6 hours. The recorded data are screened for quality and then averaged over 15, 30 or 60 seconds and graphs are subsequently generated of the specific measurements vs time. Measurements include left ventricular ejection fraction, heart rate, relative changes in end-diastolic volume, end-systolic volume, stroke volume, cardiac output and the peak filling rate as well as systolic ejection rate. This device has been used in the detection and characterization of episodes of ischaemia both silent and symptomatic as well as in our laboratory in the evaluation of ventricular function in patients with congestive heart failure before and after treatment. The recordings may be obtained at rest and during physiological activities such as eating, walking, sitting, standing or during pharmacological testing or exercise testing both on the bicycle and treadmill. This technique, however, is probably of limited value in screening for coronary artery disease in patients who are asymptomatic because of the infrequent occurrences of both symptomatic and asymptomatic ischaemia in such patients.

References

1. Iskandrian AS. Thallium-201 myocardial imaging and radionuclide ventriculography: theory, technical considerations and interpretation. In: AS Iskandrian (ed), Nuclear Cardiac Imaging: Principles and Applications, F.A. Davis Co., Philadelphia, 1986.
2. Iskandrian AS, Hakki AH. Thallium-201 myocardial scintigraphy. Am Heart J 1985; 109:113.
3. Hadjimiltiades S, Watson R, Hakki AH, Heo J, Iskandrian AS. Relation between myocardial thallium-201 kinetics during exercise and quantitative coronary angiography in patients with one-vessel coronary artery disease. J Am Coll Cardiol 1989; 13:1301.
4. Iskandrian AS, Heo J, Askenase A, Segal BL, Helfant RH. Thallium imaging with single photon emission computed tomography. Am Heart J 1987; 114:852.
5. Iskandrian AS, Heo J, Kong B, Lyons E. The effect of exercise level on the ability of thallium-201 tomographic imaging in detecting coronary artery disease: analysis of 461 patients. J Am Coll Cardiol 1989; 14:1477.

6. Iskandrian AS, Heo J, Askenase A, Segal BL, Auerbach N. Dipyridamole cardiac imaging. Am Heart J 1988; 115:432.
7. Beer SG, Heo J, Kong B, Lyons E, Iskandrian AS. Use of oral dipyridamole SPECT thallium-201 imaging in detection of coronary artery disease. Am Heart J 1989; 118:1022.
8. Heo J, Hermann GA, Iskandrian AS, Askenase A, Segal BL. New myocardial perfusion imaging agents: description and applications. Am Heart J 1988; 115:1111.
9. Iskandrian AS, Heo K, Kong B, Lyons E, Marsch S. Use of technetium-99m isonitrile (RP-30A) in assessing left ventricular perfusion and function at rest and during exercise in coronary artery disease and comparison with coronary arteriography and exercise thallium-201 SPECT imaging. Am J Cardiol 1989; 64:270.
10. Blumgart HL, Weiss S. Studies on the velocity of blood flow: VIII the pulmonary circulation time in normal resting individuals. J Clin Invest 1927; 4:399.
11. Prinzmetal M, Corday E, Bergman HC, Schwartz L, Spritzler RJ. Radiocardiography: a new method for studying the blood flow through the chambers of the heart in human beings. Science 1948; 108:340.
12. Iskandrian AS, Hakki AH, Depace NL, Manno B, Segal BL. Evaluation of left ventricular function during exercise in normal subjects and in patients with chronic coronary heart disease. J Am Coll Cardiol 1983; 1:1518.
13. Hakki A-H, Iskandrian AS. Effect of gender on left ventricular function during exercise in patients with coronary artery disease. Am Heart J 1986; 111:543.
14. Iskandrian AS, Heo J. Left ventricular pressure/volume relationship in coronary artery disease. Am Heart J 1986; 112:375.
15. Iskandrian AS, Heo J, Askenase A, Helfant RH, Segal BL. Factors affecting exercise left ventricular performance in patients free of obstructive coronary artery disease. Am J Cardiol 1987; 60:1173.
16. Iskandrian AS, Heo J, Hakki AH. The degree of left ventricular dysfunction in silent myocardial ischaemia. Am J Noninvas Cardiol 1988; 2:255.
17. Iskandrian AS, Hakki A-H, Newman D. The relation between myocardial ischaemia and the ejection fraction response to exercise in patients with normal or abnormal resting left ventricular function. Am Heart J 1985; 109:1253.
18. Heo J, Iskandrian AS, Hakki A-H. Relation between left ventricular diastolic function and exercise tolerance in patients with left ventricular dysfunction. Cathet Cardiovasc Diag 1986; 12:311.
19. Heo J, Thompson WO, Iskandrian AS. Prognostic implications of normal exercise thallium images. Am J Noninvas Cardiol 1987; 1:209.
20. Iskandrian AS, Hakki A-H, Kane-Marsch S. Prognostic implications of exercise thallium-201 scintigraphy in patients with suspected or known coronary artery disease. Am Heart J 1985; 110:135.
21. Iskandrian AS, Hakki A-H, Goel IP, Mundth ED, Kane-Marsch SA, Schenk CL. The use of rest and exercise radionuclide ventriculography in risk stratification in patients with suspected coronary artery disease. Am Heart J 1985; 110:864.
22. Felsher J, Meissner D, Hakki A-H, Heo J, Kane S, Iskandrian AS. Exercise thallium imaging in patients with diabetes mellitus prognostic implications. Arch Int Med 1987; 147:313.
23. Iskandrian AS, Heo J. The ambulatory nuclear monitor for assessment of left ventricular function. Journal of Myocardial Ischaemia 1989; 1:82.

10. Echocardiography in the diagnosis and assessment of occult coronary artery disease

PETROS NIHOYANNOPOULOS

Atherosclerotic coronary artery disease remains one of the leading causes of death in western civilization. The severity of coronary atherosclerosis however found in patients who die suddenly shows a remarkable variability suggesting that other factors superimposed on a variable degree of atherosclerosis may substantially contribute to sudden death [1]. Acute myocardial ischaemia is by itself responsible for the fatal event, whereas the anatomic lesions of the coronary arteries may only favour or predispose the development of such ischaemia [2].

Angina is only one of the possible manifestations of acute myocardial ischaemia, which can be totally asymptomatic or appear as sudden and unexplained acute left ventricular failure or as arrhythmias. Yet it is the symptom that constitutes the 'alarm' signal of myocardial ischaemia obliging the patient to undertake action and stop the pain and therefore the myocardial ischaemia.

In order to determine the anatomical distribution of obstructive coronary arterial lesion, coronary angiography is required. However, the latter is insufficient as it provides no information regarding the amount of blood supplied and therefore oxygen upon the myocardium. To ascertain the physiologic significance of coronary arterial narrowing, namely the presence and distribution of ischaemia, the use of a stress test is necessary. The current traditional modes of stress testing utilise graded treadmill or bicycle protocols with measurement of heart rate, blood pressure and electrocardiographic parameters, aiming to reproduce the patients clinical symptoms, namely the anginal pain. However, observations during exercise stress testing occasionally show the development of typical ischaemic electrocardiographic changes in the absence of anginal pain or long before its appearance (see chapters 6 & 8). Therefore these superficial measurements only constitute the 'tip of the iceberg' of myocardial ischaemia.

Echocardiography is perhaps the most readily available technique to

A.-M. Salmasi and A. N. Nicolaides (eds.), Occult Atherosclerotic Disease, 139–151.

provide the clinician with a complete assessment of left ventricular systolic performance by directly imaging the myocardial contractility. Furthermore, a rapidly developing area of cardiac ultrasound that is of great interest, is the use of ultrasound contrast techniques to determine myocardial perfusion and coronary risk areas.

Exercise echocardiography

Exercise stress testing is widely used in the diagnosis and assessment of patients with known or suspected coronary artery disease. The haemodynamic response to a maximal symptom-limited treadmill exercise stress test in a normal subject includes a one-and-a-half-fold increase in stroke volume and a three-fold increase in heart rate. The systolic arterial pressure increases on average by 60–80 mmHg and the diastolic arterial pressure decreases by about 10–20 mmHg [3].

Stress or exercise two-dimensional echocardiography has been demonstrated to be effective in eliciting new regional wall motion abnormalities by multiple investigators. These wall motion abnormalities correlate well with corresponding coronary artery atherosclerotic lesions. A wide variety of stress tests have been utilised. Handgrip, cold pressor test, supine bicycle exercise, upright bicycle exercise, treadmill exercise as well as pharmacologic interventions and pacing have all been used. Handgrip exercise did not produce ischaemic changes with sufficient frequency to be practical. Cold pressor tests are extremely painful and are not tolerated well by the patient. In addition, it too does not produce ischaemia with sufficient frequency. Supine bicycle exercise offers a problem with leg fatigue which limits the ability of the patient to generate a sufficient heart rate to produce ischaemia. Upright bicycle exercise is an excellent technique for performing echocardiograms during exercise. This examination is perhaps best done if the patient's upper body is supported in some fashion so that is remains immobile during cycling.

An increasingly popular technique is obtaining a two-dimensional echocardiogram immediately post-treadmill exercise. There was however an initial concern that the wall motion abnormalities would revert back to normal too rapidly to permit clinically useful information. However, subsequent experience demonstrated that such concerns were unfounded; several investigators including ourselves, have now demonstrated that this is not the case. Wall motion abnormalities persist for several minutes so that there is plenty of time for the patient to lie on a couch still connected with the epicardial 12 lead electrocardiogram and obtain optimal two-dimensional echocardiographic images.

Technique and image characteristics

Although M-mode echocardiography has been used in previous studies to define left ventricular contraction both at rest and during exercise, the technique has major limitations of spatial resolution in its ability to record echocardiographic images from the same region of the ventricle over a

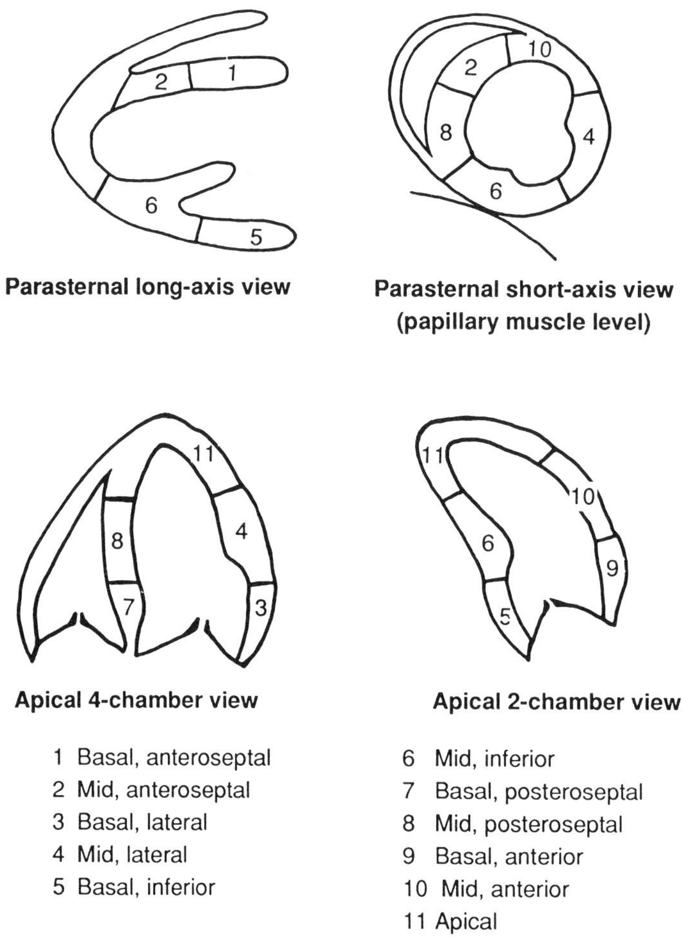

Figure 10.1. Left ventricular segmentation and the respective nomenclature used in our laboratory. The left ventricle is divided in 11 segments using both the apical long axis and parasternal short axis projections at mitral valve level (basal), mid-papillary muscles and apex.

period of time necessary for such a study. In addition, it is only possible to examine a small area of the left ventricle at any one time. Furthermore, the majority of the septum and antero-lateral wall cannot be accurately assessed as the endocardial surface of these regions of the ventricle will necessarily pan obliquely through the M-mode beam path. The resulting recordings may be uninterpretable or may erroneously suggest exaggerated endocardial excursion. Using two-dimensional echocardiography the left ventricle should be divided into segments for the careful analysis of regional dysfunction. Several investigators have divided the left ventricle differently. We chose to divide the left ventricle into 11 segments (Figure 10.1) so that each segment is sufficiently large to adequately describe its contraction. The division of left ventricle into 11 segments is based on the coronary artery distribution. Briefly, the right coronary artery distribution is defined as the inferior wall of the left ventricle and the posterior septum at all three levels (segments 6, 7, and 8) the left anterior descending coronary artery distribution as the anterior septum and anterior free wall (segments 1, 2, 9, 10, and 11). The lateral wall (segments 3, 4, and 5) is considered as the territory of the left circumflex artery distribution.

The ability of two-dimensional echocardiography to visualise the entire left ventricular wall in any given phase and to reliably reproduce images of the same tomographic section of the ventricle over any period of time, is due to the methods obligatory use of internal reference points. It is not uncommon for a patient with occult atherosclerotic coronary artery disease to present to his physician the sole symptom of shortness of breath. This patient may be treated for lung disease or congestive heart failure and even be given a blind diagnosis of cardiomyopathy. A simple two-dimensional echocardiographic examination can however instantly reveal the presence of an abnormal left ventricular function at rest, which could by itself raise the suspicion of caronary artery disease. In our experience such patients often have extensive coronary artery disease going-on for many years undiagnosed, simply because the patient does not complain of the 'alarming' symptom of chest pain.

Several studies have proved the usefulness of two-dimensional echocardiography as a non-invasive tool of diagnosing transient myocardial ischaemia in patients suspected to have atherosclerotic coronary artery disease. The success rate of obtaining technically adequate images ranges from 71% to 100%. With recent technological advances in imaging acquisition and computerised regional left ventricular wall motion analysis an even higher success rate has been obtained.

Although echocardiography could be considered routine when performed at rest, it becomes an expert procedure when performed during or after exercise. The problems posed by technical difficulties as a result of body habitus and signal attenuation are inevitable and despite the recent marketing of computerised wall motion analysis for exercise echocardiography, it cannot overcome the problems involved in data acquisition.

Transducer locations

All of the commonly used transducer locations have been utilised during a stress test to assess left ventricular function. The type and position of exercise usually dictate the transducer window to be used. While parasternal short axis views have been used successfully during treadmill or bicycle exercise they can be difficult to obtain because of exaggerated chest wall movements. The parasternal short axis views are usually recorded at three planes. These include the parasternal short axis at the apex, mid-papillary muscle and mitral valve levels. The apical two and four chamber views have become the most frequently used views during either bicycle or treadmill exercise. There, the transducer is directly located over the cardiac apex and providing tomographic sections of the left ventricle along its long axis, either horizontally (four-chamber) or perpendicularly (two-chamber). Thus these images provide a biplane evaluation of left ventricular function and data from both images can be acquired in a short period of time.

Subcostal views offer alternatives to the parasternal short axis and apical four chamber views when either of these are not obtainable. These can also be used when the exercise stress-test is performed in supine or semi-recumbent positions.

Assessment of left ventricular function

Several experimental studies have assessed regional wall motion changes in response to ischaemia using two-dimensional echocardiography [4–7]. They demonstrated a linear reduction in regional wall thickness. The extent and velocity of shortening during graded ischaemia roughly paralleling an increase in local lactate production indices of global left ventricular function were affected only with more severe ischaemia and electrocardiographic changes are even absent with milder degrees of ischaemia. These studies substantiate the sensitivity of regional wall motion changes as markers of ischaemia.

Regional myocardial function is assessed by motion of the endocardial and epicardial surfaces between sequentially recorded images. As the ventricle contracts the endocardial surface move inward towards the centre of the left ventricle (endocardial excursion). The cavity area decreases (area shrinkage), the cavity perimeter becomes smaller and the distance between the endocardial and epicardial surfaces increases (wall thickening). Following myocardial ischaemia a decrease in the amplitude of endocardial excursion and subjacent wall thickening becomes apparent within seconds in the area supplied by the diseased vessel. In the previously normal ventricle

Hammersmith Hospital
Echocardiography Laboratory
Exercise echocardiography - stress test wall motion analysis

Patients name **Hospital No**

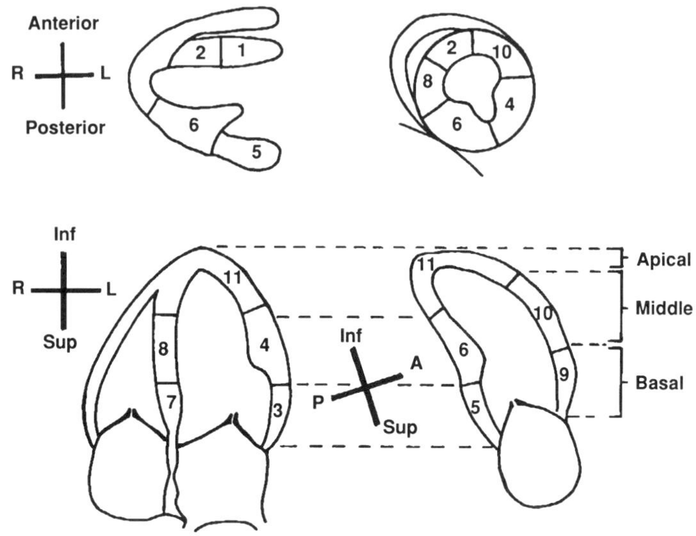

Wall motion abnormalities detection				
Segment	**Rest**		**Post-stress**	
	Basal	Middle	Basal	Middle
Anterior IVS	1.	2.	1.	2.
Lateral	3.	4.	3.	4.
Inferior	5.	6.	5.	6.
Post. IVS	7.	8.	7.	8.
Ant. Free Wall	9.	10.	9.	10.
Apex	11.		11.	
Score: Normokinetic = 1 Hypokinetic = 2 Akinetic = 3 Dyskinetic = 4				

Total wall motion score = [ ] Index (per No. of segments) = [ ]

Figure 10.2. The left ventricle is now divided into 11 segments. Note that the cardiac apex is not divided, allowing for an easier assessment of the apical contraction during or immediately after the stress test.

these changes are sufficiently distinct that they can be easily visualised in comparison with the adjacent normally contracting muscle. Once established, the severity of the contraction abnormality can be defined semiquantitatively as hypokinetic (normal direction but reduced magnitude), akinetic (absent) or dyskinetic (systolic expansion). The extent of abnormal wall motion within a single tomographic section can also be determined visually by defining the junctional points between the normally moving myocardium and the abnormal segment.

Assessment of wall motion

If two-dimensional echocardiography is to be clinically useful in patients with suspected coronary artery disease, the echocardiographer must pay particular attention to complete recording of the endocardium in all myocardial segments. Investigators have employed a variety of methods to divide and assess the left ventricular contraction [8–10]. We chose to divide the left ventricle into 11 segments (Figure 10.2). Here we prefer not to divide the cardiac apex, in order to have a larger myocardial segment and therefore a better assessment of apical contractility, following the exercise test. The obtain complete two-dimensional echocardiographic views of all 11 segments, multiple views must be obtained from the left parasternal, apical, and subcostal transducer positions. Visual definition of the extent of abnormal wall motion from a real-time display is the simplest approach. The tomographic section, i.e. a short axis view of the left ventricle, can be divided into several segments (Figure 10.2) and the function can be determined semiquantitatively (normal, hypokinetic, akinetic, and dyskinetic) at rest and after exercise. Despite the attractive simplicity of this approach, it is strongly dependent upon the skill and experience of the operator and therefore may lack objectivity. For this reason a variety of quantitative approaches for measuring regional wall motion abnormalities have been developed.

The first step in any quantitative analysis of wall motion or thickening is to define the endocardial and epicardial interfaces from which all quantitative parameters are derived. Then the interfaces will be traced using an electronically directed cursor [11, 12] or using an automated border tracking algorithm [13], (Figure 10.3). Once the endocardial and epicardial interfaces have been stored in a digital format, function can be assessed from their motion and separation. The two primary quantitative descriptions of regional function are wall motion (endocardial excursion) and wall thickening (interface separation).

For identification of the presence or absence of a contraction abnormality either motion or thickening, analysis is adequate. When quantitation of

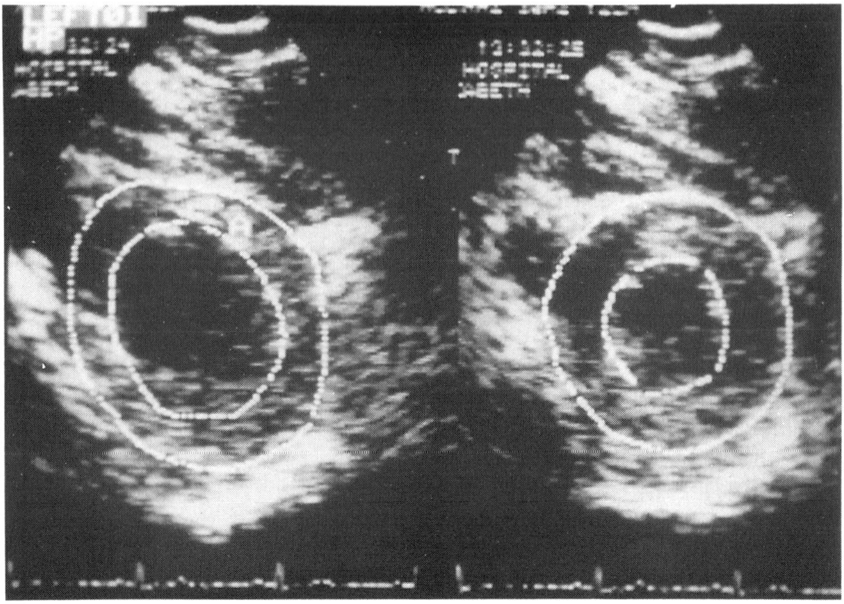

Figure 10.3. Parasternal short axis view during diastole (left) and systole (right) showing the mode of endocardial and epicardial tracing.

ischaemic regions or infarct size is required and two-dimensional echocardiogram is of insufficiently high quality and causes less over-estimating of ischaemic region size. Short axis tomographic sections are ideally suited to more detailed manual or computer analysis. Because short axis motion is directed radially toward or away from the centre of the ventricle, analysis is generally based on some form of radial coordinate system.

The next choice to be made is between types of measurement. These are radial endocardial excursion, radial wall thickening or change in cavity area (Figure 10.4). Parisi *et al.* [14] showed a clear advantage of area methods in the parasternal short axis view more reproducible, less variability, greater accuracy. There are not many data on the number of measurements to make (number of left ventricular subdivisions). Fewer subdivisions should be more prone to miss small regional wall motion abnormalities. Area octants are no more sensitive than area quadrants in one study [14], and in another, further subdivision down to five intervals (72 segments) with areas or radii was no better than octants [12]. It is our practice to divide the entire left ventricle into 11 segments (Figure 10.2). One segment for the cardiac apex and two segments (middle and upper third) for the anterior, lateral, inferior, anteroseptal and inferoseptal walls for any, qualitative or quantitative wall motion

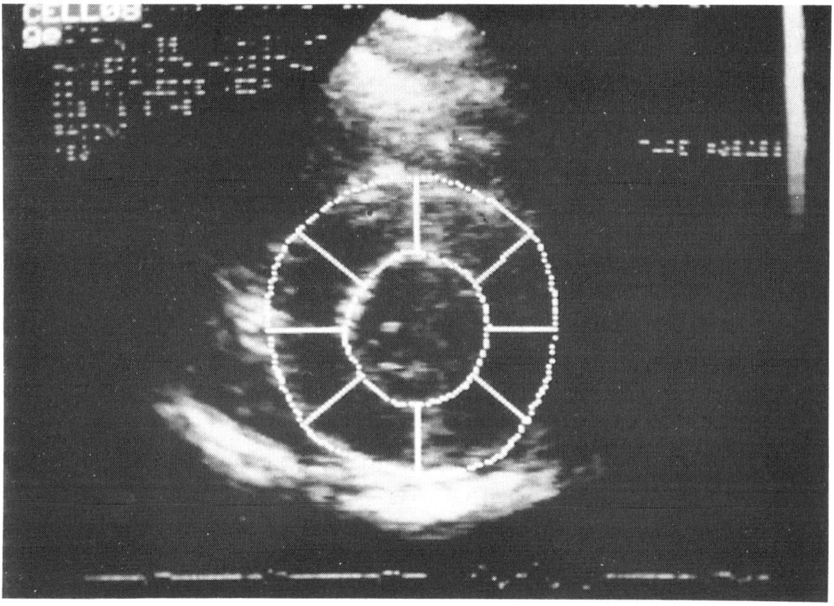

Figure 10.4. Radial wall thickening type of measurement from a patient with suspected coronary artery disease.

analysis. Wall motion is then radially sampled at 45 degrees intervals around the circumference of the left ventricle (using preferably short axis projections) and a three dimensional plot is constructed, describing the amplitude and timing of excursion at each point from end-diastole and end-systole (Figure 10.5).

Clinical studies comparing echocardiography to angiography at rest have demonstrated the ability of echocardiography to accurately identify abnormally contracting segments seen during angiography. Comparison of two-dimensional echocardiography to thallium-201 scintigraphy during exercise in patients with coronary artery disease indicates that there is a high degree of correlation between areas of wall motion abnormality demonstrated by echocardiography with areas of hypoperfusion seen on thallium-201 scintigraphy [15]. These data support the concept of wall motion abnormality as a manifestation of ischaemia induced contractile dysfunction and provide a reliable marker for detecting atherosclerotic coronary artery disease even in asymptomatic patients, using echocardiography. When a wall motion abnormality already exists, it is more difficult to accurately assess ischaemia. If however a new wall motion abnormality arises in an area remote to the pre-existing abnormal segment, it is likely to represent ischaemia in that

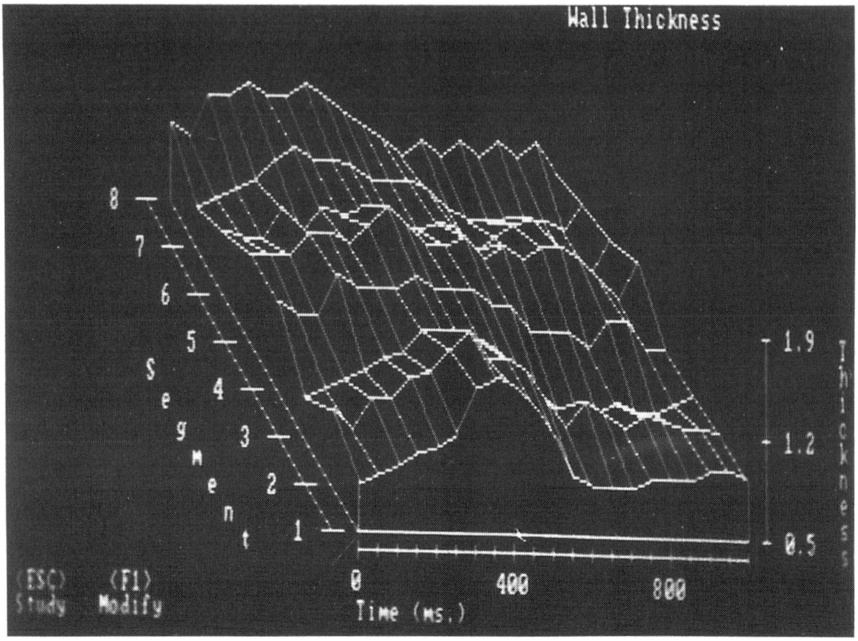

Figure 10.5. Three dimensional display of the myocardial thickening from individual points at 45-degree intervals (octants) around the circumference of the ventricle obtained from digitised data. This plot depicts the change of myocardial thickness from end-diastole (left) to end systole (right) at points along each of the eight segments.

region. The variability of detecting regional wall motion abnormalities reflects the influence of the extent of coronary artery disease but also the degree of ischaemia elicited by the exercise protocol. It therefore becomes apparent that the detection of new or worsening wall motion abnormalities detected with exercise echocardiography is highly specific for identifying the presence of atherosclerotic coronary artery disease. However, the absence of this finding however does not necessarily exclude the presence of coronary artery disease but does make its presence unlikely.

Echocardiographic assessment of myocardial perfusion

Recent advances in the field of acoustic contrast have expanded the role of two-dimensional echocardiography to include the direct assessment of myocardial perfusion. Inherent image contrast in an echocardiogram is related to regional variations in ultrasound backscatter. The backscatter from well perfused regions of myocardium can be substantially increased by injecting a variety of substances into the vascular system. These substances will increase the amplitude of echoes returning from blood, a technique termed contrast echocardiography [16].

Since De Maria's original report that the intracoronary injection of either CO2 or microbubbles resulted in contrast enhancement of the canine myocardium [17], a variety of contrast agents have been employed to provide reproducible definition of coronary arterial perfusion beds. Thus, myocardial contrast echocardiography has rapidly become established as an invaluable tool in the experimental study of myocardial ischaemia. Newer agents allow injection of high concentration of small stable microbubbles thus enhancing the myocardial definition. This myocardial contrast effect is presumed due to the presence of microbubbles flowing to all regions of myocardium and increasing the reflectance of the myocardium by their presence in the arteriolar or capillary bed. To obtain this myocardial contrast effect the contrast material had to be injected directly into the coronary arteries or coronary sinuses of the aortic root so that the highest concentration into the myocardium can be obtained. When injected peripherally, these microbubbles dissipate into the pulmonary capillary bed [18]. Several attempts have been made to produce agents with sufficiently small size microbubbles to pass through the pulmonary capillary bed. The amount of contrast however, appeared insufficient for myocardial blood flow analysis.

Relation to myocardial flow

Both static and dynamic analyses have been used to assess myocardial perfusion. Kaul and associates [19] demonstrated that myocardial contrast echocardiography can accurately determine the 'area at risk' for the entire left ventricle as well as for a single tomographic section. Dynamic analysis of the kinetics of myocardial contrast agents as they traverse the myocardium are being actively investigated as a method of myocardial perfusion is that the ultrasound contrast agent behaves as a blood flow indicator, that is that the ultrasound targets are uniformly distributed through the blood pool and their downstream concentration is directly related to the distribution and quantity of blood flow. Consequently the analysis of perfusion studies will involve a number of acquired tomographic images of the left ventricle before, during and after injection of the ultrasound contrast agent into the coronary arteries. Then selected image frames from this sequence will be digitised and a time-intensity curve generated from the myocardial region of interest. Parameters that can be measured after generations of such a curve include peak intensity, intensity change from baseline, time to peak intensity, slope of initial appearance and parameters of disappearance from the myocardium, such as half-time of washout of total area under the curve of ultrasound contrast intensity versus time [20]. Further studies [21] using sonicated dextrose have identified parameters other than the contrast half-time that distinguish state of hyper perfusion, hypo-perfusion and normal perfusion. These include the closely related exponential decay rate and the time to 20% washout. Although attempts have been made to separate degrees of ischaemia of 25%, 50%, 75% and 90% reduction in flow using contrast kinetics, these have been only partially successful. Presumably the pattern of contrast disappearance is dependent not only on myocardial perfusion but on the ability of the microbubbles contained within the contrast agent to traverse the capillary bed.

Summary

In summary, the ability of contrast echocardiography to define myocardial areas at risk is now well established. By application of indicator dilution techniques or quantitative assessment of coronary blood flow has been successfully performed using a variety of easily prepared agents by direct intracoronary and/or intra-aortic injections. The use of this technique to quantitate perfusion however is still in the developmental stage and its application is initially dependent on microbubble size and therefore best performed with agents containing uniformly small micro-bubbles.

References

1. Goldstein S. Sudden death and coronary heart disease. Futura Publishing Co. Mount Kisco, New York, 1974.
2. Maseri A. Pathogenetic mechanisms of angina pectoris: Expanding views. Br Heart J 1980; 43:648.
3. Bardsley WT, Mankin HT. Exercise testing. In: RO Brandenburg, V Fuster, ER Giuliani, DC McGoon (eds), Cardiology: Fundamentals and practice. Chicago, 1987; 369.
4. Goldstein S, de Jong JW. Changes in left ventricular wall dimensions during regional myocardial ischaemia. Am J Cardiol 1974; 34:56.
5. Theroux P, Franklin D, Ross J Jr *et al.* Regional myocardial function during acute coronary artery occlusion and its modification by pharmacologic agents in the dog. Circ Res 1974; 35:896.
6. Kerber RE, Marcus ML, Ehrhardt J *et al.* Correlation between echocardiographically demonstrated segmental dyskinesis and regional myocardial perfusion. Circulation 1975; 52:1097.
7. Battler A, Froelicher VF, Gallagher KP *et al.* Dissociation between regional myocardial dysfunction and ECG changes during ischaemia in the conscious dog. Circulation 1980; 62:735.
8. Visser CA, Lie KI, Kan G, Meltzer R, Durrer D. Detection and quantification of acute, isolated myocardial infarction by two-dimensional echocardiography. Am J Cardiol 1981; 47:1020.
9. Heger JJ, Weyman AE, Wann LS, Dillon JC, Feigenbaum H. Cross-sectional echocar-

diography in acute myocardial infarction: detection and localisation of regional left ventricular asynergy. Circulation 1979; 60:531.
10. Morganroth J, Chen CC, David D, Sawin HS, Naito M, Parrotto C, Meixell L. Exercise cross-sectional echocardiographic diagnosis of coronary artery disease. Am J Cardiol 1981; 47:20.
11. Gillam LD, Hogan RD, Foale RA *et al.* A comparison of quantitative echocardiographic methods for delineating infarct-induced abnormal wall motion. Circulation 1984; 70:112.
12. Schnittger I, Fitzgerarld PJ, Gordon EP *et al.* Computerised quantitative analysis of left ventricular wall motion by two-dimensional echocardiography. Circulation 1984; 70:242.
13. Oliver L, Geiser E, Zhang L *et al.* Evaluation of an automated border detection algorithm in two-dimensional echocardiographic images of varying quality: observer vs computer variability. J Am Coll Cariol 1984; 3:564.
14. Parisi AF, Moynihan PF, Folland ED *et al.* Quantitative detection of regional left ventricular contraction abnormalities by two-dimensional echocardiography. II. Accuracy in coronary artery disease. Circulation 1981; 63:761.
15. Maurer G, Nanda NC. Two-dimensional echocardiographic evaluation of exercise-induced left and right ventricular asynergy. Correlation with Thallium scanning. Am J Cardiol 1981; 48:720.
16. Feinstein SB, Lang RM, Dick C *et al.* Contrast echocardiographic perfusion studies in humans. Am J Cardiac Imaging 1986; 1:29.
17. De Maria AN, Bommer WJ, Riggs K *et al.* Echocardiographic visualisation of myocardial perfusion by left heart and intracoronary injections of echo-contrast agents. Circulation 1980; 62:III, (suppl 3):143.
18. Feinstein SB, Shah PM, Bing RJ *et al.* Microbubble dynamics visualised in the intact capillary circulation. J Am Coll Cardiol 1984; 3:595.
19. Kaul S, Pandian NG, Okada RD *et al.* Contrast echocardiography in acute myocardial ischaemia: I. *In vivo* determination of total left ventricular 'are at risk'. J Am Coll Cardiol 1984; 4:1272.
20. Armstrong WF. Assessment of myocardial perfusion with contrast enhanced echocardiography. Echocardiography 1986; 3:355.
21. Ten Cate FG, Drury JK, Meerbaum S *et al.* Myocardial contrast two-dimensional echocardiography: Experimental examination at different coronary flow levels. J Am Coll Cardiol 1984; 3:1219.

11. Doppler ultrasound in the diagnosis and assessment of occult coronary artery disease

PETROS NIHOYANNOPOULOS and PETER MAZEIKA

In clinical practice the ejection fraction is frequently used to assess left ventricular systolic function and the left ventricular end-diastolic pressure at cardiac catheterisation to assess diastolic function. Echocardiography and nuclear scintigraphic techniques are two of the non-invasive approaches used to determine ventricular function [1]. The use of aortic and mitral flow profiles obtained with Doppler ultrasonography to evaluate global left ventricular systolic and diastolic function in patients with coronary artery disease has been intensively studied. Doppler ultrasound-determined peak aortic velocity and maximum aortic systolic acceleration at rest have been shown to be sensitive indices in the detection of ischaemic left ventricular dysfunction and correlate well with ejection fraction [2]. Comparison of Doppler echocardiographic assessment of left ventricular diastolic filling with cineangiography and radionuclide ventriculography has shown a good agreement in filling indices between these methods [3, 4]. This and much other work supports the value of Doppler analysis of aortic and mitral flow in the evaluation of left ventricular function.

Assessment of ischaemic heart disease

Assessment of left ventricular performance

Myocardial ischaemia causes regional and global, systolic and diastolic left ventricular dysfunction which can be detected on two-dimensional echocardiography by the development of regional wall motion and systolic wall thickening abnormalities. Can Doppler ultrasound detect myocardial ischaemia? One study evaluated left ventricular systolic function using Doppler echocardiography during transient myocardial ischaemia induced by coronary angioplasty and was able to detect ischaemia-induced diastolic

A.-M. Salmasi and A. N. Nicolaides (eds.), Occult Atherosclerotic Disease, 153–163.

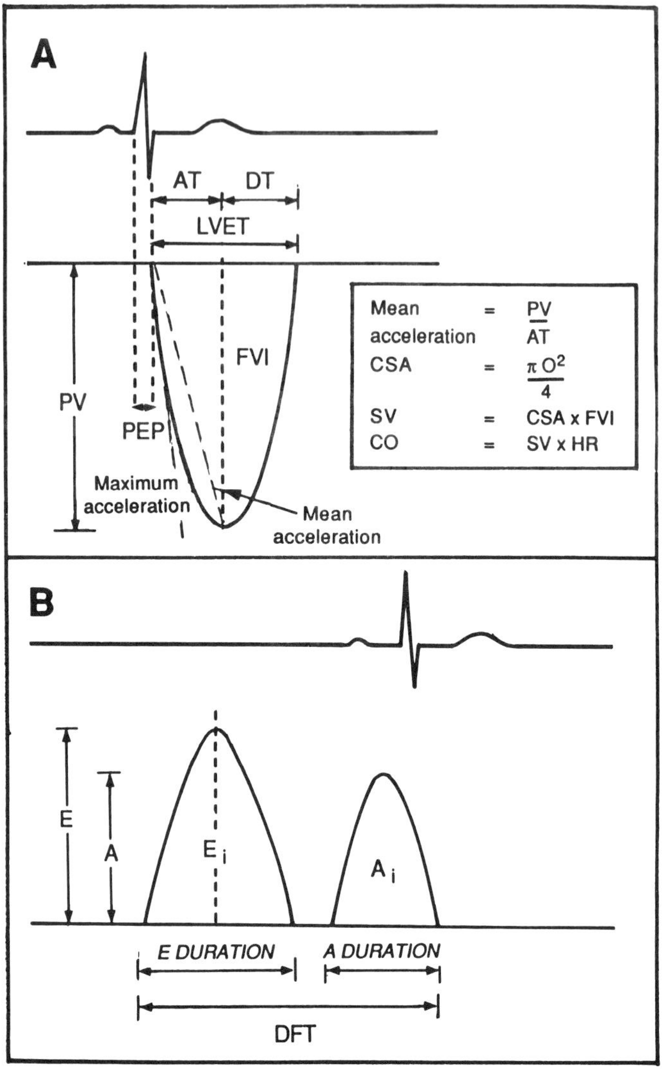

Figure 11.1. Aortic and mitral flow profiles and the parameters which can be measured from the Doppler recordings. PEP = pre-ejection period; LVET = left ventricular ejection time; AT = acceleration time; DT = deceleration time; PV = peak aortic velocity; FVI = aortic flow velocity integral; D = diameter at the sample volume site; CSA = cross-sectional area at the sample volume site; SV = stroke volume; CO = cardiac output; HR = Heart rate; E = peak velocity of the early diastolic filling wave; A = peak velocity of the atrial filling wave; DFT = diastolic filling time; O = diameter.

dysfunction with this approach which was noted to occur before ECG changes, systolic impairment and angina [5].

Several parameters can be derived from the aortic and mitral waveforms including measurements of the cardiac output (Figure 11.1). If Doppler ultrasound methods are to be used to assess ventricular function, reference values for the measured parameters in normal subjects must be established in each laboratory and reproducibility fully determined [6, 7].

Doppler ultrasound interrogation of blood flow within the ascending aorta can provide several types of data which would reflect the left ventricular systolic performance, including measurements of cardiac output at well as acceleration and peak velocity to flow. Acceleration and peak velocity are related to the contractile state of the left ventricle. Loeppky *et al.* [8] first used Doppler echocardiography to measure stroke volume during exercise in normal subjects. They compared responses to supine versus upright exercise in eight healthy volunteers measuring the stroke velocity integral using pulsed Doppler. The aortic diameter is only measured at rest and assumed not to change during exercise. In this study, resting stroke volume was found to be significantly higher in the supine versus the upright posture and rose significantly during exercise in the upright but not the supine position. These differences between the supine and upright positions are presumed to be due to the differences in venous return from the legs. It was later that Salmasi and associates [9] produced the first report on characterising global left ventricular function in patients with coronary artery disease using Doppler ultrasound measurement of aortic blood velocity during exercise.

Myocardial relaxation is altered in patients with coronary artery disease, even in those with relatively well preserved systolic function. In normal subjects, diastolic mitral flow velocities are affected by both age and phase of the respiratory cycle but not by body surface area, gender, or blood pressure in the normal range [10]. In patients with coronary artery disease and severe left ventricular damage the E to A ratio is decreased as the passive ventricular filling is impaired [11]. This pattern however can be seen in any patient with poor left ventricular function and is not specific for coronary artery disease [12]. Figure 11.2 is from a 52 year old patient with extensive coronary artery disease. Note that the early filling wave ('E' wave) is reduced and smaller than the late filling wave ('A' wave).

Exercise Doppler echocardiography

Several investigators have used Doppler echocardiography to detect manifestations of ischaemic heart disease during exercise [9, 13–15]. Rassi *et al.* [16] studied the mechanisms of increased blood flow at the mitral and aortic valves during graded bicycles exercise in normal subjects. The mitral valve

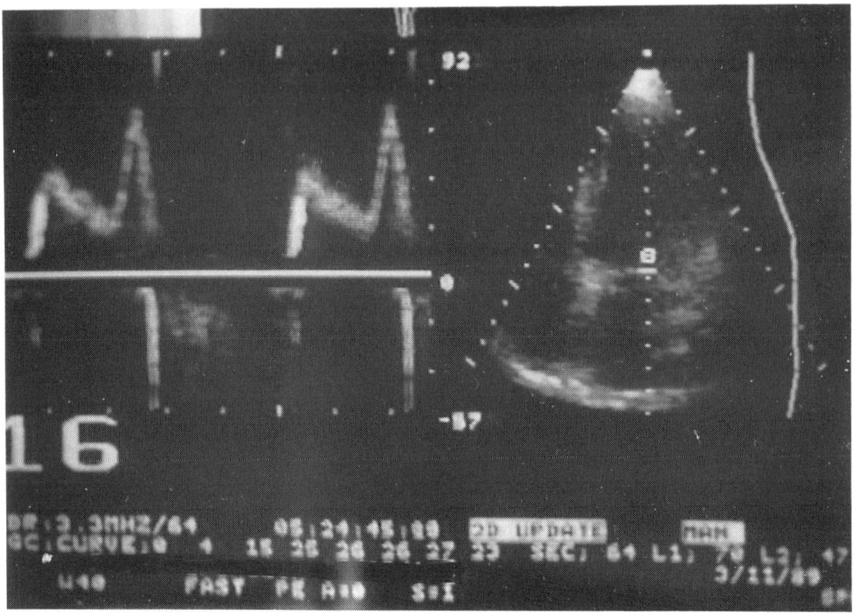

Figure 11.2. Left ventricular filling profile in patients with left ventricular dysfunction due to coronary artery disease demonstrating a reduced early filling velocity ('E' wave) when compared with the late filling velocity ('A' wave).

flow increases, largely by an increase in the valve orifice area, whereas at the aortic valve an increase in the flow velocity integral occurs with little change in the cross-sectional area. Doppler ultrasound measurements of aortic flow have documented significant increases in stroke volume, peak velocity and mean acceleration during exercise in normal subjects [17]. One study documented a 45% increase in peak velocity from 1.09±0.16 m/s at rest to 1.58±0.21 m/s during early recovery [18]. Doppler ascending aortic blood flow parameters differ at baseline and during exercise in normals depending on whether exercise is performed supine or upright. Stroke volume and peak velocity at rest are lower in the upright position but equalize in the supine position at maximal exercise whereas there is no difference in mean aortic acceleration at baseline and during exercise between the two positions.

Doppler ultrasound measurement of aortic blood velocity during exercise has proven very useful in assessing the effect of coronary artery bypass grafting [19]. Salmasi and associates [19, 20] reported an increase in the peak velocity, systolic velocity integral and systolic acceleration at peak exercise rather than at rest after coronary artery bypass grafting.

Doppler ultrasound assessment of mitral blood flow in normal subjects during exercise reveals that the period of diastasis progressively shortens as the heart rate increases until the E and A waves overlap; with further increases in heart rate the two waves fuse to form a single diastolic filling wave [16]. This renders interpretation of conventional Doppler parameters of diastolic function difficult if not impossible.

Exercise is able to induce myocardial ischaemia in patients with significant coronary artery disease. Mehta *et al.* [21] performed exercise Doppler echocardiographic studies of aortic flow in 165 patients three to four weeks after acute myocardial infarction. Peak flow velocity, peak acceleration and stroke volume were all significantly lower in those patients with positive ST-segment response to exercise. Since Doppler evaluation of aortic and mitral blood flow provides a non-invasive beat-to-beat assessment of left ventricular function, it offers the potential to detect ischaemia and can be used to study the haemodynamic changes induced by exercise in this group of patients. Unfortunately, many other factors can affect the Doppler data apart from exercise-induced myocardial ischaemia. These include: changes in preload, afterload, heart rate and contractility with exercise, the patient's age; the exercise stage reached; whether or not the patients are taking cardioactive therapy such as beta-blockers; and resting left ventricular function. For example, the effects of a cold pressor test on transmitral velocities in 11 healthy volunteers showed that the large acute increases in arterial pressure induced by this test has not consistent effect on the transmitral velocity profile [22]. However, small changes in heart rate from 70 to 80 beats/minute increased the A to E ratio by about 30%, mainly by increasing the A wave. Decreases in preload reduce the E to A ratio and increase the percentage of filling occurring during atrial contraction. Similarly, aortic flow is affected more by changes in afterload than preload.

Despite these reservations, experimental work in dogs has shown Doppler measurements of peak aortic blood velocity and mean acceleration to be an effective means of assessment short term changes in left ventricular performance under conditions of varying preload heart rate and inotropic state [23].

Doppler examination of ascending aortic blood flow during exercise is generally performed with the transducer in the suprasternal notch [24]. The transducer angulation is adjusted using the audio signal and spectral display as a guide until the highest velocity spectral recording with a clear velocity envelope is obtained. Use of continuous wave Doppler may be preferable to pulsed wave during exercise because of difficulties in maintaining a constant sample volume site throughout exertion and the possibility of 'aliasing' at very high flow rates. The effects of respiration on the Doppler signal may be a problem in some patients and excessive motion during exercise limited the examination beyond stage four of the Bruce protocol in one study [25]. Doppler devices intended for exercise studies are commercially available, e.g. Exerdop, AH Robins. The latter is a continuous wave instrument which operates at 3 MHz, samples every 5 msec and measures model velocity. Peak acceleration and flow velocity integral are accurately derived internally and the device provides a digital printout of the results but lacks the capability of a full spectral tracing.

Recent studies have investigated the haemodynamic effects of exercise in patients with coronary artery disease and whether or not myocardial ischaemia can be detected by Doppler examination of ascending aortic blood flow [21–23]. Unfortunately, qualitatively similar responses in Doppler aortic flow parameters occur in normal subjects during exercise. In one study [25] aortic flow velocity integral was found to be of no value in identifying coronary artery disease. No significane difference in the mean change in maximal aortic velocity achieved with exercise was found between a group of 37 patients with scintigraphic evidence of ischaemia compared with a similarly aged group of 25 patients with normal thallium perfusion scans. There was also no significant difference in the mean change in peak aortic acceleration between these two groups when only those patients who achieved 85% of their age-predicted maximal heart rate were analyzed [25]. However, repeated analysis of peak aortic disease in the ischaemia-positive group showed a smaller rise in this Doppler parameter in these patients which was significant at the 0.01 level. The authors tentatively concluded that the inability to reach a peak acceleration in excess of 30 m/s/s in a patient who can exercise to 85% of their age-predicted maximal heart rate may be of value in detecting advanced stages of coronary artery disease [25]. The left ventricular functional response to exercise shortly after acute myocardial infarction has been assessed using Doppler measurement of ascending aortic flow: peak velocity and maximal acceleration were significantly lower in patients with three-vessel disease than in those with one- and two-vessel disease [21].

The effect of upright bicycle exercise on left ventricular filling determined using pulsed-wave Doppler has also been studied [26–28]. At rest, the ratio of the early filling velocity integral to the late filling velocity integral is greater in normals compared to the coronary disease patients; this ratio remains largely unchanged in the normals during exercise but decreased significantly by 34% in the coronary artery disease patients. Transient mitral regurgitation with exercise has also been frequently observed.

Difficulties in maintaining a constant sample volume location with increasing heart rates and respiratory rates are noted and it is very difficult if not impossible to obtain adequate Doppler ultrasound signals above a heart rate of 130 beats/minute. Recording the Doppler spectral display on videotape at a fast speed improves the accuracy of Doppler measurements at higher heart rates.

In summary, Doppler echocardiography is able to study changes in global left ventricular systolic function at rest and during exercise in patients with coronary artery disease but has not been shown to be able to reliably detect myocardial ischaemia in this setting.

Pharmacological stress

(1) *Dipyridamole.* Intravenous dipyridamole stress testing (most commonly using doses of 0.56 mg/kg over 4 minutes or 0.75 mg/kg over 10 minutes) with or without exercise, has been used in conjunction with the 12 lead ECG [29], thallium-201 imaging [30] and two-dimensional echocardiography [31, 32] in the diagnosis and assessment of patients with suspected coronary artery disease. The dipyridamole two-dimensional echocardiography test is useful in this setting especially with being proposed to be high dose and faster administration of the drug, a manoeuvre which does not compromise patient safety. Since the test relies on the identification of ischaemia-induced endocardial wall motion and systolic wall thickening abnormalities, all anti-anginal medication, an antagonist at adenosine receptors and nitrates can be used to reverse ischaemia if necessary. Drinks containing theophylline, a dipyridamole antagonist present in tea, coffee and cola must also be avoided prior to testing. Despite the enthusiasm of dipyridamole two-dimensional echocardiography from the Italian group, others including ourselves have failed to reproduce their high sensitivity of this technique [33].

The effect of intravenous dipyridamole on Doppler-derived indices of aortic and mitral flow has recently been reported [34]. The hypothesis being tested by these studies is that dipyridamole-induced transient ischaemic systolic and diastolic left ventricular dysfunction may be detected by Doppler-documented changes in aortic and mitral blood flow and that this information may improve the accuracy of dipyridamole two-dimensional echocardiography in the diagnosis of coronary artery disease. Intravenous dipyridamole causes some vasodilatation of systemic arterioles with a slight decrease in systolic and diastolic arterial pressure and reflex increase in heart rate and cardiac output; these changes in haemodynamics will also alter aortic and mitral flow patterns and are potentially confounding when using Doppler ultrasound to detect myocardial ischaemia. Labovitz *et al.* [30] measured changes in aortic blood flow using Doppler during intravenous dipyridamole-thallium imaging. There was a statistically significant difference in percent change from baseline to peak dipyridamole effect in peak aortic velocity and acceleration between 41 patients with normal and 53 patients with abnormal thallium perfusion images. The combination of two-dimensional and Doppler echocardiographic parameters increased the sensitivity in the detection of coronary artery disease from 64% (two-dimensional echocardiography alone) to 85%. One recent study however concluded that intravenous dipyridamole-Doppler echocardiography (of mitral and aortic flow) could not reliably detect ischaemia or significant coronary artery stenoses [35].

(2) *Dobutamine.* Dobutamine is a sympathomimetic amine which exerts its

effects via stimulation of beta-1, beta-2 and alpha-1 receptors [36]. Dobutamine is relatively more inotropic than chronotropic and studies have shown that it is able to induce echocardiographically detectable myocardial ischaemia in areas supplied by significantly stenosed coronary arteries which it does primarily by increasing myocardial oxygen demand [37]. Recent reports of the value of dobutamine stress two-dimensional echocardiography in the evaluation of patients with coronary artery disease have been promising [38, 39]. Mannering *et al.* [38] compared the dobutamine stress test with exercise testing in 50 patients three weeks after acute myocardial infarction. The heart rate and double product increased more during exercise than during dobutamine infusion, while maximum acceleration of aortic flow in the ascending aorta, measured using a continuous wave Doppler transducer in the suprasternal notch, increased more during dobutamine infusion than during exercise. Ischaemia was induced in a similar proportion of patients with the two tests suggesting that dobutamine-induced ischaemia is due mainly to the increased inotropic state of the myocardium rather than to an increase in heart rate. Further work is needed to establish the value of Doppler echocardiographic information during dobutamine stress testing.

(3) *Ergonovine.* Coronary artery vasospasm frequently occurs at the site of coronary artery stenoses. Administration of ergonovine is the standard way of provoking spasm and the use of two-dimensional echocardiography in conjunction with intravenous ergonovine to document ischaemia-induced regional wall motion abnormalities has not been fully investigated. Doppler monitoring of transmitral flow in six spontaneous attacks of prinzmetal's angina [12] showed reduction in the peak velocity of the early ('E' wave) and late ('A' wave) ratio and occurred before electrocardiographic ST-segment elevation.

Conclusion

Although Doppler echocardiography is capable of detecting myocardial ischaemia in certain circumstances, no Doppler-based stress test exists to date which can reliably detect myocardial ischaemia, thereby aiding in the diagnosis of coronary artery disease and most investigative efforts in this area to date have been negative. Doppler echocardiography is of value in assessing global left ventricular systolic and diastolic function and can accurately determine cardiac output at rest and during exercise in coronary artery disease patients. Further work is needed to fully realize the potential of Doppler ultrasound techniques in the evaluation of this patient group, (see chapter 7 for further details and applications).

References

1. Harizi R C, Bianco J A, Alpert J S. Diastolic function of the heart in clinical cardiology. Arch intern Med 1988; 148:99.
2. Sabbah B S, Khaja F, Brymer J F *et al.* Non-invasive evaluation of left ventricular performance based on peak aortic blood acceleration measured with a continuous wave Doppler velocity meter. Circulation 1986; 74:323.
3. Rokey R, Kuo L C, Zoghbi W A, Limacher M C, Quinones M A. Determination of parameters of left ventricular disastolic filling with pulsed doppler echocardiography: comparison with cineangiography. Circulation 1985; 71:543.
4. Friedman B J, Drinkovic N, Miles H, Shih W J, Mazzoleni A, DeMaria A N. Assessment of left ventricular diastolic function: comparison of doppler echocardiography and gated blood pool scintigraphy. J Am Coll Cardiol 1986; 8:1348.
5. Labovitz A J, Lewen M K, Kern M, Vandormael M, Deligonal U, Kennedy H L. Evaluation of left ventricular systolic and diastolic dysfunction during transient myocardial ischaemia produced by angioplasty. J Am Coll Cardiol 1987; 10:748.
6. Wilson N, Goldberg S J, Dickinson D F, Scott O. Normal intracardiac and great artery blood velocity measurements by pulsed doppler echocardiography. Br Heart J 1985; 53:451.
7. Spirito P, Maron B J, Verter I, Merill J S. Reproducibility of Doppler echocardiographic measurements of left ventricular diastolic function. Eur Heart J 1988; 9:879.
8. Loeppky J A, Greene E R, Hoekenga E D *et al.* Beat-to-beat stroke volume assessment by pulsed-Doppler in upright and supine exercise. J Appl Physiol 1981; 50:1173.
9. Salmasi S N, Salmasi A M, Hendry W G *et al.* Exercise-induced changes in stroke volume measured non-invasively in coronary artery disease. Ultrasound Med Biol 1982; 8(a):170.
10. Bryg R J, Williams G A, Labovitz A J. Effect of aging on left ventricular diastolic filling in normal subjects. Am J Cardiol 1987; 59:971.
11. Fugii J, Yazaki Y, Sawada H, Aizawa T, Watanabe H, Kato K. Non-invasive assessment of left and right ventricular filling in myocardial infarction with a two-dimensional Doppler echocardiographic method. J Am Coll Cardiol 1985; 5:1155.
12. Moscarelli E, Distante A, Rovai D, Lombardi M, Morales M A. Changes in mitral flow induced by transient myocardial ischaemia produced by angioplasty. J Am Coll Cardiol 1986; 74:11.
13. Salmasi A M, Salmasi S N, Nicolaides A N *et al.* Non-invasive assessment of left ventricular function in coronary artery disease by Doppler stress testing. J Cardiovasc Surg 1987; 28(3):313.
14. Daley P J, Sagar K B, Collier B D, Kalbfleisch J, Wann L S. Detection of exercise induced changes in left ventricular performance by Doppler echocardiography. Br Heart J 1987; 58:447.
15. Maeda M, Yokota M, Iwase M, Miyahara T, Hayashi H, Sotobata I. Accuracy of cardiac output measured by continuous wave Doppler echocardiography during dynamic exercise testing in the supine position in patients with coronary artery disease. Am J Cardiol 1989; 13:76.
16. Rassi A, Crawford M H, Richards K L, Miller J F. Differing mechanisms of exercise flow augmentation at the mitral and aortic valves. Circulation 1988; 77:543.
17. Daley P J, Sagar K B, Wann L S. Doppler echocardiographic measurement of flow velocity in the ascending aorta during supine and upright exercise. Br Heart J 1985; 54:562.
18. Gardin J M, Kozlowski J, Dabestani A *et al.* Studies of Doppler aortic flow velocity during supine bicycle exercise. Am J Cardiol 1986; 57:327.
19. Salmasi A M, Salmasi S N, Nicolaides A N, Dore C, Kidner P H. Assessment of the effect

of coronary artery bypass grafting on left ventricular performance by Doppler measurement of the aortic blood velocity during exercise. J Cardiovasc Surg 1988; 29(1):89.
20. Salmasi AM. Assessment of the effect of coronary artery bypass grafting on left ventricular function by stress Doppler echocardiography. In: stress Doppler Echocardiography. Ed., SM Teague. Kluwer Academic Publishers. Dordrecht/Holland. 1990; pp. 137.
21. Mehta N, Bennett D, Mannering D, Dawkins K, Ward DE. Usefulness of non-invasive Doppler measurement of ascendind aortic blood velocity and acceleration in detecting impairment of the left ventricular functional response to exercise three weeks after acute myocardial infarction. Am J Cardiol. 1986; 58:879.
22. Smith SA, Stoner JE, Russel AE, Sheppard JM, Aylward PE. Transmitral velocities measured by pulsed Doppler in healthy volunteers: effects of acute changes in blood pressure and heart rate. Br Heart J 1989; 61:344.
23. Wallmeyer K, Wann LS, Sagar KB, Kalbfleisch J, Klopfenstein HS. The influence of preload and heart rate on Doppler echocardiographic indices of left ventricular performance: comparison with invasive indices in an experimental preparation. Circulation. 1986; 74:181.
24. Bennett ED, Barkley SA, Davis AL, Mannering D, Mehta N. Ascending aortic blood velocity and acceleration using Doppler ultrasound in the assessment of left ventricular function. Cardiovasc Res 1984; 18:632–8.
25. Harrison MR, Smith MD, Friedman BJ, De Maria AN. Uses and limitations of exercise Doppler echocardiography in the diagnosis of ischaemic heart disease. J Am Coll Cardiol 1987; 10:809.
26. Bryg RJ, Labovitz AJ, Mehdirad AA, Williams GA, Chaitman BR. Effect of coronary artery disease on Doppler-derived parameters of aortic flow during upright exercise. Am J Cardiol 1986; 58:14.
27. Kuecherer HF, Ruffman K, Schaefer E, Kuebler W. Doppler echocardiographic assessment of left ventricular filling dynamics in patients with coronary heart disease and normal systolic function. Eur Heart J 1988; 9:649.
28. Mehdirad AA, Williams GA, Labovitz AJ, Bryg RJ, Chaitman BR. Evaluation of left ventricular function during upright exercise: correlation of exercise Doppler with post-exercise two-dimensional echocardiographic results. Circulation 1987; 75:413.
29. Tavazzi L, Previtali M, Salerno JA *et al.* Dipyridamole test in angina pectoris: diagnostic value and pathophysiological implications. Cardiology 1982; 69:34.
30. Taillefer R, Lette J, Phaneuf DC, Leveille J, Lemire F, Essiambre R. Thallium-201 myocardial imaging during pharmacologic coronary vasidilatation: comparison of oral and intravenous administration of dipyridamole. J Am Coll Cardiol 1986; 8:76.
31. Picano E, Lattanzi F, Masini M, Distante A, L'Abbate A. High dose dipyridamole echocardiography test in effort angina pectoris. J Am Coll Cardiol 1986; 8:848.
32. Picano E, Lattanzi F, Masini M, Distante A, L'Abbate A. Usefulness of the dipyridamole-exercise echocardiography test for the diagnosis of coronary artery disease. Am J Cardiol 1988; 62:67.
33. Margonatto A, Chierchia S, Cianflone D *et al.* Limitations of dipyridamole-echocardiography in effort angina pectoris. Am J Cardiol 1987; 59:225.
34. Labovitz AJ, Pearson AC, Chaitman BR. Doppler and two-dimensional echocardiographic assessment of left ventricular function before and after intracenous dipyridamole stress testing for detection of coronary artery disease. Am J Cardiol 1988; 62:1180.
35. Grayburn PA, Popma JJ, Pryor SL, Walker BS, Simon TR, Smitherman TC. Dipyridamole-Doppler echocardiography: comparison to thallium-201 imaging and quantitative coronary arteriography (abstract). J Am Coll Cardiol 1989; 13:159A.
36. Leier CV, Unverferth DV. Dobutamine. Ann Intern Med 1988; 99:490.
37. Fung AY, Gallagher KP, Buda AJ. The physiologic basis of dobutamine as compared

with dipyridamole stress interventions in the assessment of critical caronary stenosis. Circulation 1987; 76:943.

38. Mannering D, Cripps T, Leech G *et al.* The dobutamine stress test as an alternative to exercise testing after acute myocardial infarction. Br Heart J 1988; 59:521.
39. Berthe C, Pierard L A, Hiernaux M *et al.* predicting the extent and location of coronary artery disease in acute myocardial infarction by echocardiography during dobutamine infusion. Am J Cardiol 1986; 58:1167.

12. Prognosis and management of occult coronary artery disease

DAN TZIVONI, JESAIA BENHORIN and SHLOMO STERN

Haemodynamic significance of silent ischaemia

Ischaemic episodes during daily activities are frequent in patients with coronary artery disease [1–8]. These episodes, detected by ambulatory electrocardiographic monitoring which are mostly silent, last from a few minutes up to several hours. Treatment of patients with silent ischaemic episodes is justified only if silent ischaemia represents similar degree of ischaemia, as symptomatic one. Levy and coworkers [9] studied 19 patients with coronary artery disease who had 67 ischaemia episodes. During the 35 painful episodes the pulmonary artery diastolic pressure increased in 34, while during the 32 silent episodes it increased in 30 patients. Thus, silent and symptomatic episodes were associated with similar haemodynamic changes. In our study of 191 patients with coronary artery disease [10], patients with silent episodes had the same extent of coronary disease as patients with symptomatic episodes. The average duration of the silent episodes (15 minutes) was similar to that of the symptomatic ones (14 minutes), the heart at onset at the ischaemia was similar (94/min vs. 96/min) as well as the maximal ST depression (2.0 mm vs 2.1 mm). Similar findings were reported by von Arnim [11]. Deanfield and coworkers [12] found that the heart rate of onset of ST depression was similar during the silent and symptomatic episodes, but the symptomatic episodes were slightly longer (by a mean of 13%) than those without pain. Hirzel and coworkers [13] performed haemodynamic measurements during exercise in 36 patients with coronary artery disease. The left ventricular end diastolic pressure increased from 18 to 36 mmHg in the group with silent ischaemia during exercise and from 13 to 29 mmHg in the symptomatic group (p=NS). The left ventricular ejection fraction decreased from 59% to 50% in the silent group and from 60% to 52% in the symptomatic group (p=NS). Davies and coworkers [14] found in patients with angina at rest that transient asymptomatic ST segment

A.-M. Salmasi and A. N. Nicolaides (eds.), Occult Atherosclerotic Disease, 165–171.

shifts are consistently associated with large changes in left ventricular volume, similar to those observed during painful episodes. Wohlgelernter *et al.* [15] reported that during balloon angioplasty, echocardiographic measurements of global and regional left ventricular dysfunction were comparable in patients who were symptomatic or asymptomatic during the balloon inflations. These studies suggest that silent and symptomatic ischaemic episodes represent the same degree of myocardial ischaemia, and that patients with silent ischaemia have the same extent of coronary disease, as patients with painful ischaemia.

Repeated exercise induced ischaemia has been shown to be associated with changes in myocardial structure. Hess and coworkers [16] performed myocardial biopsies during coronary bypass surgery in 15 patients with documented exercise-induced wall motion abnormalities without previous infarction. Biopsies taken from the ischaemic regions showed higher concentration of fibrous tissue and more muscle fibre hypertrophy compared to normal regions. These changes were more pronounced in the subendocardial than in the subepicardial areas. These authors concluded therefore that repeated ischaemia was responsible for the permanent myocardial changes. Other authors have shown that myocardial dysfunction persisted after exercise induced ischaemia [17]. Thus, repeated exercise induced ischaemia and therefore probably also ischaemia during daily life is associated with prolonged functional and permanent structural changes.

Prognosis of silent ischaemia during exercise

Falcone *et al.* [18] compared 269 patients with painful ischaemia during exercise with 204 patients with silent ischaemia during exercise. The frequency of single, double or triple coronary artery disease was identical in the two groups. There was no difference in survival between those with silent or symptomatic exercise induced ischaemia. Weiner and coworkers [19] compared 424 patients with silent positive stress tests from the Coronary Artery Surgery Study to 456 patients who had both ST depression and anginal pain during exercise. Patients with silent and patients with symptomatic ischaemia had a similar risk of developing an acute myocardial infarction or sudden death.

Callaham and coworkers [20] assessed the prognosis of 1743 patients who had treadmill stress tests. The overall 1-year mortality was 6% in patients with silent ischaemia during exercise and 7% in those with symptomatic ischaemia, while patients with negative stress test, had only 3% mortality. The prognosis was related to the degree of ST depression and not to the presence or absence of pain.

Prognostic significance of silent ischaemia in patients with unstable angina

Silent ischaemic episodes were shown by Gottlieb *et al.* [21] and by Nademanee *et al.* [22] to be associated with worse short and long term prognosis in patients hospitalized with unstable angina. In the study of Gottlieb *et al.* [21] the 37 patients who had ischaemic episodes had higher rate of myocardial infarction, bypass surgery or balloon angioplasty within one month, compared to 33 patients without ischaemic episodes. Multivariate analysis showed that silent ischaemia was the best predictor for outcome among the 15 variable tested. Patients who had more than 60 minutes of ischaemia per 24 hours had worse prognosis than those with shorter duration of ischaemia. A follow up of these patients revealed that the adverse outcome of silent ischaemic episodes persisted for a 2-year period [23]. In the study of Nademanee and coworkers [22] the short term follow-up of those with unstable angina and ischaemic episodes was markedly worse than those without ischaemia. They had higher frequency of triple coronary disease and more proximal disease in their coronary arteries.

Prognostic significance of silent ischaemia in patients with stable ischaemic heart disease

In patients with stable angina pectoris Rocco *et al.* [24] found ischaemic episodes in 49 of 86 patients with positive exercise tests. These patients had a total of 426 ischaemic episodes, only 14% of them were symptomatic. During a 12 months follow-up period, there were 2 cardiac deaths, 4 myocardial infarctions, 4 hospitalizations for unstable angina and 11 revascularization procedures. All but one of these events occurred in the group of patients with ischaemic changes on Holter monitoring ($p<0.003$). Multivariate analysis revealed that the presence of ischaemic episodes on Holter monitoring was a significant predictor for outcome while exercise tests characteristics were not. In our earlier study of 1974 [1] the 37 patients who had ischaemic changes on Holter monitoring had higher frequency of worsening of their symptoms and/or development of ECG ST-T abnormalities compared to 43 patients without ischaemic changes. Recently we assessed the prognostic significance of ischaemic changes during daily activities in 224 low risk post infarction patients [25]. Seventy-four of the patients had ischaemic episodes. During the 28 months of follow-up the frequency of cardiac events (cardiac death, reinfarction, hospitalization for unstable angina, balloon angioplasty or coronary bypass surgery) was 51% among those with ischaemic episodes compared with 12% in those without such changes ($p<0.0001$). The difference in event rate reached statistical significance only for hospitalizations for unstable angina ($p=0.005$) or for coronary angioplasty or bypass surgery ($p=0.0001$). The 74 patients who were positive on both exercise tests and on Holter had 51% event rate compared to 20% in patients with positive exercise tests but negative Holter monitoring ($p<0.0001$). Thus, the presence of ischaemic changes on Holter contributed to the prognostic assessment of these patients beyond the results of exercise testing. Patients who were negative on both exercise tests and on Holter had the lowest event rate (8.5%). The presence of ischaemic episodes contributed to the prognostic assessments of these patients beyond the left ventricular function, as in the groups with good (>40%) or reduced (<40%) left ventricular ejection fraction, those with ischaemic changes had worse prognosis than those without. A similar event rate was found in patients with only silent, only symptomatic or with silent and symptomatic ischaemic episodes.

Another group of 56 patients with severe stable angina was recently studied by us [26]. All patients had angiographically proven coronary artery disease without previous myocardial infarction and a positive stress test. During a 23 months of follow-up period the frequency of cardiac death or myocardial infarction was 28% in the 43 patients with ischaemic changes compared to none among the 13 patients without such changes.

Aronow and Epstein [27] studied by Holter monitoring 185 coronary patients. During a 26 months follow-up new cardiac events (non fatal or fatal myocardial infarction, primary ventricular fibrillation or sudden cardiac death) occurred in 65% of patients with ischaemic episodes compared to 32% of patients free of such episodes ($p<0.001$).

Ischaemia, arrhythmia and sudden cardiac death

Garan and coworkers [28] studied 15 patients with coronary artery disease, who had ventricular tachycardia or fibrillation. All patients developed ventricular tachycardia during electrophysiological stimulation. After coronary bypass surgery in only 7 of the 15 patients, ventricular tachycardia could be induced by electrophysiological stimulation. The authors concluded therefore, that pacing-induced ischaemia played an important role in the genesis of ventricular tachycardia. Morady *et al.* [29] found lactate production in the coronary sinus 1 minute prior the electrophysiologic stimulation-induced ventricular tachycardia in 6 patients, 5 of them did not develop ventricular tachycardia when ischaemia was not present. Carboni *et al.* [30] found ventricular arrhythmia in 11 of 32 patients with ischaemic episodes on Holter. Arrhythmia was associated with ischaemia in 40 out of the 115 episodes (35%). In our recent study [31] increased ventricular ectopic activities was present in 11 of 75 patients with ischaemic episodes. In these patients the increased ectopy was present in 27% of the episodes. There are several case reports of patients who died during Holter monitoring in which ischaemia preceded the development of fatal ventricular arrhythmia [32, 33]. From the above literature it seems that when ventricular arrhythmia occurs in the setup of ischaemia, it tends to be more dangerous, while in other patients ischaemia can be the cause of the arrhythmia.

Therapy of silent ischaemia

Anti-anginal therapy is guided mainly by patients' symptoms. Patients with severe and frequent symptoms receive more intensive anti-anginal therapy, whereas patients with occasional symptoms usually receive only minimal therapy. This traditional concept that one can judge the activity of the disease by patients' symptoms has been challenged by many reports that have shown that most ischaemic episodes are silent. Several authors have reported that nitrates [33, 34] beta-adrenergic blocking agents [35, 36] and calcium antagonists [37, 38] are effective in reducing the frequency of both symptomatic and silent ischaemic episodes.

Since both silent and symptomatic ischaemia are associated with a similar amount of myocardium at jeopardy, and since the extent of coronary disease is similar in patients with silent and symptomatic ischaemia, it is not surprising that patients with silent and symptomatic ischaemia have similar prognoses. It seems that repeated ischaemic episodes aggravate prognosis beyond the extent of coronary disease and left ventricular function. We believe that of two patients with identical coronary pathology and left ventricular function, the one with frequent ischaemic episodes is at higher risk compared to one with rare episodes. It seems therefore, that all effort should be made to prevent these episodes. Anti-ischaemic therapy should be guided by the presence or absence of ischaemia either on exercise or during daily activity. It is not clear whether asymptomatic patients should be submitted to coronary bypass surgery or balloon angioplasty, yet many patients with advanced coronary disease are being submitted today to interventions according to the severity of the disease and not according the symptoms.

References

1. Stern S, Tzivoni D. Early detection of silent ischaemic heart disease by 24-hour electrocardiographic monitoring of active subjects. Brit Heart J 1974; 36:481.
2. Stern S, Tzivoni D, Stern Z. Diagnostic accuracy of ambulatory ECG monitoring in ischaemic heart disease. Circulation 1975; 52:1045.

3. Allen RD, Gettes LS, Phalan C, Avington DM. Painless ST-segment depression in patients with angina pectoris. Chest 1976; 69:467.
4. Schang SJ, Pepine CJ. Transient asymptomatic ST segment depression during daily activity. Am J Cardiol 1977; 39:396.
5. Deanfield JE, Shea M, Ribiero P, de Landshere CM, Wilson RA, Horlock P, Selwyn AP. Transient ST-segment depression as a maker of myocardial ischaemia during daily life. Am J Cardiol 1984; 54:1195.
6. Cohn PF, Lawson WE. Characteristics of silent myocardial ischaemia during out-of-hospital activities in asymptomatic angiographically documented coronary artery disease. Am J Cardiol 1987; 59:746.
7. Tzivoni D, Gavish A, Benhorin J, Keren A, Stern S. Myocardial Ischemia during daily activities and stress. Am J Cardiol 1986; 58:47b.
8. Campbell S, Barry J, Rebecca GS, Rocco MB, Nabel EG, Wayne RR, Selwyn AP. Active transient myocardial ischaemia during daily life in asymptomatic patients with positive exercise tests and coronary artery disease. Am J Cardiol 1986; 57:1010.
9. Levy RD, Shapiro LM, Wright C, Mockus L, Fox K. The haemodynamic significance of asymptomatic ST segment depression assessed by ambulatory pulmonary artery pressure monitoring. Br Heart J 1986; 56:526.
10. Stern S, Gavish A, Weisz G, Benhorin J, Keren A, Tzivoni D. Characteristics of silent and symptomatic myocardial ischaemia during daily activities. Am J Cardiol 1988; 61:1223.
11. von Arnim T, Hofling B, Schreiber M. Characteristics of episodes of ST elevation or ST depression during ambulatory monitoring in patients subsequently undergoing coronary angiography. Brit Heart J 1985; 54:484.
12. Deanfield JE, Selwyn AP, Chierchia S, Maseri A, Ribiero P, Krikler S, Morgan M. Myocardial ischaemia during daily life in patients with stable angina: Its relation to symptoms and heart rate changes. The Lancet 1983; 753.
13. Hirzel HO, Leutwyler R, Krayenbuehl HP. Silent myocardial ischaemia: hemodynamic changes during dynamic exercise in patients with proven coronary artery disease despite absence of angina pectoris. J Am Cardiol 1985; 6:275.
14. Davies GJ, Bencivelli W, Fragasso G, Chierchia S, Crea F, Crow J, Cream PA, Pratt T, Morgan M, Maseri A. Sequence and magnitude of ventricular volume changes in painful and painless myocardial ischaemia. Circulation 1988; 78:310.
15. Wohgelernter D, Jaffe CC, Cabin HS, Yeatman LA, Cleman M. Silent ischaemia during coronary occlusion produced by balloon inflation: relation to regional myocardial dysfunction. J Am Coll Cardiol 1987; 10:491.
16. Hess OM, Schneider J, Nonogi H, Carroll JD, Schneider K, Turina M, Krayenbuehl HP. Myocardial structure in patients with exercise-induced ischaemia. Circulation 1988; 77:967.
17. Homans DC, Sublett E, Dai XZ, Bache RJ. Persistence of regional left ventricular dysfunction after exercise-induced myocardial ischaemia. J Clin Invest 1986; 77:66.
18. Falcone C, de Servi Stefano, Poma E, Campana C, Scire A, Montemartini C, Specchia G. Clinical significance of exercise-induced silent myocardial ischaemia in patient with coronary artery disease. J Am Coll Cardiol 1987; 9:295.
19. Weiner DA, Ryan TJ, McCabe CH, Ng G, Chaitman BR, Sheffield TL, Tristani FE, Fisher LD. Risk of developing an acute myocardial infarction or sudden coronary death in patients with exercise-induced silent myocardial ischaemia. A report from the coronary artery surgery study (CASS) registry. Am J Cardiol 1988; 62:1155.
20. Callaham P, Dubach P, Klein J, Rish M, Froelicher V. Prognostic significance of silent myocardial ischaemia discovered during exercise testing. J Am Coll Cardiol (Abstr) 1988; 11:24.
21. Gottlieb SO, Weisfeldt ML, Ouyang P, Mellits DE, Gerstenblith G. Silent ischaemia as a marker for early unfavorable outcomes in patients with unstable angina. N Engl J Med 1986; 314:1214.

22. Nademanee K, Intarachot V, Josephson MA, Reiders D, Moody FV, Singh BN. Prognostic significance of silent myocardial ischaemia in patients with unstable angina. J Am Coll Cardiol 1987; 10:1.
23. Gottlieb SO, Weisfeldt ML, Ouyang P, Mellitus ED, Gerstenblith G. Silent ischaemia predicts infarction and death during 2 year follow-up of unstable angina. J Am Coll Cardiol 1987; 10:756.
24. Rocco MB, Nabel EG, Campbell S, Goldman L, Barry J, Mead K, Selwyn AP. Prognostic importance of myocardial ischaemia detected by ambulatory monitoring in patients with stable coronary artery disease. Circulation 1988; 78:877.
25. Tzivoni D, Gavish A, Zin D, Gottlieb S, Moreil M, Keren A, Banai S, Stern S. Prognostic significance of ischaemic episodes in patients with previous myocardial infarction. Am J Cardiol 1988; 62:661.
26. Tzivoni D, Weisz G, Gavish A, Zin D, Keren A, Stern S. Comparison of mortality and myocardial infarction rates in stable angina pectoris with and without ischaemic episodes during daily activities. Am J Cardiol 1989; 63:273.
27. Aronow WS, Epstein S. Usefulness of silent myocardial ischaemia detected by ambulatory electrocardiographic monitoring in predicting new coronary events in Elderly patients. Am J Cardiol 1988; 62:1295.
28. Garan H, Ruskin JN, DiMarco JP, Derkac WM, Akins CW, Daggett WM, Austen WG, Buckley MJ. Electrophysiologic studies before and after myocardial revascularization in patients with life-threatening ventricular arrhythmias. Am J Cardiol 1983; 51:519.
29. Morady F, DiCarlo LA, Krol RB, Annesley TM, O'Neill WW, de Buitleir Michael, Baerman JM, Kou WH. Role of myocardial ischaemia during programmed stimulation in survivors of cardiac arrest with coronary artery disease. J Am Coll Cardiol 1987; 9:1004.
30. Carboni GP, Lahiri A, Cashman PM, Raftery EB. Mechanism of arrhythmias accompanying ST-segment depression on ambulatory monitoring in stable angina pectoris. Am J Cardiol 1987; 60:1246.
31. Banai S, Stern S, Keren A, Tzivoni D. Increased ventricular extopic activity during ischaemic episodes in ambulatory patients J Am Coll Cardiol (Abstr) 1989; 13:33A.
32. Gradman AH, Bell PA, DeBusk RF. Sudden death during ambulatory monitoring: clinical and electrocardiographic correlations: report of a case. Circulation 1977, 55:210.
33. Shell WE. Mechanism and therapy of silent myocardial ischaemia and the effects of transdemal nitroglycerin. Am J Cardiol 1985; 56:231.
34. Amsterdam EA. Relation of silent myocardial ischaemia to ventricular arrhythmias and sudden death. Am J Cardiol 1988; 62:24.
35. von Arnim T, Erath A. Nitrates and calcium antagonists for silent myocardial ischaemia. Am J Cardiol 1988; 61:15.
36. Khurmi NS, Bowles MJ, O'Hara MJ. Effect of propranolol on indices of intermittent myocardial ischaemia, assessed by exercise testing and ambulatory ST-segment monitoring. Clin Cardiol 1986; 9:391.
37. Quyyumi AA, Wright CM, Mockus LJ, Fox KM. Effect of partial agonist activity in B blockers in severe angina pectoris: a double blind comparison of pindolol and antenolol. Br Med J 1984; 289:951.
38. Cohn PF, Lawson WE, Gennaro V, Brady D. Effect of nifedipine on out-of-hospital silent myocardial ischaemia in asymptomatic men with coronary artery disease. Am J Cardiol 1988; 61:908.
39. Banai S, Stern S, Tzivoni D. Effect of nisoldipine on myocardial ischaemia: Evaluation by Holter monitoring. In: Nisoldipine 1987. PG Hugenholtz, J Meyer, eds. Springer-Verlag Berlin, Heidelberg 1987, p. 276.

13. Occult myocardial infarction

PETER F. COHN

That myocardial infarctions can occur without pain or other recognizable symptoms is not a new concept; in fact, one of the pioneers in clinical cardiology, Herrick, noted it in his landmark paper published in 1912 [1]. Anecdotal reports throughout the 1930s and 1940s from Kennedy, [2] Boyde and Weblow, [3] Gorham and Martin, [4] and Stroud and Wagner, [5] maintained interest in this seeming paradox [2–5]. Roseman [6] reviewed the literature in 1954 and found that 220 cases of this syndrome had been reported, some in more detail than others.

Definition and prevalence

It is obvious that one of the problems in discussing occult infarctions is in its *definition*. Unlike transient episodes of silent myocardial ischaemia that can be well-documented during exercise tests, radionuclide procedures, Holter monitoring, etc., unrecognized myocardial infarctions are not witnessed at the time they occur. More recently, there have been exceptions to this statement; namely, the few evolving myocardial infarctions that are detected via use of 24-hour ambulatory electrocardiographic monitoring.

Reliance on patients' memory of possible cardiac symptoms is not the best type of data, nor are physician's office notes sufficient. In the final analysis, we are usually left with electrocardiographic evidence of a transmural myocardial infarction (T wave changes alone may or may not indicate a prior non-Q wave infarction) that occurred at some point between two standard ECG examinations.

Several groups of investigators have attempted to assess the prevalence of this phenomenon using ECG tracings. One such survey was the Framingham Heart Study, a long-term prospective study of cardiovascular disease which began in 1948 in Framingham, Massachusetts, under the auspices of the

A.-M. Salmasi and A. N. Nicolaides (eds.), Occult Atherosclerotic Disease, 173–181.

National Institutes of Health. In this survey, a standard cardiovascular examination was performed twice a year on 5209 subjects who ranged from 30 to 62 years at time of entry into the study. Cardiovascular end-points were noted on these examinations, as well as by reviewing admission lists at the town's only hospital. The initial report on unrecognized infarctions was published in 1970 [7] and supplemented in 1973, [8] 1984 [9] and 1986 [10]. The last report represents a 30-year follow-up. At that time, over 28% of infarctions in men and 35% in women were unrecognized (Table 13.1). Of these, half were truly silent, while in the other half some atypical symptoms were present but were not sufficient for either the patient or physician to consider that a myocardial infarction was occurring or had occurred. What this last report also shows is that these unrecognized infarctions were uncommon in patients with prior angina. More recently, in a preliminary report concerning unrecognized infarction in the Framingham age group between 65 to 94 years, Vokonas and colleagues [11] found that 33% of infarctions in men and 36% in women were unrecognized, figures consistent with the Framingham population as a whole.

Table 13.1. Prevalence of presenting symptoms of recognized acute myocardial infarction and of unrecognized healed myocardial infarction in 110 documented myocardial infarctions in elderly patients

	n	(%)
Chest pain	24	(22)
Dyspnea	38	(35)
Neurological symptoms	20	(18)
Gastrointestinal symptoms	5	(4)
Unrecognized Q-wave myocardial infarction	23	(21)

Source: W.S. Aronow. *Am. J. Cardiol., 60*:1182, 1987. Reproduced with permission.

Other groups have also documented the figures of occult infarctions in specific populations. The Multiple Risk Factor Intervention Trial (MRFIT) was a primary risk prevention study involving 12,866 men between the ages of 35 and 57. The goal of the study was to evaluate the effect of a multifactor intervention program on mortality from coronary heart disease. Patients were randomly assigned to a program of aggressive risk factor modification or were referred to the usual sources of health care in the community. In this study, 25% of myocardial infarctions were clinically unrecognized and detected only by serial ECG changes [12]. Another large survey, that of the Western Collaborative Group, found a 30% rate of unrecognized infarction [13]. These types of studies are not confined to the United States. Medalie and Goldbourt [14] performed a prospective analysis of myocardial infarctions in 9509 healthy government employees in Israel.

Almost 40% of the subsequent 427 infarctions in this group were unrecognized. Like the Framingham Study, half of the unrecognized infarctions were totally silent. Also, like the Framingham Study [15], increasing age and blood pressure were significantly associated with the development of unrecognized infarctions.

In analyzing the age issue more closely, Aronow initially reported that 68% of infarctions in an elderly population (64–100 years) were unrecognized [16]. This is a higher percentage than reported by the Framingham investigators [11]. Aronow subsequently revised this figure to 21% in a prospective study (Table 13.1) when physicians were instructed to look more carefully for non-pain presentations (dyspnoea, neurological symptoms, etc.) [17]. This is important, since signs and symptoms due to the complications of silent infarctions – such as pulmonary oedema or dyspnoea [18, 19] – can be the first clues to the underlying problem. The figures that he reported in his latest survey are closer to that of Vokonas, *et at.* [11] than his earlier study.

It must be remembered that these reports deal only with transmural (Q-wave) infarctions; no data is available concerning the frequency of unrecognized non-Q-wave infarctions.

Pathological findings

In addition to the clinical reports from the 1930s to the 1950s cited earlier [2–6], interesting pathological studies have been made available more recently comparing the extent of coronary narrowing to the size of the healed infarct in these patients.

In 1982, Cabin and Roberts [20] reported on studies in 61 patients with a healed transmural myocardial infarction. Medical records were reviewed in detail and the patients were divided into two groups according the presence or absence of a clinical history of acute myocardial infarction; 33 patients were in the former group and 28 patients in the latter group. Patients with equivocal or inadequate histories were excluded. The 28 patients with unrecognized infarcts had a significantly higher prevalence of death from non-cardiac causes (Table 13.2). They also had more posterior wall infarcts that those with recognized infarctions, smaller infarctions as determined by post-mortem measurements, and a higher incidence of diabetes. However, the extent of narrowing of the coronary arteries was similar, as was the involvement of the various vessels. The authors also addressed the question of whether patients with unrecognized infarcts had prior angina less frequently than did patients with symptomatic infarctions. Their results suggested this was the case, but the differences were not statistically significant.

Table 13.2. Clinical findings in 33 patients with clinically recognized and in 28 with clinically unrecognized acute myocardial infarction (MI) and healed transmural infarction at necropsy

	Clinically recognized acute MI (33 patients)		Clinically unrecognized acute MI (28 patients)		
	n	%	*n*	%	*p* value
Age (yr)					
Mean	61	—	60	—	NS
Range	27–81	—	25–82	—	
Male-female ratio	25:8	—	21:7	—	NS
Angina pectoris	14	42	6	21	NS
Chronic congestive heart failure	14	42	9	32	NS
Systemic hypertension	11	33	12	43	NS
Diabetes mellitus (adult onset)	5	15	12	43	0.05
Mode of death					
Sudden	13	39	6	21	NS
Acute MI	8	24	7	25	NS
Chronic congestive heart failure	5	15	1	4	NS
Cardiac operation	2[a]	6	2[b]	7	NS
Cardiac catheterization	2	6	1	4	NS
Noncardiac	3	9	11	39	0.01

[a] Coronary artery bypass grafting in one and left ventricular aneurysmectomy in one.
[b] Coronary artery bypass grafting in both.
Source: H. S. Cabin and W. C. Roberts. *Am. J. Cardiol.*, *50*:677, 1982. Reproduced with permission.

Pathogenesis and pathophysiology

The search for clues to the pathogenesis of this syndrome has largely been unsuccessful. This is unlike the situation in patients with unrecognized myocardial ischaemia, where there are a host of studies on mechanism. Perhaps the most notable of the infarction studies is that of Procacci, *et al.* [21] who studied 18 subjects with occult infarctions. These investigators tested cutaneous pain thresholds in the arm and found them to be significantly higher than in normal controls, but not higher than in patients with painful infarctions. They also studied upper-limb ischaemia via cuff inflation techniques and again found a different onset of pain and altered pain patterns compared to normals. They chose the arm because of the similar peripheral innervation found in 'referred' cardiac pain.

Procacci, and associates did not evaluate the effect of diabetes mellitus but others have. For example, Bradley and Schonfeld [22] reported that 42 of 100 nondiabetic patients had painless infarctions compared with 6 of 100 nondiabetic patients. This relationship was confirmed in the previously cited autopsy study of Cabin and Roberts [2]. In that study, there was a significantly increased prevalence of diabetes mellitus among the patients in the unrecognized infarct group (43%) compared with those in the recognized infarct group. However, in two epidemiologic studies noted earlier [9, 13] the association of diabetes with unrecognized myocardial infarction did not reach a statistically significant level.

Pathological involvement of the autonomic nervous system by diabetes was demonstrated by Faerman, *et al.* [23]. Abnormal morphology was found in cardiac sympathetic and parasympathetic nerves. None of the changes were found in specimens taken from a control group.

These findings of a visceral neuropathy may help to explain the absence of pain during transient ischaemia as well as during infarction. A clinical example is presented in the case report by Raper, *et al.* [19] who postulated that diabetes was responsible for painless infarction in one of four cases that they reported as presenting to the hospital with acute life-threatening cardiac illness. These patients came to the hospital because of complications of cardiac ischaemia (such as pulmonary oedema) but were pain-free.

Prognosis after occult myocardial infarction

As noted earlier, in the Framingham Study myocardial infarctions were designated as 'unrecognized' and then further subdivided into atypical or silent, depending on whether patients – in retrospect – could identify any complaints as having possibly been compatible with an acute myocardial infarction. (About half of the 108 infarctions were of the truly silent type.) The 3-year mortality rates for both unrecognized and recognized myocardial infarctions were similar. (In the Israeli study of Medalie and Goldbourt, the mortality following unrecognized myocardial infarctions was markedly lower

Table 13.3. Proportion of ECG-documented myocardial infarctions (MI) followed by angina pectoris (AP) in subjects aged 30–62 years on entry. Framingham study, 22-year follow-up

	Number with MI	Followed by AP *n*	Followed by AP %
Unrecognized	98	18	18
Recognized	190	113	59
Total	288	114	45

Eighty-nine patients had prior angina pectoris or died and were eliminated from consideration.

Source: W.B. Kannel and R.D. Abbott. In *Silent Myocardial Ischemia* (W. Rutishauser and H. Roskamm, eds), Springer-Verlag, Berlin, 1984, pp. 131–137. Reproduced with permission.

than after recognized myocardial infarctions – unlike the Framingham experience.)

In their most recent report (30-year follow-up), the Framingham investigators have updated their results. As before, there are no data available on prognosis in the immediate convalescent period since, by definition, these patients are not identified until the next routine ECG is performed. However, in those who survived the initial period, the mortality statistics are available. Unrecognized infarctions are just as lethal as the recognized ones. Thus, ten years after an infarction, 45% of patients with unrecognized infarctions and 39% of those with recognized infarctions were dead. Sudden deaths occurred with equal frequency, and at about nine times the rate seen in the general population. Although less prone to angina (18% vs. 59%) (Table 13.3), patients with unrecognized infarctions develop congestive heart failure just as often (Table 13.4). Reinfarction is also common (3% per year in men and 10% per year in women). About 50% of the recurrences are fatal.

Table 13.4. Proportion of ECG-documented myocardial infarctions followed by cardiac failure in subjects 30–62 years of age at entry. Framingham study, 22-year follow-up

		Followed by cardiac failure	
	Number	*n*	%
Unrecognized	100	21	21
Recognized	221	55	25
Total	321	76	24

Source: W. B. Kannel and R. D. Abbott. In *Silent Myocardial Ischemia* (W. Rutishauser and H. Roskamm, eds), Springer-Verlag, Berlin, 1984, pp. 131–137. Reproduced with permission.

In the elderly population in the Framingham Study, patients with recognized and unrecognized infarctions also had similar mortality rates. Aronow, in the most recent follow-up of very elderly patients that he has been studying, also found that the incidence of new coronary events was also similar for patients with recognized versus unrecognized infarction (Table 13.5) [24].

In addition to overt coronary events, occult infarction can also be followed by silent ischaemia either on the exercise test, Holter monitoring, or both. We have seen several such patients at our hospital. One patient had an unrecognized inferior myocardial infarction, triple vessel disease on coronary arteriography, and both a positive exercise test and frequent episodes of silent ischaemia on 48 hour Holter monitoring (Table 13.6) [25].

Table 13.5. Incidence of new coronary events at four-year follow-up in elderly patients with recognized or unrecognized myocardial infarction (MI)

	New Coronary Events	
	No. Events/ Total Pts	%
Women with recognized MI (mean age 82)	19/29	66
Women with unrecognized MI (mean age 82)	29/53	55
Men with recognized MI (mean age 82)	5/8	63
Men with unrecognized MI (mean age 82)	15/25	60

Source: W. S. Aronow. AM J Cardiol 1989; 63:621. Reproduced with permission.

To assess the frequency of silent ischaemia in a population with unrecognized infarctions, Hands, *et al.* [26] used Holter monitoring to study 13 surviving patients of an unrecognized Q-wave myocardial infarction. Two patients had a total of three episodes during 24 hour ambulatory ECG monitoring. Therefore, the authors concluded that silent myocardial ischaemia is uncommon in patients with unrecognized myocardial infarction.

Whether patients who experience an unrecognized infarction are more likely to have another unrecognized infarct (rather than a symptomatic one) is not clear from present data.

Table 13.6. Episodes of silent myocardial ischaemia over a 48-hour period

Episodes (day-event)	Max ST ↓ (mm)	HR at Onset of ST ↓ (beats/min)	Duration (min)
1–1	1.5	90	4
1–2	1	105	5
1–3	1	110	4
1–4	3	110	5
1–5	3	90	4
1–6	2.5	105	8
1–7	1	100	4
1–8	3	115	3
1–9	3	110	3
1–10	4	120	12
2–1	1	110	6
2–2	4.5	105	23
2–3	4.5	110	15
2–4	2.5	95	4
2–5	1	100	4
2–6	1	110	6
2–7	3	110	10
Mean ± SD	2.4 ± 1.2	105 ± 7.7	7.0 ± 5.5

Source: P. F. Cohn, *et al.* J Am Coll Cardiol 1986; 8:982. Reproduced with permission.

Treatment

Theoretically, there should be no difference in treatment between painful and occult myocardial infarctions except for the use of analgesics. However, in practice, by the time it is realized that an occult infarct has occurred, most of the usual measures that we employ for an acute event (thrombolytic therapy, anti-arrhythmic therapy, etc.) are no longer appropriate. If the infarct is recognized early enough in the recovery period (within 21 days), then beta-blockers should be utilized prophylactically as they are in patients with symptomatic infarctions.

Risk factor modification should also be employed and periodic exercise tests used to document recurrent ischaemia. This in turn will dictate therapy with anti-ischaemic agents or the need for coronary angiography.

Conclusions

It is apparent from both historical data, on-going epidemiologic studies and evidence from recent Holter monitoring studies that occult myocardial infarctions are real events and are not uncommon. About 25% of transmural (Q-wave) myocardial infarctions are unrecognized at time of their occurrence. Aside from the possible presence of a visceral neuropathy in diabetics, no plausible explanation for the lack of pain has been offerred. Prognosis after these events appears to be the same as that following a symptomatic infarction. With the increasing use of Holter monitoring, it can be expected that more evolving infarctions (both Q-wave and non-Q-wave) will be documented as they occur. This should prove invaluable in increasing our knowledge of this puzzling, and ubiquitous, phenomenon.

References

1. Herrick J B. Clinical features of sudden obstruction of the coronary arteries. JAMA 1912; 59:2015.
2. Kennedy J A. The incidence of myocardial infarction without pain in autopsied cases. Am Heart J 1937; 14:703.
3. Boyde L D and Weblow S C. Coronary thrombosis without pain. Am J Med Sci 1937; 194:814.
4. Gorham L E and Martin S J. Coronary artery occulsion with and without pain. Arch Intern Med 1938; 112:812.
5. Stroud W D and Wagner J A. Silent or atypical coronary occlusion. Ann Intern Med 1941; 15:25.
6. Roseman M D. Painless myocardial infarction: A review of the literature and analysis of 220 cases. Ann Intern Med 1954; 41:1.

7. Kannel W B, McNamara P M, Feinleib M *et al.* The unrecognized myocardial infarction: 14 year follow-up experience in the Framingham study. Geriatrics 1970, 25:75.
8. Margolis J R, Kannel W B, Feinleib M *et al.* Clinical features of unrecognized myocardial infarction: 18 year follow-up: The Framingham study. Am J Cardiol 1973; 32:1.
9. Kannel W B and Abbott R D. Incidence and prognosis of unrecognized myocardial infarction. Based on 26 years follow-up on the Framingham study. In: Silent Myocardial Ischaemia, Rutishauser W. and Roskamm H., eds., Berlin: Springer-Verlag, 1984, p. 131.
10. Kannel W B. Silent myocardial ischaemia and infarction: Insights from the Framingham Study. Cardiol Clin 1986; 4:583.
11. Vokonas, P S, Kannel W B, and Cupples L A. Incidence and prognosis of unrecognized myocardial infarction in the elderly, The Framingham Study. J Am Coll Cardiol 1988; 11:51A.
12. Grimm R H, Jr., Tillinghast S, Daniels K, Neaton J D, Mascoli S, Crow R, Pritzker, M, Prineas R J. Unrecognized myocardial infarction: Experience in the Multiple Risk Factor Intervention Trial (MRFIT). Circulation, 1987; 75(Suppl II):6.
13. Rosenman R H, Friedman M, Jenkins C D *et al.* Clinically unrecognized infarction in the Western Collaborative Study. Am J Cardiol 1967; 19:776.
14. Medalie J H and Goldbourt U. Unrecognized myocardial infarction: Five-year incidence, mortality, and risk factors. Ann Intern Med 1976; 84:526.
15. Kannel W B, Dannenberg A L, and Abbott R D. Unrecognized myocardial infarction and hypertension. The Framingham Study. Am Heart J 1985; 109:581.
16. Aronow W S, Starling L, Etienne F, D'Alba P, Edward M, Lee N H and Parungao R F. Unrecognized Q-wave myocardial infarction in patients older than 64 years in a long-term health-care facility. Am J Cardiol 1985; 56:483.
17. Aronow W S. Prevalence of presenting symptoms of recognized acute myocardial infarction and of unrecognized healed myocardial infarction in elderly patients. Am J Cardiol 1987; 60:1182.
18. Brush J E, Cabin H S, Wohlgelernter D, Hammond G L, and Cohen L S. Ventricular septal rupture following a clinically unrecognized myocardial infarction. Am Heart J 1985; 110:667.
19. Raper A J, Hastillo A, and Paulsen W J. The syndrome of sudden severe painless myocardial ischaemia. Am Heart J 1984; 197:813.
20. Cabin H S and Roberts W C. Quantitative comparison of extent of coronary narrowing and size of healed myocardial infarct in 33 necropsy patients with clinically recognized and in 28 with clinical unrecognized ('silent') previous acute myocardial infarction. Am J Cardiol 1982; 59:677.
21. Procacci P, Zoppi M, Padeletti L, and Maresca M. Myocardial infarction without pain. A study of the sensory function of the upper limbs. Pain 1976; 2:309.
22. Bradley R F and Schonfeld A. Diminished pain in diabetic patients with myocardial infarction. Geriatrics 1962; 17:322.
23. Faerman I, Faccio E, Milei J, Nunez R, Jadzinsky M, Fox D, and Rapaport M. Autonomic neuropathy and painless myocardial infarction in diabetic patients: Histologic evidence of their relationship. Diabetics 1977; 26:1147.
24. Aronow W S. New coronary events at four-year follow-up in elderly patients with recognized or unrecognized myocardial infarction. Am J Cardiol 1989; 63:621.
25. Cohn P F, Sodums M T, Lawson W E, Vlay S C, and Brown, E J Jr. Frequent episodes of silent myocardial ischaemia after apparently uncomplicated myocardial infarction. J Am Coll Cardiol 1986; 8:982.
26. Hands M E, Sia S T B, Shook T L, Anderson K, Stone P H, Levy D, Castelli W P, Rutherford J D, and the Framingham Heart Study Group. Silent myocardial ischaemia in asymptomatic survivors of unrecognized myocardial infarction and matched controls. Am Heart J 1988; 116:1488.

PART FOUR

Occult atherosclerotic disease of the aorta and arteries of the lower limbs

14. Epidemiology of occult atherosclerosis in the lower limbs

F. GERRY R. FOWKES

During the last thirty years epidemiological research into atherosclerotic disease has concentrated on coronary artery disease and stroke because of their high mortality and morbility. Consequently peripheral atherosclerosis affecting the lower limbs has been overshadowed and largely ignored for epidemiological study. Most epidemiological research into peripheral arterial disease has been simply an adjunct to major studies of coronary artery disease in which questions on intermittent claudication have been included in cardiovascular questionnaires. Unfortunately very few studies have attempted to employ non-invasive measurement techniques used commonly in clinical practice to diagnose peripheral arterial disease. This is particularly disappointing as the arteries in the lower limb are relatively accessible to non-invasive measurement and offer considerable potential for the study of asymptomatic disease. Knowledge of the epidemiology of occult atherosclerosis in the lower limbs is thus somewhat limited due to the dearth of studies in this field.

What is occult atherosclerotic disease of the lower limbs? In western countries almost every adult has pathological evidence of atherosclerosis affecting their peripheral arteries, and so it is difficult to classify individuals meaningfully as simply diseased or non-diseased on the basis of pathological findings. A description of disease based on the degree of atherosclerosis is more appropriate. Angiography has traditionally been used as the best method of assessing this in living subjects, but such a hazardous investigation cannot be used ethically to study asymptomatic subjects. Recent innovations in non-invasive imaging techniques, such as duplex scanning, have not been assessed adequately as to their value in measuring the extent of disease. Thus, measurement of occult disease, at least in living subjects, must rely on indirect non-invasive measures of the effects of disease. This then has a bearing on how we define occult disease, at least for the purposes of epidemiological research [1]. In practice, significant occult atherosclerosis is

A.-M. Salmasi and A. N. Nicolaides (eds.), Occult Atherosclerotic Disease, 185–204.

usually considered to be present when there is a measurable disruption to blood flow without clinical symptoms.

Epidemiological measurement

In asymptomatic individuals, the presence of significant occult atherosclerosis in the lower limbs can be assessed by palpation of peripheral pulses, measurement of the ankle brachial systolic pressure ratio, and stress tests such as measurement of the ankle pressure after exercise or during reactive hyperaemia. Autopsy studies may also be useful. Each of these techniques however has limitations in the assessment of occult disease.

Palpation of peripheral pulses

In around 20 per cent of the adult population, at least one pulse is not detected when the femoral, posterior tibial and dorsalis pedis arteries are palpated [2, 3]. This is due not only to arterial disease but to obesity and other factors making detection difficult. Also, the dorsalis pedis artery is congenitally absent in four to twelve percent of the population; the posterior tibial artery on the other hand in invariably present [4, 5]. Despite these findings, palpation of the peripheral pulses is reasonably specific in only identifying significant disease, but the sensitivity (that is, the ability to detect cases) is quite poor. When evaluated against other measures of peripheral arterial disease, such as ankle brachial systolic pressure ratios, an absent pulse in one or more arteries was found in one study to be only 48% sensitive and 96% specific [2]. In another study diminished or absent pulses were found to be 77% sensitive and 86% specific [3]. As might be expected, considerable inter- and intra-observer variability occurs in the detection of pulses [6, 7]. Furthermore, palpation of the peripheral pulses does not easily allow a graded response but simply an indication of a pulse present or absent, so that its usefulness in measuring the extent of occult disease is severely limited.

Ankle brachial systolic pressure ratio

The results of studies based on small numbers of subjects have suggested that an ankle brachial systolic pressure ratio of less than 0.9 is up to 95% sensitive in detecting angiogram positive disease and a ratio of 0.9 or higher is almost 100% specific in identifying supposedly healthy subjects [8–11]. Also, the magnitude of this ratio (the ankle brachial pressure index) would appear to correlate with the severity of disease [10, 12]. However these studies have mostly used selected hospital patients who were symptomatic.

Table 14.1. 95% Confidence limits of brachial and ankle systolic pressures and ankle brachial ratios measured under given conditions

	Brachial systolic pressure (± mmHg)		Ankle systolic pressure (± mmHg)		Ankle brachial ratio (± %)	
Mean of:	Normals	Diseased	Normals	Diseased	Normals	Diseased
One observer, one measurement	14.0	23.8	15.7	25.8	16.4	16.9
One observer, two repeat measurements	12.5	22.9	14.0	25.0	14.4	16.0
Two observers, one measurement each (same day)	10.7	18.4	12.5	22.0	12.1	13.6
Two observers, two measurements each (all on same day)	9.7	17.8	11.5	21.5	10.8	13.0
Two observers, two measurements each (one on one day and another on a different day)	8.9	16.2	9.9	17.6	10.2	11.3

Reprinted with permission from Fowkes *et al.*, J Epidem and Comm Health [13].

It is not known how ratios in the general population would correlate with the extent of occult peripheral arterial disease, but it is likely that the results among those with severe occult disease would be similar to those found in hospital patients. Also the distribution of the ratio in a population should give some indication of the occurrence of disease although the significance of a value in an individual subject must be open to doubt.

The variability in measuring ankle pressure has been examined in a few studies. In one study which we conducted in Edinburgh, 36 subjects had repeat measurements taken by four observers on two separate days using a Doppler probe and random zero sphygmomanometer [13]. The 95% confidence limits of one measurement of the ankle brachial ratio was estimated to be ± 16%, reducing to ± 10% for the mean of four measurements by two observers on two days (Table 14.1). Analysis of variance indicated that the variability in the measurement of ankle brachial ratios attributable to observers, different days, timing of measurements on the same day, and repeat measurements was considerably less than the 'biological' variability between subjects and between legs. This suggests that the ankle brachial systolic pressure ratio is a useful measure in assessing the epidemiology of occult disease, but does not negate the caution which must be exercised in using the ratio as a measure of disease in an individual subject.

Stress tests

In some patients known to have significant peripheral arterial disease, blood flows and pressures may be normal at rest but may become abnormal after exercise or an equivalent stress such as that caused by obstructing blood flow (reactive hyperaemia test).

A standard amount of exercise in patients with peripheral arterial disease demonstrated by angiography will produce a significantly greater fall in ankle pressure and longer recovery time than in normal subjects [11, 14–16]. Also, in these patients the reduction in ankle systolic pressure is related to the severity of disease [17]. However, it is not known the extent to which an exercise test when used in an epidemiological study in the general population would improve the detection of occult disease. In one small study, Carter conducted an exercise test on 18 patients with 'questionable' peripheral arterial disease and found that 11 patients had a fall in pressure equivalent to patients with known mild peripheral arterial disease suggesting that the exercise test was detecting disease in individuals who on other grounds might be classified as normal [14].

In a typical reactive hyperaemia test, blood flow is occluded at the upper thigh or above the knee, and the ankle systolic pressure measured on releasing the obstruction. The systolic pressure in patients with peripheral arterial disease is reduced two to three times further and takes longer to return to pre-occlusion levels than in healthy subjects [18–20]. However, as with an exercise test, the extent to which a reactive hyperaemia test improves diagnostic sensitivity of occult disease in the general population is not clearly known. In one study on hospital patients in which reactive hyperaemia and exercise tests were compared, reactive hyperaemia was marginally less sensitive but this may have been because the patients in each group were not strictly comparable [21]. When a reactive hyperaemia test was used in combination with other non-invasive tests on one population which included a high proportion of subjects with hyperlipidaemia, an additional 16% of subjects (who had normal ankle pressures at rest) had results which would be considered abnormal in clinical patients [22]. Thus it is likely that the reactive hyperaemia test may be useful in detecting significant occult disease. The variability of the reactive hyperaemia test has been shown to be comparable to resting ankle brachial systolic ratios [23].

Duplex ultra sound scanning

The more sophisticated non invasive tests which have been developed in recent years for the assessment of peripheral arterial disease in clinical practice include Doppler wave form analysis, Duplex ultrasound scanning and nuclear magnetic resonance. Duplex scanning offers considerable potential to visualise peripheral vessels by means of pulse echo imaging and to simultaneously measure blood flow by means of Doppler wave form analysis. This is being used with some success in assessment of carotid artery stenosis, but has proved difficult in assessing disease of the lower limbs because of the more diffuse nature of the atherosclerotic lesions [24]. In Edinburgh, we are currently examining the validity and reliability of this technique, and are hopeful that it may prove to be a useful tool in the assessment of occult disease.

Incidence and prevalence

Autopsy atherosclerosis

A systematic revue of autopsies is a relatively simple method of obtaining information on the prevalence of atherosclerosis but may be limited in the assessment of occult disease because there may be no information on whether the subjects had symptoms. Also subjects coming to post mortem are often a highly selected group and not typical of the population as a whole. Unfortunately, very few autopsy studies of atherosclerosis have included an examination of the peripheral arteries, and those that have done so have limited their observations to specific sites in the arterial tree.

However, in a study of 293 unselected adult necropsy cases in Oxford, Mitchell and Schwartz examined the iliac arteries and found that severe atherosclerosis was common [25]. In about half the common iliac arteries, more than 50% of the surface was affected by lesions. Fifteen per cent of men and 5% of women had severe disease resulting in stenosis of more than half the diameter of at least one artery. None of the men and only one woman were free of atherosclerotic plaques in their common iliac arteries. The internal iliac arteries were usually affected to a similar extent as the common iliac arteries, but the external iliac arteries were less severely affected. A comparable study of 500 consecutive adults who had died in a general hospital in Pittsburg also found that the iliac arteries were invariably affected by atherosclerosis [26]. Among subjects who had not died of an 'atherosclerotic catastrophy', atherosclerosis in the common iliac arteries, which was graded according to the percentage of the surface area affected and the severity of lesions at the worst site, was as extensive as disease elsewhere in the vascular tree.

In Malmo, Sweden, an autopsy study of 1486 subjects aged between 30–79 years, which included 66% of all deaths in the city, found similar results to those in Oxford and Pittsburg [27]. But in this study the disease was generally more severe in the right than left common iliac arteries suggesting that haemodynamic factors may be important in pathogenesis, particularly as the femoral arteries were equally affected. As expected, the degree of atherosclerosis increased with age and was greater in males than females, but not significantly so after 70 years of age. Although no information is provided in these surveys of the proportion of subjects that were symptomatic, numerous cardiovascular surveys examining the prevalence of intermittent claudication during the last 25 years [28] have shown a prevalence ranging from 0.3% (among 40–59 year old male telephone employees in the United States) [29] to 7.7% (among 55–74 year old men in rural Finland) [30]. These rates are much lower than disease rates detected at post mortem; thus many subjects with substantial atherosclerosis at post mortem would undoubtedly have had occult disease.

Non-invasive measurement of populations

Non-invasive measures of haemodynamic disturbance due to peripheral arterial disease have not been used widely in epidemiological surveys. In a major study in Basle, analysis of pulse wave forms identified on oscillography was included as a screening test for the disruption of peripheral blood flow [31]. Among men the prevalence of occlusion, confirmed by arteriography, increased from 0.4% at age 20–24 years to 7.5% at age 60–64 years. Among women, occlusion occurred rarely at younger ages, but over 50 years of age the prevalence was about half that occurring in men. In Glostrup,

Denmark, a population survey of 60 year old people born in 1914 found that 14% had peripheral arterial disease manifest by an ankle brachial pressure ratio of <0.9 [2]. In a recent study in the United States using a combination of non-invasive tests which included systolic blood pressures, arterial wave forms, and a reactive hyperaemia test, the prevalence of large vessel disease increased progressively with age from 3% at less than 60 years of age to more than 20% at age 75 years and older [22].

In the Edinburgh Artery Study, ankle brachial systolic pressure ratios were measured in a random sample of 1592 men and women aged 55–74 years. Preliminary results indicate that the ankle brachial systolic pressure ratio (minimum in right or left leg) was distributed normally around a mean of 1.03. The cummulative percentage distribution showed that 6% had a ratio of <0.7, 9% had ratio of <0.8 and 18% had ratio of <0.9. Thus, on the basis of a single ankle brachial pressure ratio, a large percentage of the population would theoretically have disease if the convential clinical level of 0.9 were accepted as the cut off point between normality and abnormality. About 4.6% had intermittent claudication and, as shown in Figure 14.1, many of these subjects had a low ankle brachial pressure ratio (<.85). However, 7.6% had a low ratio and no symptoms suggesting that for every subject with intermittent claudication, there may be about two subjects with atherosclerosis severe enough to cause a disruption to resting blood flow.

In addition to the measurement of resting ankle brachial ratios, most subjects in the Edinburgh Artery Study had a reactive hyperaemia test performed on each leg. Arterial blood flow was occluded above the knee at 50 mm Hg above systolic pressure for four minutes using a sphygmomanometer cuff. Fifteen seconds after releasing the obstruction, ankle systolic pressure was measured using a random zero sphygmomanometer and

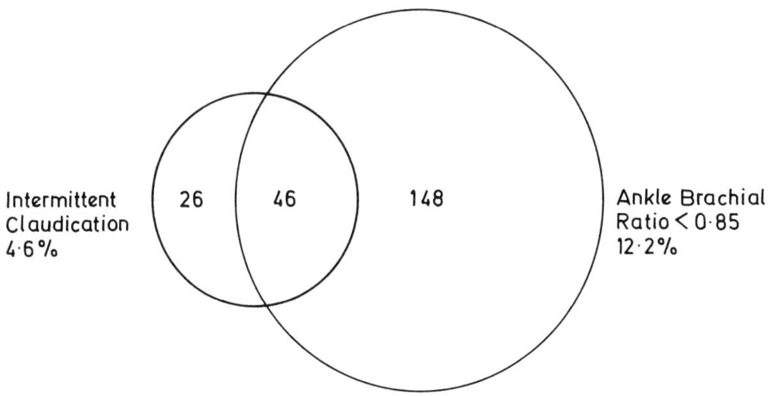

Figure 14.1. Edinburgh Artery Study: Prevalence of intermittent claudication and low ankle brachial systolic pressure ratio.

Table 14.2. Prevalence of 'occult' peripheral arterial disease in population surveys

Study Location	Author	Year	Population	Prevalence of Peripheral Arterial Disease (%) Intermittent Claudication (%)	'Occult' disease[a] (%)
Belgium	De Backer *et al.* [32]	1979	Men 40–59 yrs	1.4	4.3
Glostrup,	Schroll & Munck [2]	1981	Men 60 yrs	5.8	)
Denmark			Women	1.3	)10.5
Lipid Research	Criqui *et al.* [22]	1985	Men 38–82 yrs	2.2	)
Clinics, USA			Women	1.7	) 9.0
Edinburgh, UK	Fowkes *et al.*	1989	Men 55–74 yrs	4.4	)
	(unpublished)		Women	4.7	) 7.6

[a] 'Occult' disease is defined as an abnormal ankle brachial ratio and/or abnormalities of flow velocity as stated in each study and excludes those with symptoms of peripheral arterial disease.

Doppler probe. Preliminary results in the first 822 subjects participating in the study showed that 56 subjects (7%) had a normal pre-occlusion ankle brachial ratio of ≥ 0.8 and a low post occlusion ratio of < 0.8. Although further analysis is required on the whole population, examining in particular the reduction in pressure during hyperaemia, these 56 subjects had a high prevalence of other cardiovascular diseases suggesting that the reactive hyperaemia test was indeed detecting additional occult disease in a small percentage of the population.

Table 14.2 summarises the results of four population based studies which have examined both intermittant claudication and occult disease by means of Doppler pressure and flow analysis. The results vary because of the differing age, sex, and nationalities of the populations and definitions of 'occult disease'. Despite these limitations, a reasonably consistent picture emerges with about two to four times the number of symptomatic subjects having occult disease. The prevalence of occult disease might indeed have been greater if stress tests, such as an exercise or reactive hyperaemia test, had been applied to each population.

The incidence of disease detected by non-invasive procedures shows similar age and sex patterns to prevalence. In the Basle Study, the 5-year cummulative incidence of occlusive disease was 4% in men aged 35–44 years and 18% in those 65 years and over [33]. Of these subjects, approximately one-third developed intermittent claudication and more than two-thirds acquired haemodynamic abnormalities detected on non-invasive testing.

Aetiology

Smoking

Knowledge about the aetiology of occult peripheral atherosclerosis is hampered by the lack of studies examining asymptomatic subjects. However, there are a few studies which have examined the relationship between risk factors and non-invasive measures of disease. These, in combination with studies examining claudication in the general population (indicating bias towards milder forms of disease than in hospital studies) should give some indication about the aetiology of occult disease.

Smoking is undoubtedly an important risk factor for peripheral atherosclerosis. Among patients attending out-patient clinics or requiring vascular surgery, 90–100% were current or recent smokers [34, 36]. These patients, however, were at the severe end of the spectrum of disease. Cross-sectional studies in the general population of patients with intermittent claudication have provided somewhat different estimates of the overall risks. Table 14.3

Table 14.3. Risks associated with cigarette smoking in population studies of peripheral arterial disease.

Author	Location	Study population	Definition of smoker	Relative risk of smoking	Population attributable fraction: Due to smokers	Population attributable fraction: Due to smokers & ex-smokers
Higgins & Kjelsberg (1967) [37]	Tecumseh, Michigan	Men 20–79 yrs	Current smoker	1.9	53%	59%
Kannel & Shurtleff (1973) [38]	Framingham	Men 35–62 yrs Women 35–62 yrs	Smoker at date of entry	2.9[a]	78%	—
Bothig *et al.* (1976) [39]	Moscow & Berlin	Men 50–54 yrs	10 + cigarettes per day	1.4[a]	18%	—
Heliovaara *et al.* (1978) [30]	Rural Finland	Men 55–74 yrs	1 + cigarettes per day	7.4	36%	76%
Hughson *et al.* (1978) [40]	Oxford	Men 45–69 yrs Women 50–69 yrs	1 + cigarettes per day	7.5	39%	42%
De Backer *et al.* (1979) [32]	Belgium	Men 40–45 yrs	Current smoker	1.4	14%	22%
Reunanen *et al.* (1982) [41]	Finland	Men 30–59 yrs	Current smoker	1.7[a]	30%	—

[a] Relative risk of smoker v non-smoker and ex-smoker

NB All studies are cross-sectional except the Framingham Study.

Reprinted with permission from Fowkes, Eu J Vasc Surg [28]

shows that the relative risk of peripheral arterial disease in smokers compared to non-smokers ranged from 1.4 to 7.5. Despite the considerable variation in results, these studies indicate the substantial risks associated with smoking, but also that many cases were not related to smoking. It may be that the influence of smoking is not so important with less severe forms of disease. The results of studies examining occult atherosclerosis, however, suggest that smoking is still a major risk factor [2, 32]. In the Danish study of ankle blood pressure measurements in a population of 60 year old men and women, smoking habits were related both cross-sectionally and longitudinally to the ankle arm systolic pressure ratio [2]. In a major cardiovascular survey in Belgium, the proportion of current smokers in those with an ankle arm ratio <0.9 was slightly, but not significantly, higher than those with a ratio >1.0 [32].

Preliminary results on the smoking habits of the first 931 subjects of the Edinburgh Artery Study are shown in Table 14.4. As expected, more subjects with intermittent claudication and occult disease (defined as an ankle brachial ratio of <0.9) had smoked compared to normal subjects. But in keeping with other population based studies [30, 32, 37–41] and in contrast to most hospital based studies [34–36], a sizeable proportion of those with both overt and occult disease had never smoked. More subjects with occult disease were current cigarette smokers than those with intermittent claudication. Indeed, current levels of cigarette smoking among those with intermittent claudication were similar to those without peripheral arterial disease; one interpretation is that many with overt disease had given up cigarettes for a pipe or cigars, in contrast to those with occult disease who may have had no medical advice to stop smoking.

Table 14.4. Edinburgh Artery Study: Smoking in Sub-sample of 931 Subjects according to Intermittent Claudication and low ankle brachial systolic pressure ratio

	Smoking habits (% subjects)				
Peripheral Arterial Disease	Current cigarette	Current pipe or cigars	Ex-cigarette	Never smoked	Total
Intermittent Claudication	19	16	35	29	100
Ankle brachial ratio <0.9	35	8	33	24	100
None	18	13	28	41	100

Blood pressure

The importance of blood pressure as a risk factor for lower limb arterial disease has been examined in several studies in the general population.

Cross-sectional studies have demonstrated associations with systolic and diastolic pressure [40, 42] and with only systolic pressure [2, 32, 43]. Others have produced conflicting results [39] or shown no association [41]. Likewise longitudinal studies have not produced consistent findings. In the Framingham study, hypertension imposed a three-fold increased risk of intermittent claudication at 26 years of follow-up; systolic pressure was more closely related to the level of risk than diastolic pressure [44]. The follow-up study in Denmark of 50 year old men and women showed significant correlations between initial systolic and diastolic pressures and occult disease as measured by ankle brachial pressure induced 10 years later [2]. In the longitudinal study in Basle, however, systolic blood pressure was not independently related to the development of intermittent claudication [45]. In many of these studies, the methods of measuring blood pressure and defining hypertension were not adequately reported and some results may have been prone to considerable bias. Nevertheless, the evidence on balance would indicate that blood pressure, and particularly systolic pressure, may be an independent risk factor for the development of both symptomatic and occult peripheral arterial disease.

Glucose intolerance

Clinicians have known for many years that patients with diabetes mellitus are at particularly high risk of developing peripheral arterial disease [46]. But the extent to which impaired glucose intolerance in the general population is a risk factor for occult or symptomatic peripheral arterial disease is less obvious. In a cross-sectional study in Moscow and Berlin, impaired glucose tolerance occurred more commonly in individuals who had intermittent claudication than in those who did not [39]. At 16 years of follow up in the Framingham study, the age adjusted incidence of intermittent claudication in diabetics was 4.5 times that in non-diabetics with no significant differences between males and females [47]. This risk was maintained during subsequent years: at 26 years of follow-up every indicator of impaired glucose tolerance, including elevated casual blood glucose or glycosuria, was associated with an increased risk [44]. Also, blood glucose had an independent effect when other risk factors were taken into account.

Conflicting results, however, have been obtained in other population studies. In Oxford, Hughson *et al.* [40] found that individuals with intermittent claudication did not have a higher fasting blood glucose than controls. In Finland, the prevalence of intermittent claudication in a population of 11,000 was not related to blood glucose measured after an 'oral glucose load' [41]. Similar results have been obtained in the Basle and Danish longitudinal studies. Indeed, in the Basle study, an inverse association was found between the degree of glucose intolerance (fasting blood glucose or two hours after oral load) and the occurrence of disease [45]. In the Danish study initial fasting blood glucose levels did not correlate with later ankle-brachial pressure indices(2). Thus there is no clear evidence of a relationship between glucose intolerance and occult atherosclerosis in the general population.

Lipids

Serum levels of cholesterol and triglycerides and peripheral arterial disease have been examined in over 20 clinical and epidemiological studies. In all but one study, serum triglycerides were found to be higher in cases than in controls. However, relationships with other risk factors have often not been considered and, as is the case with ischaemic heart disease, the risks associated with an elevated triglyceride might well disappear. Indeed, in the Danish study a significant univariate inverse association was noted between the fasting serum triglyceride and the ankle brachial ratio both cross-sectionally and longitudinally [2]. But on multivariate analysis, serum triglyceride was not significantly associated longitudinally with the ankle brachial ratio.

Cross-sectional studies in the community examining total serum cholesterol and peripheral arterial disease have produced variable results. Significant elevations of serum cholesterol were found in cases in Finland [41] and Denmark [2], but not in Sweden [43], Belgium [32] or Oxford [40]. Positive associations have however been found in the two longitudinal studies relating serum cholesterol at entry to later occurrence of peripheral arterial disease. Serum cholesterol was found to be a significant, but weak risk factor for intermittent claudication after 26 years of follow-up in Framingham [44]. Similarly, in the Danish study examining occult disease, serum cholesterol at age 50 years was found to correlate with ankle brachial pressure indices 10 years later and to be independently related [2]. This latter relationship persisted on multivariate analysis, suggesting that serum cholesterol is indeed a risk factor for occult peripheral atherosclerosis. Preliminary analysis of data on 1592 subjects in the Edinburgh Artery Study also confirms this relationship. Figure 14.2 shows the univariate relationship between total serum cholesterol and ankle brachial ratio.

The relationship between HDL cholesterol and peripheral arterial disease has not been widely investigated. In two studies lower mean levels were found in cases than controls [48, 49] but in another, this difference occurred only in men and not women [50]. A third study found no difference between

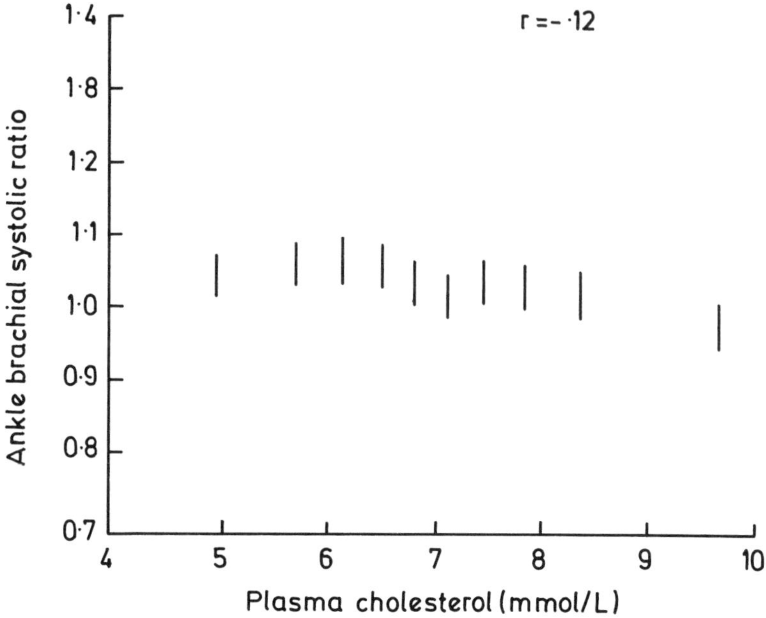

Figure 14.2 Edinburgh Artery Study: 95% confidence limits of ankle brachial systolic pressure ratio by total plasma cholesterol.

cases and controls [51] except that the HDL ratio of HDL cholesterol ÷ (total-HDL cholesterol) was significantly reduced in both males and females. Low HDL cholesterol may well be a risk factor for peripheral arterial disease, but it has not been investigated in a community based study, nor in the longitudinal studies in Framingham [44] Basle [45] and Denmark [2].

There is some suggestion that apolipoprotein rather than lipid or lipoprotein levels may be a better discriminator of cases of peripheral arterial disease and normal subjects [52]. Apolipoprotein B levels in very low density lipoprotein (VLDL) and low density lipoprotein (LDL) have been shown to be higher in hospital cases than controls [53, 54], but this was not confirmed in another study [55], and has not been tested in the community.

Haemostatic factors

In recent years, attention has been given to the role of haemostatic factors, particularly serum fibrinogen, in the aetiology and pathogenesis of peripheral arterial disease (and other atherosclerotic diseases). In a random sample of the general population in Oxford, Hughson *et al.* [40] found a significantly higher plasma fibrinogen level in subjects with intermittent claudication than in an age and sex matched control group ($p<0.001$). Raised fibrinogen levels might however have been due to increased smoking among diseased subjects [56, 57]. Higher fibrinogen levels have been shown to be predictive of occlusion occurring in peripheral arterial grafts [58, 59] but the relationship between fibrinogen levels and incidence of peripheral arterial disease, whether overt or occult, has not been investigated in longitudinal studies.

Serum uric acid has also been studied as a potential risk factor since hyperuricaemia may increase platelet aggregability [60]. In the Oxford study [40] a level greater than 0.36 m.mol per litre was associated with a relative risk of intermittent claudication of 2.6 (95% confidence limits of 1.3–5.3). But this association was not confirmed for occult disease in the Danish longitudinal study in which the serum uric acid at age 50 years did not correlate with ankle brachial pressure ratios 10 years later [2].

In the Framingham study, raised haematocrit was not associated with a greater risk of intermittent claudication [44], although hospital studies have shown patients to have higher haematocrits than controls [56, 61] and haematocrit has been shown to be predictive of future occlusion of peripheral arterial grafts [62]. However, some of these differences may well be due to an association between smoking and haematocrit levels [56, 57].

Blood viscosity has likewise been shown to be higher in subjects with intermittent claudication than controls [56, 63, 64] but, as with haematocrit and fibrinogen, the association can be attributed to differences in smoking levels [56, 57]. Also, blood viscosity is related to haematocrit, fibrinogen and other possible risk factors for peripheral arterial disease such as age, male sex, blood pressure, hyperlipidaemia, and diabetes [65].

There have been a few studies examining coagulation factors such as factors VII, VIII and antithrombin III, but to date these have provided variable results. Clearly, further research is required to elucidate the role of haemostatic factors in the pathogenesis of peripheral arterial disease, paying particular attention to the inter-relationship between factors, to the influence of other risk factors such as smoking, and to determining the extent to which elevated levels are the cause or effects of disease, or both.

Prognosis

Although there have been many studies examining the prognosis of intermittent claudication, the natural history of occult atherosclerosis is not clearly known. It can be assumed that many subjects with atherosclerosis severe enough to cause a disruption to peripheral blood flow will progress to symptomatic disease, but the rate of progression and annual incidence is unknown.

It might be expected that individuals with occult atherosclerosis would have a worse prognosis than a comparable healthy population since there is some evidence that those with occult disease have a relatively high prevalence of coronary artery disease. In the Edinburgh Artery Study we found that subjects with a low ankle brachial ratio had a higher prevalence of angina and of occult coronary artery disease as measured by resting ECG, compared to those with normal ankle brachial ratios. Table 14.5 for example, shows some preliminary results indicating that higher proportions of subjects with ankle brachial ratios <0.9 had a history or ECG evidence of coronary artery disease than those with higher ratios. It would thus be expected that those subjects with occult atherosclerosis would be at a higher risk of having a myocardial infarction or cardiovascular death in the future. In the cohort phase of the Edinburgh Artery Study we are following up this population to determine these risks more precisely.

Table 14.5. Edinburgh Artery Study: History or ECG evidence of coronary artery disease according to ankle brachial systolic pressure ratio

		Coronary Artery Disease	
		History	ECG ischaemia (no history)
Ankle Brachial Systolic Ratio	<0.9 (*n*=289)	86 (30%)	63 (22%)
	≥0.9 (*n*=1292)	277 (21%)	171 (13%)
Intermittent Claudication	(*n*=73)	38 (52%)	13 (18%)

Follow-up studies of intermittent claudication in the community can provide some insights into the likely progress of occult disease, at least in terms of mortality. There have been four such population studies: Framingham [38, 44], Basle [66], London Whitehall [67], and in Finland [41]. Five year cumulative mortality rates ranged from 4.8% [67] to 17% [38]. Ischaemic heart disease is the commonest cause of mortality contributing to around 50% of deaths [66, 68]. Cerebrovascular disease causes about 10% and other vascular diseases about 8% of deaths [66, 68]. Very few deaths are due directly to peripheral arterial disease except for the high operative mortality associated with amputations. Population follow-up studies have shown that the relative risk of death from ischaemic heart disease is approximately three times that in comparable populations without intermittent claudication [41, 67, 69]. In patients with occult peripheral atherosclerosis the relative risks are probably not as high as for subjects with intermittent claudication – preliminary data from the Edinburgh Artery Study (Table 14.5) suggests that subjects with intermittent claudication have more evidence of coronary artery disease than those with only a low ankle brachial ratio.

Survival is adversely affected by the presence of coronary or cerebrovascular disease [40, 41, 44]. Indeed in the Framingham study, survival rates in subjects with intermittent claudication and no evidence of coronary or cerebrovascular disease were similar to the general population free of these cardiovascular impairments [38]. Multiple logistic analysis of prognostic factors on death in the Finnish study suggested that most, but not all, of the excess mortality in subjects with intermittent claudication was due to other concomitant cardiovascular disease [41].

Certain prognostic factors have been associated with increased mortality, for example, cigarette smoking [40, 41, 66] blood pressure [41, 66, 70] serum cholesterol [41] and diabetes mellitus [66]. There is little doubt that smoking has a profound prognostic effect with relative risks of between 1.5 and 3.0 for smokers compared to non-smokers [41, 66], and improved survival among subjects who stop smoking [71]. But, increased risks have not been found to be universally associated with blood pressure [40] serum cholesterol [71] and diabetes mellitus [40, 70]. These conflicting results may have arisen because not all studies attempted to analyse the independent effects of prognostic factors on mortality. There is no reason to believe, however, that these factors do not also have an influence on the prognosis of occult disease. Indeed one of the great merits of studying occult disease in the lower limbs is that it may help us to identify, in combination with other risk factors, those who are apparently healthy, but who are at particularly high risk of sustaining a major cardiovascular event in the future.

References

1. Fowkes FGR. The measurement of atherosclerotic peripheral arterial disease in epidemiological surveys. Int J Epidemiol 1988; 17:248.
2. Schroll M, Munck O. Estimation of peripheral arteriosclerotic disease by ankle blood pressure measurements in a population study of 60 year old men and women. J Chron Dis 1981; 34:261.
3. Criqui MH, Fronek A, Klauber MR, Barrett-Conner E, Gabriel S. The sensitivity, specificity and predictive value of traditional clinical evaluation of peripheral arterial disease: results from noninvasive testing in a defined population. Circulation 1985; 71:516.
4. Barnhorst DA, Barner HB. Prevalence of congenitally absent pedal pulses. N Eng J Med 1968; 278:264.
5. Ison JW. Palpation of dorsals pedis pulse. JAMA 1968; 206:2745.
6. Ludbrook J, Clarke AM, McKenzie JK. Significance of absent ankle pulse. Br Med J 1962; 1:1724.
7. Meade TW, Gardner MJ, Cannon P *et al.* Observer variability in reading the peripheral pulses. Br Heart J 1968; 30:661.
8. Winsor T. Influence of arterial disease on the systolic blood pressure gradients of the extremity. Am J Med Sci 1950; 220:117.
9. Yao ST. New techniques of objective arterial evaluation. Arch Surg 1973; 106:600.

10. Bernstein E F, Fronek A. Current status of noninvasive tests in the diagnosis of peripheral arterial disease. Surg Clin North Am 1982; 62:473.
11. Laing S, Greenhalgh R M. The detection and progression of asymptomatic peripheral arterial disease. Br J Surg 1983; 70:628.
12. Chamberlain J, Housley E, Macpherson A I S. The relationship between ultrasound assessment and angiography in occlusive arterial disease of the lower limb. Br J Surg 1975; 62:64.
13. Fowkes F G R, Housley E, Macintyre C C A, Prescott R J, Ruckley C V. Variability of ankle and brachial systolic pressures in the measurement of atherosclerotic peripheral arterial disease. J Epidem and Comm Health 1988; 42:128.
14. Carter S A. Response of ankle systolic pressure to leg exercise in mild or questionable arterial disease. N Eng J Med 1972; 287:578.
15. Thulesius O. Systemic and ankle blood pressure before and after exercise in patients with arterial insufficiency. Angiology 1978; 29:374.
16. Osmundson P J, Chesebro J H, O'Fallon W M *et al.* A prospective study of peripheral occlusive arterial disease in diabetes II. Vascular laboratory assessment. Mayo Clin Proc 1981; 56:223.
17. Strandness D E, Bell J W. An evaluation of the haemodynamic response of the claudicating extremity to exercise. Surg Gynecol Obstet 1964; 119:1237.
18. Hummel B W, Hummel B A, Mowbry A *et al.* Reactive hyperemia vs treadmill exercise testing in arterial disease. Arch Surg Res 1978; 113:95.
19. Johnston W C. Doppler ankle pressure and reactive hyperaemia in the diagnosis of arterial insufficiency. J Surg Res 1975; 18:1771.
20. Baker J D. Post stress Doppler ankle pressures. Arch Surg 1978; 113:117.
21. Ouriel K, McDonnell A E, Metz C E, Zarins C K. A critical evaluation of stress testing in the diagnosis of peripheral vascular disease. Surgery 1982; 91:686.
22. Criqui M H, Fronek A, Barrett-Connor E. The prevalence of peripheral arterial disease in a defined population. Circulation 1985; 71:510.
23. Fowkes F G R, Housley E, Macintyre C C A, Prescott R J, Ruckley C V. Reproducibility of reactive hyperaemia test in the measurement of peripheral arterial disease. Br J Surg 1988; 75:743.
24. Wetnzer S M, Kiser J C, Bezreh J S. Doppler ultrasound imaging: vascular applications. Radiology 1984; 150:507.
25. Mitchell J R A, Schwartz C J. Arterial disease, Blackwell, Oxford, 1965.
26. Roberts J C, Moses C, Wilkins R H. Autopsy studies in atherosclerosis. 1. Distribution and severity of atherosclerosis in patients dying without morphologic evidence of atherosclerotic catastrophe. Circulation 1959; 20:511.
27. Sternby N H. Atherosclerosis in a defined population. An autopsy study in Malmo, Sweden. Acta Path Microbiol. Scand 1968; suppl. 194.
28. Fowkes F G R. Epidemiology of atherosclerotic arterial disease in the lower limbs. Eur J Vasc Surg 1988; 2:283.
29. Holland W W, Raftery E B, McPearson P, Stone R W. A cardiovascular survey of American East Coast telephone workers. Am J Epidemiol 1967; 85:61.
30. Heliovaara M, Karvonen M J, Vilhunen R, Punsar S. Smoking, carbon monoxide and atherosclerotic diseases. Br Med J 1978; 1:268.
31. Widmer L K, Greensher A, Kannel W B. Occlusion of peripheral arteries: a study of 6,400 working subjects. Circulation 1964; 30:836.
32. De Backer I G, Kornitzer M, Sobolski J, Denolin H. Intermittent claudication – epidemiology and natural history. Acta Cardiol 1979; 34:115.
33. Widmer L K, Biland L, Da Silva A. Risk profile and occlusive peripheral artery disease (OPAD) In: Proceedings of 13th International Congress of Angiology, Athens, 1985.

34. Lord J W. Cigarette smoking and peripheral atherosclerotic occlusive disease. JAMA 1965; 191:249.
35. Farid N R, Dickinson P H, MacNeal I F, Anderson J. Hyperlipoproteinaemia in peripheral arterial disease in the north of England. J Cardiovasc Surg 1974; 15:366.
36. Sirtori C R, Biasi G, Vercellio G, Agradi E, Malan E. Diet lipids and lipoproteins in patients with peripheral vascular disease. Am J Med Sci 1974; 268:325.
37. Higgins M W, Kjelsberg M. Characteristics of smokers and non-smokers in Tecumseh, Michigan. Am J Epidemiol 1967; 86:60.
38. Kannel W B, Shurtleff D. The natural history of arteriosclerosis obliterans. Cardiovasc Clin 1971; 3:37.
39. Bothig S, Metelitsa V I, Barth W *et al.* Prevalence of ischaemic heart disease, arterial hypertension and intermittent claudication, and distribution of risk factors among middle aged men in Moscow and Berlin. Cor Vasa 1976; 18:104.
40. Hughson W G, Mann J I, Garrod A. Intermittent claudication: prevalence and risk factors. Br Med J 1978; 1:1379.
41. Reunanen A, Takkunen H, Aromaa A. Prevalence of intermittent claudication and its effect on mortality. Acta Med Scand 1982; 211:249.
42. Reid D D, Holland W W, Hummerfelt S, Rose G. A cardiovascular survey of British postal workers. Lancet 1966; 1:614.
43. Isacsson S. Venous occlusion plethysmography in 55 year old men: a population study in Malmo, Sweden. Acta Med Scand 1972; 537 (Suppl):1.
44. Kannel W B, McGhee D L. Update on some epidemiological features of intermittent claudication: The Framingham Study. J Am Ger Soc 1984; 33:13.
45. Da Silva A, Widmer L K, Ziegler H W, Nissen C, Schweizwer. The Basle longitudinal study: report on the relation of initial glucose level to baseline ECG abnormalities, peripheral artery disease, and subsequent mortality. J Chronic Dis 1979; 32:797.
46. Jarrett R J, Keen H, Chakrabarti R. Diabetes, hyperglycaemia and arterial disease. In H Keen, R J Jarrett, eds. Complications of diabetes. 2nd Ed. London: Edward Arnold, 1982; 179.
47. Garcia M J, McNamara P M, Gordon T, Kannel W B. Morbidity and mortality in diabetics in the Framingham population. Sixteen year follow-up study. Diabetes 1964; 23:105.
48. Anquist K A, Johnson O, Ericsson M, Tollin C. Serum lipoproteins and apolipoproteins A1 and A11 in male patients with peripheral arterial insufficiency. Acta Clin Scand 1982; 148:675.
49. Bihari-Varga M, Szekely J, Gruber E. Plasma high density lipoproteins in coronary, cerebral and peripheral vascular diseases. The influence of various risk factors. Atherosclerosis 1981; 40:337.
50. Meerloo J M, Billimoria J D. High density lipoprotein cholesterol levels in peripheral vascular disease and in women on oral contraception. Atherosclerosis 1979; 33:267.
51. Trayner I M, Mannarino E, Clyne C A C, Thompson G R. Serum lipids and high density lipoproteins in peripheral vascular disease. Br J Surg 1980; 67:497.
52. Hertzer N R. Fatal myocardial infaction following lower extremity revascularization – two hundred and seventy three patients followed six to eleven post operative years. Am Surg 1981; 193:492.
53. Pilger E, Pristauza H, Pfeiffer K H, Kostner G M. Retrospective evaluation of risk factors for peripheral atherosclerosis by stepwise discriminant analysis. Arteriosclerosis 1983; 3:57.
54. Franceschini G, Bondioli A, Mantero M, Sirtori M, Tattoni G, Biasig, Sirtori C R. Increased apoprotein B in very low density lipoproteins of patients with peripheral vascular disease. Arteriosclerosis 1982; 2:74.
55. Carlson L A, Pauciullo P, Johansson J, Olsson A G. Modified composition of very low density lipoproteins in peripheral vascular disease: evidence for low cholestoryl ester but

normal apolipoprotein B content of small VLDL. In A Ventura, G Crepaldi, U Senin, eds. Extracoronary atherosclerosis. Monogr Atheroscler 1986; 14:31.

56. Low G D O, Saniabadi A, Turner A, Lieberman P, Pollock J, Drury J. Studies on haematocrit in peripheral arterial disease. Klin Wochenschr 1986; 64:969.
57. Dintenfass L. Elevation of blood viscosity, aggregation of red cells, haematocrit values and fibrinogen levels in cigarette smokers. Med J Australia 1975; i:617.
58. Hamer J D, Ashton F, Meynell M J. Factors influencing prognosis in the surgery of peripheral arterial disease. Br J Surg 1974; 51:984.
59. Harris P L, Harvey D R, Bliss B P. The importance of plasma lipids, glucose, insulin and fibrinogen in femoropopliteal surgery. Br J Surg 1978; 65:197.
60. Winocour P D, Turner M R, Taylor T G, Munday K A. Gout and cardiovascular disease (letter) Lancet 1977; 1:959.
61. Kallero K S, Bergentz S E, Lindell S E, Janzon L. Elevated haematocrit in patients with intermittent claudication with special regard to men below the age of 60. Biblthca Haematol 1981; 47:173.
62. Bouhoutsos J, Morris T, Chavatzas D *et al.* The influence of haemoglobin and platelet levels on the results of arterial surgery. Br J Surg 1974; 51:984.
63. Dormandy J A, Hoare E, Colley J, Arrowsmith D E, Dormandy T L. Clinical, haemodynamic, rheological and biochemical findings in 126 patients with intermittent claudication. Br Med J 1973; 4:576.
64. Stormer B, Horsch R, Kleinschmidt F *et al.* Blood viscosity in patients with peripheral vascular disease in the areas of low shear rates. J Cardiovasc Surg 1974; 15:577.
65. Lowe G D O. Blood rheology in arterial disease. Editorial review. Clinical Science 1986; 71:137.
66. Biland L, Da Silva A, Zemp E, Widmer L K. Occlusive peripheral artery disease (OPAD). Mortality and risk profile. In Proceedings of 13th International Congress of Angiology, Athens 9–14 June, 1985.
67. Rose G, McCartney P, Reid D D. Self administration of a questionnaire on chest pain and intermittent claudication. Dr J Prev Soc Med 1977; 31:42.
68. Bloor K. Natural history of arteriosclerosis of the lower extremities. Ann Roy Coll Surg Eng 1961; 28:36.
69. Kannel W B, Skinner J J, Schwartz M J, Shurtleff D. Intermittent claudication: incidence in the Framingham Study. Circulation 1970; 41:875.
70. Jelnes R, Gaardsting O, Hougard Jensen K *et al.* Fate in intermittent claudication: outcome and risk factors. Br Med J 1986; 293:1137.
71. Juergens J L, Barker N W, Hines E A. Arteriosclerosis obliterans: review of 520 cases with special reference to pathogenic and prognostic factors. Circulation 1960; 21:188.

15. Occult aortic aneurysm

JACK COLLIN

The majority of abdominal aortic aneurysms produce no symptoms until they rupture, when without skilled emergency surgery the outcome is invariably death within hours or at most days. When an aneurysm ruptures anteriorly through the posterior peritoneum there can be no tamponade of the haemorrhage and exsanguination into the peritoneal cavity is immediate. Such patients seldom reach hospital alive and have no chance of surgical rescue. In some 40% of ruptures the haemorrhage is initially contained by the retroperitoneal tissues aided by the systemic hypotension produced by blood loss. It is these relatively fortunate patients who can be rescued by emergency operation [1]. The first priority is to secure control of the bleeding by direct arterial clamping. Enthusiastic attempts to raise blood pressure by transfusion before the aorta is cross-clamped are liable to precipitate extension of the rupture into the peritoneal cavity and immediate death. Because of the parlous state of patients with contained rupture, operative mortality, even in highly specialised units, remains around 30% [2] while overall a 50% mortality would be more typical.

Since most patients with a ruptured aneurysm do not arrive in hospital alive and some of those who do are in extremis and beyond surgery, not more than one in every five or six patients will survive. The impact of any reduction which might be achieved in operative mortality on overall survival would therefore be small. If operative mortality for ruptured abdominal aortic aneurysm surgery were reduced to half the present level, overall mortality from rupture would only fall from 80% to 70%. The solution to the problem of death from ruptured aneurysm does not therefore lie with improvements in emergency surgery. In reality this is fortunate since although operative mortality for elective aortic surgery has been substantially reduced over the last 30 years, that of emergency aortic surgery has barely improved at all [3].

The most common symptom from abdominal aortic aneurysm apart from

A.-M. Salmasi and A. N. Nicolaides (eds.), Occult Atherosclerotic Disease, 205–218.

catastrophic rupture is the recognition by the patient of a pulsatile abdominal mass which may be uncomfortable when firmly palpated. The presence of marked tenderness or pain in the lumbar region is more ominous and suggestive of rapid aneurysm expansion, although an inflammatory aneurysm can also produce these symptoms. Only occasionally is an aortic aneurysm directly responsible for symptoms of occlusive arterial disease either from embolism or thrombosis. Part of the mural thrombus which invariably lines the wall of all but the smallest aneurysms may become detached and embolise distally producing acute ischaemia of one or both legs. Such an event, which may follow abdominal trauma, requires emergency embolectomy to prevent infarction and gangrene of the limbs. It may be impossible clinically to differentiate a saddle embolus where the embolic material straddles the aortic bifurcation from aortic occlusion by thrombosis of the aneurysm. The distinction can be made by angiography which in addition will supply useful information about the condition of the femoral arteries. After acute aortic aneurysm thrombosis there will usually be no alternative to reconstructive arterial surgery by either an aorto-bifemoral or an axillo bifemoral bypass operation. In some patients in whom the stenosis of the aneurysm lumen has been slowly progressive over several months an adequate collateral arterial supply to the legs may have developed so that the final occlusion may not produce further symptoms.

The clinical presentation of an aortic aneurysm is likely to involve an immediate and substantial threat to life or limb with the exception of those cases detected incidentally by the patient or his doctor. If any improvement in the outcome for patients with abdominal aortic aneurysm is to occur it can only follow improved detection rates in totally asymptomatic patients with occult disease. An abdominal aortic aneurysm has been likened to a U-boat in the belly but this author is inclined to describe it as a time bomb which will inevitably explode at some time in the future. All that can save the patient from rupture of the aneurysm is elective surgery or prior death from some other disease.

Definition of an aortic aneurysm

The first requirement of any programme for the detection of an occult disease is to have a clear and precise definition of the criteria for diagnosis. Unfortunately there is no agreed definition of what constitutes an aortic aneurysm. The standard surgical textbook description of an aneurysm as a dilatation of the aorta begs the subsidiary questions of how much dilatation, and relative to what? Such a definition was acceptable when the principal means of clinical diagnosis was abdominal palpation and when elective operative mortality was so high that only the very large, obvious and immediately threatening aneurysms were considered for prophylactic surgical treatment. Radiography, ultrasonography and computerised tomography allow accurate measurement of anteroposterior and transverse external diameter of the aorta together with the length of any dilated segment and its luminal diameter if required. In addition elective operative mortality has now fallen to levels which permit consideration of prophylactic surgical resection of even quite small aneurysms. Vagueness of definition of what constitutes an aneurysm is therefore no longer acceptable and an agreed internationally approved definition is overdue.

It is by no means certain which is the more useful diameter of the aorta to measure, anteroposterior, transverse or the maximum diameter in any plane but it is clear that only the external diameter of the aorta is relevant. The diameter of the lumen or thickness of the mural thrombus has no bearing on the risk of aneurysm rupture. The anteroposterior diameter may be a better predictor of aneurysm rupture but the transverse diameter is usually greater [4]. The diameter of the aorta is likely to vary with the age, sex and ethnic origin of the population studied but for any population the aortic diameter in common with measurements of height and weight will fit into a normal distribution curve.

The most obvious definition of an aortic aneurysm would be to use an absolute measurement of external diameter so that for the infrarenal aorta an aneurysm could be said to be present if the maximum aortic diameter is at least 4.0 cms. A different value might have to be agreed, however, for each part of the aorta since the normal aortic diameter decreases from its origin to its bifurcation. Such a requirement would make the definition very cumbersome for general application but for the common abdominal aortic aneurysm it would have considerable practical appeal. The maximum external diameter of an aortic aneurysm is the measurement which currently best quantifies the risk of aneurysm rupture and this dimension is a major consideration in deciding whether to recommend elective aneurysm resection. A rational decision is based on a comparison of the risk of rupture with the operative mortality for elective aneurysm resection for the surgeon and institution. All vascular surgeons would recommend elective resection for abdominal aortic aneurysms over 6 cm in diameter, most for those over 5 cm, and some for those over 4 cm but very few surgeons would perform elective surgery on abdominal aortic aneurysms less than 4 cm in diameter. A pragmatic definition of an abdominal aortic aneurysm would therefore be a maximum infrarenal aortic diameter of at least 4 cm. The weakness of this definition is that as elective operative mortality rates fall and clearer risk factors for rupture are determined it could soon become outdated.

For biological measurements in general it is common practice to regard any value more than two standard deviations from the population mean as being possibly abnormal. The same criteria could be used for aortic diameter. The distribution of aortic diameters will depend on the age, sex, height, weight and possibly race of the population studied. Any definition of aortic aneurysm relying on the normal distribution of aortic diameters therefore requires the accumulation of a substantial data base. Abdominal aortic aneurysm is a disease of men, is rare in the young and its prevalence increases rapidly after age 55 so that it is present in 5.3% of men aged 65–74 [5]. It follows that young women with an aortic diameter more than two standard deviations from the mean for their age and sex will not have an abdominal aortic aneurysm while a number of old men with an aortic diameter within two standard deviations of the mean will. Another problem is that a man with an aortic diameter on the fifth percentile could double his aortic diameter yet still be below the 95th percentile.

If it was known that the diameter of one part of the aorta was normal the diameter of the abnormal length of aorta might be related to it. It seems improbable, however, that the normality of other parts of the aorta could be relied on in the presence of disease elsewhere in the same vessel. Sterpetti [6] has suggested that the ratio of infrarenal and suprarenal aortic diameters may be a better indicator of rupture risk than the actual size of an abdominal aortic aneurysm. An aortic index would individualise the definition of an abdominal aortic aneurysm by relating it to the patient's normal aorta assuming that the suprarenal aorta is not itself abnormally dilated. Another problem is illustrated by examining how the definition would apply at opposite ends of the normal distribution curve for suprarenal aortic diameter [5]. At one extreme one and a half times suprarenal diameter would be 1.8 cm and at the other 4.5 cm representing aortic dilatations of 0.6 cm and 1.5 cm respectively. No vascular surgeon would recommend elective aneurysm resection for the first but many would for the second, though arguably the risk of rupture might be the same for both.

The aorta normally progressively tapers from its origin to its bifurcation as branches are given off and the volume of blood it carries is thereby reduced. If the diameter of a section of aorta is greater than that of the aorta proximal to it an aneurysm is likely to be present provided the measurement is reliable. An infrarenal aorta with a diameter 0.5 cm greater than the suprarenal abdominal aorta is undoubtedly dilated and the measurements are within the capability of existing technology. The weakness of the definition is that it takes no account of the relatively common situation in which the whole abdominal aorta is uniformly dilated. Such an aorta is described as being either ectatic or aneurysmal depending on personal whim and absolute diameter.

The introduction of a definition of aortic aneurysm which will meet all requirements and apply equally to all parts of the aorta clearly presents considerable difficulties and a composite definition may be required to include all varieties of aortic dilatation. An agreed definition is certainly overdue since scientific study and clinical understanding of this fascinating and difficult disease is not helped by idiosyncrasy and imprecision. For our own studies of abdominal aortic aneurysm we have used this definition: 'An abdominal aortic aneurysm is present when the maximum external diameter of the infrarenal aorta is either greater than 4.0 cm or exceeds the maximum diameter of the suprarenal aorta by at least 0.5 cm'.

Detection

Over the last two decades medical services for the elderly have improved markedly both at primary and hospital care levels. In part these improvements have occurred as a consequence of the large increase in the number of elderly people in the population of Northern European countries and the need to organise services for them more rationally. Routine contacts of the elderly with primary care physicians and specialist geriatricians are now common and the opportunities for detection of the common diseases from which they suffer are more numerous. The first requirement for the detection of an occult aortic aneurysm is that the disease should be thought of and known to be common and curable. Clinical examination by palpation of the epigastrium will be sufficient to detect large abdominal aortic aneurysms in thin patients but in obese patients and when the aneurysm is small this will be unreliable. The normal abdominal aorta can be felt and its pulsation detected but in a patient of average girth this examination needs to be performed carefully if it is to be successful. All too often in patients presenting with a ruptured abdominal aortic aneurysm perusal of the case notes of a previous hospital admission will unearth the legend 'abdominal aorta easily palpable'. The 'easily palpable abdominal aorta' should be regarded as aneurysmal until this diagnosis has been positively excluded by ultrasonography or computerized tomography (CT) scanning of the vessels. As well as dilatation there is usually elongation of an aneurysmal artery. In the abdominal aorta such elongation tends to displace the aortic bifurcation downwards. This can be detected clinically by palpation in the midline of the abdomen an inch below the umbilicus. If the aortic pulse is felt at this level then an aneurysm should be suspected.

Atheromatous arteries often have enough calcium deposited in their walls to allow their visualisation on plain radiographs. Because of this some aortic aneurysms are detected radiologically during routine examination for some other reason particularly if a lateral film is taken. Approximately 40% of abdominal aortic aneurysms could be detected in this way. In the chest the enlargement of the soft tissue shadows of the aorta alone may be sufficient to suggest the diagnosis even if calcification is not present.

A large part of the increase in referrals of patients with abdominal aortic aneurysms which has been noted by vascular units around the world can undoubtedly be attributed to the growth of ultrasonography as a primary and almost routine examination of any patient with abdominal symptoms. Accurate measurement of the abdominal aorta by a skilled ultrasonographer is quick, simple and reliable and forms part of the routine abdominal examination by this technique.

Computerized tomography is occasionally useful but has little role in the routine detection of abdominal aortic aneurysms. Its main use is in defining the extent of the aortic dilatation particularly with suprarenal or thoraco-abdominal aneurysms. It can produce confusing information when the aorta is tortuous since the plane of the tomographic cut may not be at right angles to the aorta and aortic diameter can thereby be overestimated. Its role in the detection of occult aortic aneurysm is likely to remain limited because of the expense and time of the investigation and consequent restricted general availability.

Epidemiology

In the last 30 years there has been a linear increase in the number of recorded deaths from aortic aneurysm in England and Wales. In part this can be explained by the progressive growth in the number of elderly in the population but age specific death rates for aortic aneurysm have also increased over the age of 60 [7]. Some of the increase may be real but much of the apparent change may be due to enhanced awareness of the disease, improved diagnosis and altered referral patterns associated with the establishment of specialist vascular units. This issue is difficult to resolve because of the unreliability of National records of cause of death which ultimately depend on the diagnostic acumen of the reporting doctor seldom supported by autopsy evidence. In the United States a similar but more rapid increase in age adjusted mortality for aortic aneurysm occurred between 1951 and 1968 but recorded deaths then plateaued and in white males have declined at 2% per annum since 1976 [8]. These differences between England and the United States are best explained by dissimilar health care provision in the two countries. The seminal world event was the first successful resection of an abdominal aortic aneurysm by Dubost in 1951 [9]. The growth in Vascular surgical services in the United States was rapid to both create and satisfy the free market for this operation. In the United Kingdom Vascular surgical provision is still slowly improving as local initiatives and constant pressure gradually overcome the inertia of a centrally financed health service. In the United States 39,000 aortic aneurysmorraphies were performed in 1983 [8], while the operation rate in England was less than a third of this level.

The changing pattern of the diagnosis of aortic aneurysm has been recorded in the extensively studied and documented population resident in the city of Rochester, Minnesota [10]. The incidence of abdominal aortic aneurysm (AAA) increased seven-fold between 1951 and 1980 while newly diagnosed cases of thoracic aortic aneurysm declined. The greatest increase occurred in small, asymptomatic and uncomplicated aneurysms suggesting that improved diagnosis and the introduction of effective therapy were the most important factors. Elsewhere rapid increases in hospital admissions for abdominal aortic aneurysm have occurred in response to both administrative change and local enthusiasm [2, 11].

Age, sex and race

In contrast to occlusive arterial disease aortic aneurysm is almost exclusively confined to the elderly. There are few deaths from ruptured abdominal aortic aneurysm before 60 and the disease becomes commoner with advancing years. The annual risk of death from abdominal aortic aneurysm for a man aged 87 is 0.23% and for a woman 0.07%. In men total deaths from AAA reach a peak in the 70–74 age group while in women the peak occurs a decade later [12]. A man aged 67 is ten times more likely to die from this disease than a woman of the same age.

There is some uncertainty over the importance of racial factors in the prevalence of aortic aneurysm. Brindley and Stembridge [13] reviewed 369 necropsy cases of aortic aneurysm at all sites over the period 1892–1953 in Galveston, Texas and found that 61% occurred in negroes. Modern reports reveal a reversed pattern for abdominal aortic aneurysm with a white to black incidence ratio of two to one in North Carolina [14] and six to one in South Africa [15]. All of these studies have failed to provide convincing evidence of a true racial difference in the prevalence of AAA. In the early study [13], 54% of the cases were syphilitic in origin and only 11% of the aneurysms were of the abdominal aorta. The most likely explanation for the apparently higher incidence of abdominal aortic aneurysm in whites reported in recent years is the different age structures of the two populations. In the study from Durban [15], the black patients were on average 20 years younger than whites, while in the American study [14], no information on the age structure of the black and white population of North Carolina is given.

Aortic aneurysm and occlusive disease

Tilson has made a detailed comparison between patients with AAA and those with occlusive aorto iliac disease [16]. He found that the aneurysm patients were 9 times more likely to be male, were on average 11 years older and much less likely to have had previous arterial surgery. Patients with occlusive disease were 16 times more likely to require reoperation after aortic surgery. In addition aneurysm patients were on average more than two inches taller than patients with occlusive arterial disease and had a significantly greater body surface area [17]. Despite these differences occlusive and aneurysmal arterial disease frequently coexist and routine ultrasound examination has shown an incidence of AAA of 13.8% in men attending Vascular clinics with symptoms from occlusive arterial disease [18]. Our own clinical experience suggests that aneurysms in patients with occlusive disease are in general smaller and may therefore be less likely to rupture than in patients without gross atherosclerosis. Support for this view is provided by Sterpetti [19] who has shown that mean growth rates for small AAA's are 50% faster in the absence of obvious occlusive arterial disease.

Prevalence of aortic aneurysm

Attempts to define the prevalence of this disease in population studies have been confined to abdominal aortic aneurysm since this condition is more common and much more amenable to curative surgical treatment than thoracic aortic aneurysms. Death statistics clearly show that abdominal aortic aneurysm is predominantly a disease of men and increases rapidly with advancing age. The prevalence found in any study must therefore be interpreted by careful reference to the age and sex of the population studied as well as any selection based on likely risk factors for the disease.

In the specific population subgroup of healthy men aged 65–74 years the total prevalence of this disease has been shown to be 5.4% and aneurysms of 4 cm or more in diameter are present in 2.3% [5]. Scott [20] screened a general practice population of people aged 65–80 and found the prevalence of aortas with a diameter of at least 3.5 cms to be only 2.6% but more than half the individuals examined for this predominantly male disease were women. Others have screened patients being treated for diseases known to be associated with abdominal aortic aneurysm and found high aneurysm prevalence rates in these selected populations. Twomey [21] examined 200 male hypertensives over age 50 and found an AAA prevalence of 7%, while in Birmingham [22] 7.4% of hypertensive men over 65 had an AAA. In North America the case for early detection of AAA has been made but screening studies in defined population groups at risk have been slow to start. In Oregon, Thurmond [23] examined 90 men attending a cardiology follow up clinic and found 6 (6.7%) abdominal aortic aneurysms 4 cm or more in diameter. In patients who did not have an aneurysm aortic diameter was significantly greater in men than women and among men significantly greater in smokers, hypertensives and patients who had undergone coronary artery bypass surgery.

The low prevalence of abdominal aortic aneurysm found in Sweden [24] when a relatively young and predominantly female population was screened emphasizes the importance of carefully identifying the population at risk if screening for this disease is to be cost effective. The inclusion of women in any planned programme is likely to be unproductive since the disease does not become common until an advanced age. In men it seems sensible to screen a population old enough for aneurysms to be relatively prevalent but still young enough to benefit from prophylactic elective surgery. It is also known that the response rate of the very elderly to invitations is low [25]. Selecting groups for screening because they have associated diseases like hypertension or coronary and peripheral arterial occlusive disease will undoubtedly increase the aneurysm yield but such individuals will generally be worse candidates for major arterial surgery.

Familial aortic aneurysms

Attention was first drawn to a familial grouping of abdominal aortic aneurysm by Clifton who reported the cases of 3 brothers all of whom underwent surgery for previously asymptomatic ruptured aneurysm [26]. Tilson [27] has reported on fifty families from across the United States with abdominal aortic aneurysm in two or more first order relatives but in 23 families only one member other than the patient was known to be affected. In Northern Sweden the 87 patients treated for abdominal aortic aneurysm who responded to a postal questionnaire reported that 7 (3.4%) of their 204 deceased brothers and sisters had died from ruptured aneurysm [28]. No controls were included in this study but the reported incidence of ruptured aneurysm in siblings of affected patients is more than twice the population incidence discovered by routine autopsy in the south of Sweden [29]. Johansen [30] compared the family histories of 250 patients with AAA and 250 controls half of whom were faculty members of the University of Washington School of Medicine. Eight times as many patients as controls reported having a first degree relative with an aneurysm. Unfortunately the validity of this observation is open to question since on average patients were 15 years older than controls and would therefore be expected to have many more siblings old enough to have also developed this disease of the elderly.

There are a number of problems which make it particularly difficult to discover the true extent of the familial ingredient in the aetiology of aortic aneurysm. Because of the advanced age of onset of the disease we need to know the lifetime incidence of abdominal aortic aneurysm in both study and control populations which should contain equal numbers of men and women with similar lifespans. Like cardinals and bishops patients with aortic aneurysm have already been preselected by longevity for their condition and anility is often familial. Unlike the fashionable heart attack there is no vulgar name for aortic aneurysm which is therefore unfamiliar to the general public and in the absence of an autopsy usually undiagnosed by the physician. To overcome some of these problems we have examined by ultrasonography the abdominal aorta of brothers over 50 years of age of patients treated for abdominal aortic aneurysm. The prevalence of abdominal aortic aneurysm in these screened first degree male relatives was 29% [31].

Management of the patient with an abdominal aortic aneurysm

The purpose of treatment for aortic aneurysm is to prevent rupture and premature death which is the ultimate outcome in all patients unless they die from some other disease first. The relief of symptoms is seldom a consideration since most patients with this disease are asymptomatic and by definition all those with an occult aneurysm are free of symptoms. The only treatment which is known to be effective is surgical resection and replacement of the diseased artery with a synthetic graft. The decision to treat any individual patient is based on a careful assessment of the mortality and morbidity of elective surgery compared with the natural history of the disease. The factors to consider are the location of the aneurysm, its diameter and the general state of health of the patient.

The anatomical position of the aneurysm is the single most important factor affecting operative mortality and morbidity. Resection of abdominal aortic aneurysms confined to the infrarenal aorta can now be accomplished with a mortality of under 5% in the majority of specialist vascular units around the world although in less specialised hospitals the mortality may still be as high as 10% [32]. If the aneurysm involves the aorta above the origin of the renal arteries and the main blood supply to the abdominal viscera from the coeliac and superior mesenteric arteries the mortality risk is increased at least three-fold. When the aneurysm is thoracoabdominal, the operative mortality even in the handful of centres in the world where the operation is commonly performed is 10% [33], while in other hands a 75% mortality is still being reported. The most serious morbidity attached to the operation is the risk of paraplegia or paraparesis which may occur if the blood supply to the spinal cord is compromised. This risk is less than one in every two hundred cases for infrarenal aortic aneurysm rising to 15% for resection of thoracoabdominal aneurysms [34]. The high mortality and sometimes devastating morbidity of elective resection for thoracoabdominal aortic aneurysms has deterred most surgeons from considering this a worthwhile treatment for a disease which is likely to remain asymptomatic throughout the patients life. It is fortunate that the majority of degenerative aneurysms are confined to the infrarenal aorta while aneurysms involving only the thoracic aorta have become uncommon since the virtual elimination of tertiary syphilis.

The risk of any aneurysm rupturing is related to its external diameter. Post mortem studies have shown that for aneurysms of 7 to 10 cm in diameter measured after death 46% will have ruptured and caused death [35]. Such studies are likely to substantially underestimate the risk posed to the living patient by an aneurysm of the same size since death confers complete protection against rupture of an aneurysm which is still intact at that time. In a patient with an occult aneurysm of constant diameter the daily risk of rupture is the same so that the cumulative risk of rupture increases with time. In addition most aneurysms tend to expand at a rate which increases incrementally as expected from Laplace's law. Aneurysms less than 5 cm in diameter have been shown to expand at a mean of 0.2 cm per annum [36] while for those over 6 cm in diameter the mean rate is 0.5 cm per annum [37]. The only way in which the annual risk of rupture for aneurysms of different sizes could be accurately determined would be to follow up untreated patients until their aneurysms ruptured or they died from some other cause. There is general agreement that such a study would be unethical for patients with aneurysms of 5 cm or more in diameter and a strong case has been made for elective surgery in healthy patients with 4 cm aneurysms [38].

Elective resection of an abdominal aortic aneurysm remains a major operation. There are rapid changes in peripheral resistance venous return and cardiac output associated with both initial cross clamping and subsequent unclamping of the aorta above the aneurysm. In addition there is the ever-present risk of major haemorrhage with instantaneous changes in circulating blood volume. Most patients will require or benefit from mechanical ventilation in the early post operative period and are best cared for in an intensive care unit. It is clear that if the operation is to be performed with minimal risk the patient should have a reasonable reserve of myocardial and respiratory function. Preoperative assessment is required to measure cardiac and respiratory function and in some patients renal and hepatic function also. With modern anaesthesia most patients will be found suitable for surgery although some will require control of hypertension and preoperative physiotherapy as well as specific drug therapy to maximise cardiac and respiratory function. It is interesting to note that follow up studies of patients thought to be too ill to withstand elective aneurysm surgery have shown that half die from rupture of the aneurysm and not from the disease regarded as a contraindication to surgery [39].

In the majority of patients elective surgery will provide a complete cure and several studies have shown that the life expectation following replacement of an aortic aneurysm is similar to that of a control population. There is, however, some risk of further aneurysm formation elsewhere most critically in the remaining aorta or iliac arteries. These recurrent aneurysms may be true aneurysms with the same aetiology as the original disease or false aneurysms occurring at the arterial suture lines. The risk of developing the former can be reduced by ensuring that when an infrarenal aortic aneurysm is resected the replacement graft is attached to the aorta immediately below the renal artery origin so that a long aortic neck is avoided. False aneurysms are most likely to arise when anastomoses have been made to the femoral arteries as happens when an aortobifemoral graft is used. This complication can be prevented by replacing the aortic aneurysm wherever possible with a tube graft. If common iliac aneurysms or stenosis coexist a bifurcated graft can usually be inserted distally into the external iliac arteries.

Conclusion

Occult aortic aneurysms particularly of the infrarenal abdominal aorta are common in men over the age of 60. Undetected they are likely to rupture and cause the death of half of those who have them. A recent unconfirmed report suggests that the growth rate of aneurysms may be reduced in patients who are receiving treatment with B blockers irrespective of their effect on blood pressure control [40]. The possibility therefore exists that in future the risk of rupture of an aortic aneurysm may be minimised by early detection and medical therapy. For the present in most patients elective surgery to replace the aneurysm with a synthetic graft is the only treatment which can eliminate the risk of premature death from this disease. All patients under the age of 80 with an infrarenal abdominal aortic aneurysm greater than 4 cm should be considered for elective replacement of the aneurysm. Young patients with aneurysms extending above the renal arteries but below the diaphragm will also usually be advised to undergo aneurysm replacement surgery in a centre where this operation is regularly carried out.

For most patients with asymptomatic thoracoabdominal aortic aneurysms the operative mortality and risk of paraplegia associated with aneurysm replacement will usually make elective surgery unattractive.

References

1. Ingoldby CJH, Wujanto R, Mitchell JE. The impact of vascular surgery on community mortality from ruptured aortic aneurysms. Br J Surg 1986; 73:551.
2. Jenkins AMcL, Ruckley CV, Nolan B. Ruptured abdominal aortic aneurysm Br J Surg 1986; 73:395.
3. Fielding JWL, Black J, Ashton F, Campbell DJ. Diagnosis and management of 528 abdominal aortic aneurysms Br Med J 1981; 283:355.
4. Cronenwett JL, Murphy TF, Zelenock GB *et al.* Actuarial analysis of variables associated with rupture of small abdominal aortic aneurysms. Surgery 1985; 98:472.

5. Collin J, Araujo L, Walton J, Lindsell D. Oxford screening programme for abdominal aortic aneurysm in men aged 65 to 74 years. Lancet 1988; 2:613.
6. Sterpetti AV, Schultz RD, Feldhaus RJ, Cheng SE, Peetz DJ. Factors influencing enlargement rate of small abdominal aortic aneurysms. J Surg Res 1987; 43:211.
7. Collin J. The epidemiology of abdominal aortic aneurysm. Br J Hosp Med 1988; 40:(1) 64.
8. Lilienfeld DE, Gunderson PD, Sprafka JM, Vargas C. Epidemiology of aortic aneurysms: I Mortality trends in the United States 1951–1981 Arteriosclerosis 1987; 7:637.
9. Dubost C, Allary M, Oeconomos W. Resection of aneurysm of the abdominal aorta Arch Surg 1952; 64:405.
10. Melton LJ, Bickerstaff LK, Hollier LH. Changing incidence of abdominal aortic aneurysms: A population based study. Am J Epidemiol 1984; 120:379.
11. Collin J. Abdominal aortic aneurysms Br Med J 1987; 294:1097.
12. Mortality Statistics Cause. Office of Population Censures and Surveys. England and Wales H.M.S.O. 1984; Series DH2 11.
13. Brindley P, Stembridge VA. Aneurysms of the aorta: A clinicopathologic study of 369 necropsy cases. Amer J Path 1956; 32:67.
14. Johnson G, Avery A, McDougal EG, Burnham SJ, Keagy BA. Aneurysms of the abdominal aorta. Incidence in blacks and whites in North Carolina. Arch Surg 1985; 120:1138.
15. Costa M, Robbs JV. Abdominal aneurysms in a black population: clinicopathological study Br J Surg 1986; 73:554.
16. Tilson MD, Stansel HC. Differences in results for aneurysms Vs occlusive disease after aortic bifurcation grafts. Results of 100 elective grafts. Arch Surg 1980; 115:1173.
17. Tilson MD, Dang C. Generalised arteriomegaly. A possible predisposition to the formation of abdominal aortic aneurysms. Arch Surg 1981; 116:1030.
18. Allardice JT, Allwright GT, Wafula JMC, Wyatt AP. High prevalence of abdominal aortic aneurysm in men with peripheral vascular disease: screening by ultrasonography. Br J Surg 1988; 75:240.
19. Sterpetti AV, Schultz RD, Feldhaus RJ, Peetz DJ, Fasciano AJ, McGill JE. Abdominal aortic aneurysm in elderly patients. Selective management based on clinical status and aneurysmal expansion rate. Amer J Surg 1985; 150:772.
20. Scott RAP, Ashton HA, Kay DN. Routine ultrasound screening in management of abdominal aortic aneurysm. Br Med J 1988; 296:1709.
21. Twomey A, Twomey E, Wilkins RA, Lewis JD. Unrecognised aneurysmal disease in male hypertensive patients. Inter Angio 1986; 5:269.
22. Allen PIM, Gourevitch D, McKinley J, Tudway D, Goldman M. Population screening for aortic aneurysms. Lancet 1987; 2:736.
23. Thurmond AS, Semler HJ. Abdominal aortic aneurysm: Incidence in a population at risk. J Cardiovasc Surg 1986; 27:457.
24. Lindholm L, Ejlertsson G, Forsberg L, Norgren L. Low prevalence of abdominal aortic aneurysm in hypertensive patients. Acta Med Scand 1985; 218:305.
25. Collin J, Araujo L, Lindsell D. A community screening programme for abdominal aortic aneurysms. Eur J Vasc Surg 1988; 2:83.
26. Clifton MA. Familial abdominal aortic aneurysms. Br J Surg 1977; 64:765.
27. Tilson MD, Seashore MR. Fifty families with abdominal aortic aneurysms in two or more first-order relatives. Amer J Surg 1984; 147:551.
28. Norrgard O, Rais O, Angquist KA. Familial occurrence of abdominal aortic aneurysms. Surgery 1984; 95:650.
29. Carlsson J, Sternby NH. Aortic aneurysms. Acta Chir Scand 1964; 127:466.
30. Johansen K, Koepsell T. Familial tendency for abdominal aortic aneurysms. JAMA 1986; 256:1934.

31. Collin J, Walton J. Is abdominal aortic aneurysm familial? Br Med J 1989; 299:493.
32. Gowland Hopkins NF. Abdominal aortic aneurysms Br Med J 1987; 294:790.
33. Hollier LH, Symmonds JB, Pairolero PC, Cherry KJ, Hallet JW, Gloviczki P. Thoracoabdominal aortic aneurysm repair. Analysis of postoperative morbidity. Arch Surg 1988; 123:871.
34. Crawford ES, Mizrahi EM, Hess KR, Coselli JS, Safi HJ, Patel VM. The impact of distal aortic perfusion and somatosensory evoked potential monitoring on prevention of paraplegia after aortic aneurysm operation. J Thorac Cardiovasc Surg 1988; 95:357.
35. Darling RC, Messina CR, Brewster DC, Ottinger LW. Autopsy study of unoperated abdominal aortic aneurysms. Cardiovasc Surg 1976; 56 (Suppl 2 circ.):161.
36. Collin J, Araujo L, Walton J. How fast do very small abdominal aortic aneurysms grow? Eur J Vasc Surg 1989; 3:15.
37. Delin A, Ohlsen H, Swedenborg J. Growth rate of abdominal aortic aneurysms as measured by computed tomography. Br J Surg 1985; 72:530.
38. Collin J. Elective surgery for small abdominal aortic aneurysms. Lancet 1987; 1:909.
39. Walker EM, Hopkinson BR, Makin GS. Unoperated abdominal aortic aneurysm: presentation and natural history. Ann Roy Col Surg Eng 1983; 65:311.
40. Leach SD, Toole AL, Stern H, De Natale RW, Tilson MD. Effect of B-Adrenergic blockade on the growth rate of abdominal aortic aneurysms. Arch Surg 1988; 123:606.

16. Occult atherosclerotic disease of arteries of the lower limb – incidence, pathophysiology, diagnosis and assessment

MARY PAULA COLGAN, DERMOT J. MOORE and GREGOR D. SHANIK

Although atherosclerotic occlusive disease of the lower extremities itself rarely causes death directly, it is an important marker of morbidity particularly from cardiovascular disease. If we are to continue to strive to provide better patient care, then knowledge of the prevalence and natural history of both asymptomatic and symptomatic disease is essential. Medical literature abounds in reports on the surgical outcome of patients with peripheral vascular disease, but relatively little is known of the disease in terms of prevalence and natural history.

The aim of this chapter is to discuss both the pathophysiology and incidence of asymptomatic atherosclerotic occlusive disease of the lower extremities as well as the methods available for its diagnosis. Disease prevalence will depend on the method employed for its detection and this section will therefore be addressed before prevalence is discussed.

Pathophysiology

Information relative to the lower extremities comes from three sources: 1) clinical evaluation, 2) arteriography and 3) dissection of amputated limbs. Since autopsy studies rarely include dissection of the limbs it is difficult to obtain a clear picture of the types and sites of plaque that predominate or their rate of progression.

The most comprehensive study is that of Lindbom [1] who performed lower extremity arteriography on 139 patients and 186 cadavers. X-rays were evaluated for site and extent of disease and the presence of intimal or medial calcification. In the living subjects the highest incidence of plaque occurred in the superficial femoral artery at the level of the adductor canal and in the proximal popliteal artery. Occlusion of the profunda femoris artery was found in only four percent of studies. Most of the information

A.-M. Salmasi and A. N. Nicolaides (eds.), Occult Atherosclerotic Disease, 219–225.

regarding the below knee vessels was obtained from cadaver studies. The posterior tibial artery was the most commonly occluded artery and occlusion occurred distally. In contrast the anterior tibial artery when involved was more commonly occluded at or near its origin. The peroneal artery was the least commonly occluded artery. The arteries of the foot were difficult to assess due to poor visualization. However, Edwards [2] employed post-amputation angiography in a small series of limbs and demonstrated that occlusion of the foot vessels does occur. Of interest was the fact that involvement did not appear to differ between diabetics and nondiabetics.

While the underlying disease process is identical in both diabetics and nondiabetics, the extent and distribution differ. Gensler *et al.* [3] compared vascular lesions in 305 patients, 124 of whom were diabetic. Multi-segment involvement occurred in 75% of diabetics compared to 43% of nondiabetics. Aorto-iliac involvement was seen in 13% and 25% of diabetics and non-diabetics respectively. Wheelock [4] in a review of 428 patients with diabetes and gangrene reported that 40% had a palpable popliteal pulse and absent pedal pulses signifying occlusion of the tibial vessels. This in part helps explain the higher incidence of necrosis in patients with diabetes mellitus.

The physiological principles underlying the development and progression of atherosclerosis and the associated risk factors are similar to those associated with atherosclerosis elsewhere and have previously been discussed.

Diagnosis and assessment

Several methods have been employed to determine the presence or define the incidence of disease, each with its own benefits and pitfalls. The methods used will be discussed separately and their reliability and possible usefulness outlined.

Questionnaire

Several authors have studied the incidence of intermittent claudication and of particular note is the unreliability of questionnaires. In a study by Isacsson only one-third of patients diagnosed as claudicants by questionnaire were found to have true claudication [5]. Similar findings were reported by Reunanen and co-workers [6]. Howell *et al.* in 247 consecutive patients referred with suspected peripheral disease found a normal arterial profile in 97 (39%) instances [7]. Not only is a questionnaire inaccurate in assessing the prevalence of symptomatic disease but it can in no way separate true asymptomatic patients from those with occult peripheral vascular disease.

Physical examination

An important principle in any examination is the comparison of both lower extremities. Diminished or absent pulses, bruits or limb pallor signal advanced disease which in most instances will be symptomatic. In patients with occult disease, physical examination may be normal and therefore will lead to underestimation of disease prevalence. Repeat examination following a period of exercise will lead to the detection of additional patients with occult disease but again will underestimate disease. Additionally, physical examination as a technique for determining prevalence differences between population groups with multiple examiners is likely to vary significantly depending on the experience of the examining physician.

Noninvasive testing

Noninvasive testing as the name implies lacks morbidity and is therefore the ideal tool for epidemiological work. Several methods are available for assessing the lower extremities and the most useful are:

Walking test. This requires no special equipment and simply defines the walking capacity under normal physiological conditions. Fajgela *et al.* reported a sensitivity of 76% and a specificity of 70% for this test [8]. Their patients however were pre-selected and therefore are unlikely to represent the general population. Additionally, as a screening tool a much higher sensitivity is required and further work in this area is required.

Measurement of ankle systolic pressures. Estimation of ankle systolic pressures using a Doppler ultrasound probe as a flow sensor is easily performed. An ankle/brachial index is estimated by dividing the highest ankle pressure by the higher arm pressure. This index was first described by Winsor [9] and was popularized by Yao *et al.* [10]. Its usefulness and reliability have been confirmed in many studies [11–13]. The finding of an ankle/brachial index <0.92 is considered to signify the presence of peripheral occlusive disease.

In a review article Strandness stated that all noninvasive methods are relatively insensitive to the early changes that occur with atherosclerosis [14]. Stenosis or obstruction of a lower extremity can however under certain circumstances result in an alteration of the normal pressure/flow pattern distal to the stenosis. Although flow at rest may be adequate, the increased circulatory demands caused by exercise may not be met. This physiological finding has given rise to the development of 'stress testing'. In the peripheral circulation this involves measurement of ankle systolic pressures before and after a period of exercise.

Laing and Greenhalgh have described the 'one-minute exercise test' to determine the presence of peripheral arterial occlusive disease [15]. Resting ankle/brachial indices are determined following ten minutes rest. Following a period of exercise the patient is again returned to bed and ankle systolic pressures measured at thirty seconds. During the development of this test, patients were exercised for a) one minute at four kilometers per hour, b) one minute at six kilometers per hour, c) two minutes at four kilometers per hour and d) two minutes at six kilometers per hour. The decrease in ankle pressure was similar in all instances with differences observed in the overall recovery time. Therefore an exercise regime of one minute at four kilometers per hour was chosen. They consider a pressure decrease of >30 mm Hg as indicative of the presence of peripheral occlusive disease. For full detail and application of this test see chapter 17.

Clearly the most sensitive method of uncovering occult peripheral vascular disease is the estimation of pre- and post-exercise ankle systolic pressures. As research continues in this area it is essential that methodology is clearly described and hopefully standardized.

Incidence

Although several authors have scanned asymptomatic populations for the detection of asymptomatic carotid artery disease [16–18] or indeed abdominal aortic aneurysms [19–21] few reports exist on the prevalence of asymptomatic lower extremity atherosclerotic occlusive disease. Greenhalgh and colleagues studied a group of 107 asymptomatic employees in their sixth decade and found evidence of peripheral vascular disease in 9% using the one-minute exercise test [22]. This 10% incidence is significantly higher than the incidence of haemodynamically significant asymptomatic carotid artery disease [17]. One of the authors also screened 165 consecutive patients admitted for inguinal hernia repair. Symptoms and signs of peripheral vascular disease were found in eight patients and of the remainder, 100 underwent exercise testing and results were abnormal in ten instances giving a similar incidence of 10%.

Schroll and Munch [23] in a study of 666 males and females over the age of 60 years, found decreased ankle/brachial indices in 165 of the men and 135 of the women. The incidence of intermittent claudication was much lower at 5.8% in men and 1.3% in women. Sutton *et al.* [24] studies 56 elderly adults with isolated hypertension and found evidence of peripheral vascular disease in 40%. These were almost equally divided between those who had and those who did not have symptoms. Therefore approximately 20% had evidence of occult peripheral vascular disease.

Criqui *et al.* [25] using the standardized Rose questionnaire, physical examination and noninvasive testing studied the prevalence of peripheral vascular disease in a geographically defined population. Of the 624 subjects studied, 2.2% of men and 1.7% of women had a history of claudication based on questionnaire and 21% had pulse abnormalities. Noninvasive testing however revealed evidence of peripheral occlusive disease in 28% of the population. This again emphasizes the large proportion of patients with occult disease.

We would expect the incidence to be higher in high-risk groups such as patients with coronary artery disease or diabetes. Is this the case?

Coronary artery disease

Eighty consecutive patients awaiting coronary artery bypass surgery were studies [22]. Six patients had symptoms consistent with intermittent claudication and nine were unsuitable for treadmill testing due to the severity of their heart disease. Of the remaining patients, 50 underwent exercise testing and findings were abnormal in 19 giving a 38% incidence of asymptomatic occlusive disease.

Diabetes

Two hundred and nineteen consecutive patients over the age of forty attending a diabetic clinic were studied and 24 have symptoms of claudication while an additional seven patients had an abnormal physical examination resulting in a three percent incidence of occult disease clinically [22]. One hundred patients underwent exercise testing and in 27 instances the results were abnormal. Thus a high percentage of diabetic patients over the age of forty years had evidence of occult peripheral vascular disease. A similarly high incidence was reported by Marinelli *et al.* [26]. Four hundred and fifty-eight unselected volunteers with diabetes mellitus were studied. Eleven percent gave a history compatible with intermittent claudication however 26% had a normal noninvasive arterial profile. Of those patients who did not give a history of intermittent claudication, 31% had disease detected by noninvasive tests. Combining interview and physical examination 53% were considered normal and of these 19% had abnormal noninvasive findings.

This frequency of asymptomatic peripheral occlusive disease is comparable to autopsy studies of coronary arteries in which 30% of subjects with demonstrated occlusion had no symptoms prior to death [27]. The overall incidence of asymptomatic peripheral occlusive disease in the general population over the age of fifty is probably in the region of 10% with significantly higher incidences in high-risk groups.

This emphasizes the fact that atherosclerosis is a multi-system disease which affects many organs in the body and perhaps a patient presenting with symptoms referable to one vascular area should be screened for disease elsewhere. The management of patients with asymptomatic atherosclerotic occlusive disease of the lower extremities will be fully discussed in the following chapter.

References

1. Lindbom A. Arteriosclerosis and arterial thrombosis in the lower limb. A roentological study. Acta Radiol 1950; 80 (Suppl.): 38.
2. Edwards E A. Postamputation radiographic evidence for small artery obstruction in arteriosclerosis. Ann Surg 1959; 150:177.
3. Gensler S W, Hamovici H, Hoffert P, Steinman C, Beneventano T C. Study of vascular lesions in diabetics. 1965; Arch Surg 91:617.
4. Wheelock F C Jr. Transmetatarsal surgery and arterial surgery in diabetic patients. New Eng J Med 1961; 264:316.
5. Isacsson S O. Venous occlusion plethysmography in 55-year-old men. A population study in Malmo, Sweeden. Acta Med Scand (Suppl). 1972; 537.
6. Reunanen A, Takkunen H, Aromaa A. Prevalence of intermittent claudication and its effect on mortality. Acta Med Scand 1982; 211:249.
7. Howell M A, Colgan M P, Seeger R W, Ramsey D E, Sumner D S. Relationship of severity of lower limb peripheral vascular disease to mortality and morbidity: A six year follow-up study. J Vasc Surg 1989; 9:691.
8. Fajgela A, Haeger K, Lindell S E, Olsson N M. Arteriography, plethysmography and walking test in arterial obliteration of the legs. Vasc Dis 1967; 4:280.
9. Winsor T. Influence of arterial disease on systolic blood pressure gradients of extremities. Am J Med Sci 1950; 220:117.
10. Yao S T, Hobbs J T, Irvine W T. Ankle systolic pressure measurements in arterial disease affecting the lower extremities. Br J Surg 1969; 56:676.
11. Thulesius O, Gjores J E. Use of Doppler shift detection for determining peripheral arterial blood pressures. Angiology 1971; 22:594.
12. Sumner D S. Measurement of segmental arterial pressure. In: R B Rutherford, (ed.) Vascular Surgery. 2nd. edition. Philadelphia: W B Saunders 1984; p. 109.
13. Carter S A. Clinical measurement of systolic pressures in limbs with arterial occlusive disease. JAMA 1969; 207:1869.
14. Strandness D E Jr. Pathological alterations in blood flow. Ann Rev Med 1969; 20:1.
15. Laing S P, Greenhalgh R M. Standard exercise test to assess peripheral arterial disease. Br Med J 1980; 280:13.
16. Ramsey D E, Miles R D, Lambeth A, Sumner D S. Prevalence of extracranial carotid artery disease: a survey of an asymptomatic population with noninvasive techniques. Surg 1987; 5:584.
17. Colgan M P, Strode G R, Sommer J D, Gibbs J L, Sumner D S. Prevalence of asymptomatic carotid disease: Results of duplex scanning in 348 unselected volunteers. J Vasc Surg 1988; 8:674.
18. Hennerici M, Aulich A, Sandemann W, Freund H. Incidence of asymptomatic extracranial arterial disease. Stroke 1981; 17:877.
19. Allen P I, Gourevitch D, McKinley J, Tudway D, Goldman M. Population screening for abdominal aortic aneurysms. Lancet 1987; 2:736.

20. Collin J. Screening for abdominal aortic aneurysms. Br J Surg 1985; 72:851.
21. Graham AH, Chan A. Ultrasound screening for clinically occult abdominal aortic aneurysm. Can Med Assoc J 1988; 138:627.
22. Greenhalgh RM, Laing S, Ellis M, Walton J, Baxter K, Powell JT. How do we detect early subclinical disease? In: Greenhalgh, Jamieson and Nicolaides (eds.), Vascular Surgery: Issues in current practice London, Grune and Stratton, 1986; p. 57.
23. Schroll M, Munck O. Estimation of peripheral arteriosclerotic disease by ankle blood pressure measurements in a population study of 60-year-old men and women. J Chron Dis 1981; 34:261.
24. Sutton KC, Wolfson SK Jr., Kuller LH. Carotid and lower extremity arterial disease in elderly adults with isolated systolic hypertension. Stroke 1987; 18:817.
25. Criqui MH, Fronek A, Barrett-Connor E, Klauber MR, Gabriel S, Goodman D. The prevalence of peripheral arterial disease in a defined population. Circulation 71, 1985; 510.
26. Martinelli MR, Beach KW, Glass MJ, Primozich JF, Strandness DE Jr. Noninvasive testing vs clincial evaluation of arterial disease. A prospective study. JAMA 1979; 241:2031.
27. Allison RB, Rodriguez FL, Higgins EA *et al.* Clinicopathologic correlations in coronary atherosclerosis. Four hundred and thirty patients studies with postmortem coronary angiography. Circulation 1963; 27:170.

17. The detection of occult peripheral arterial disease using the one-minute exercise test

SUSAN LAING

Peripheral arterial disease is often considered one of the less serious manifestations of atherosclerosis as it rarely causes death and the outcome for a patient presenting with symptoms of intermittent claudication is, in fact, often good. As many as 50% of patients may improve symptomatically during the first year after presentation [1] and the presence of peripheral arterial disease alone does not reduce the life expectancy of the patient [2]. However, if the atherosclerosis is more widespread their life expectancy is reduced compared with the general population, many of the patients dying as a result of their concommitant disease [1, 3, 4]. Thus, whilst fairly benign in itself, peripheral arterial disease may be indicative of more serious disease elsewhere.

The prevalence of intermittent claudication has been studied in a number of cardiovascular surveys. These have usually used a questionnaire, backed up in some cases by clinical examination or simple non-invasive tests. Hughson and co-workers [5] in Oxford reported a prevalence of 2.2% for men and 1.2% for women, and a more recent study by Criqui and co-workers [6] reported similar findings. However, in a much more elderly group Hale and co-workers [7] reported a prevalence of 14.1% in women and 14.4% in men.

The prevalence of occult peripheral arterial disease has not been widely investigated, although some idea of its distribution is essential for an understanding of the natural history of atherosclerosis. This chapter describes the development of a simple stress test for occult peripheral arterial disease which might be suitable for use in large scale epidemiological studies.

Development of a one-minute exercise test

The indirect measurement of arterial systolic pressures using a Doppler ultrasound probe and a sphygmomanometer is a well-established technique

A.-M. Salmasi and A. N. Nicolaides (eds.), Occult Atherosclerotic Disease, 227–241.

for the assessment of peripheral arterial disease [8]. In addition, as the symptoms initially develop during exercise, it is appropriate to incorporate a period of stress in the evaluation. This may be done either by exercising the patient or occluding the arterial in-flow, resulting in hyperaemic flow as the cuff is released.

Exercise tests were first used for the assessment of symptoms by Boyd and co-workers in 1949 [9]. Initially these tests were an attempt to quantify the symptoms, the time at which the patient first developed intermittent claudication, and the total walking time being the parameters measured. In practice, this test is often inconclusive, and in a consecutive series of 250 outpatients suitable for treadmill testing we showed that only 38% stopped walking as a result of intermittent claudication within a maximum period of 5 minutes. A further 35% stopped walking due to other symptoms (shortness of breath, angina, etc.), and 27% were able to complete the full 5 minutes of exercise. In addition, for those patients in whom it was possible to measure the claudication time and total walking time, these measurements were shown to be very inconsistent.

A second method of incorporating a period of treadmill exercise in the assessment of these patients is to measure the ankle pressure both before and after exercise. The changes in blood flow and pressure that occur with exercise were originally described theoretically by Daniel Bernouilli, a Swiss mathematician, in the 18th century. His theory equates the total energy of blood at two points in the same stream line, providing that flow is steady and there is no friction. Thus as the blood flow is increased the pressure is decreased. This theory has to be modified when it is applied to the circulatory system due to energy loss in both normal and diseased vessels. This energy loss is especially important as blood flows through a stenosis, and Poiseuille later demonstrated that the pressure drop across a stenosis is directly proportional to the flow. Hence, the pressure fall is dependent on both the flow and the severity of the stenosis, a fall in pressure for a given stenosis will be greater at high flow rates and reduced at low flow rates. A stenosis which may not cause a pressure drop at low flow rates may cause a pressure drop at high flow rates.

Experimental work suggests that there is a critical level of stenosis above which an increase in flow results in a significant reduction in pressure. May and co-workers, in an early publication in 1963 [10], suggested that at rest this was as much as an 80% reduction in the cross-sectional area, but at higher flow rates this critical level was correspondingly reduced. After a period of stress a 60–70% reduction in the cross-sectional area (corresponding to 40–50% lumen diameter reduction) may become critical. Furthermore, subcritical stenoses have an additive effect, although not in a linear fashion [11].

In a leg, free from functionally significant arterial disease, the ankle

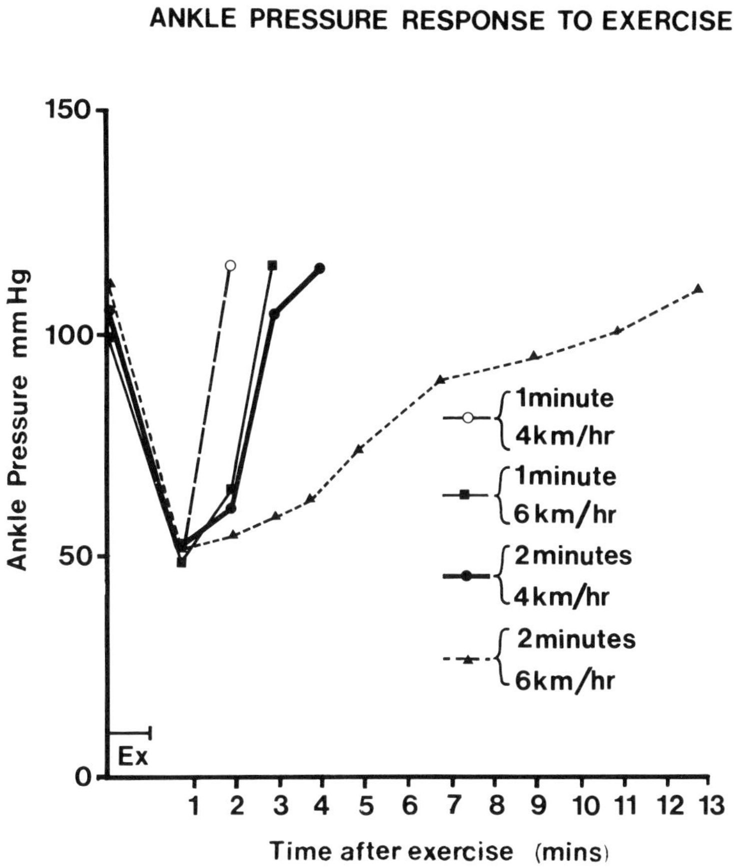

Figure 17.1. The ankle pressure response of an individual patient with peripheral arterial disease to 4 different workloads.

pressure measured 35 seconds after a period of exercise will be the same, or slightly above, the pre-exercise level. The theory suggests that even in a normal leg an initial small fall in ankle pressure may occur, but this is not usual in clinical practice and has only been observed under extreme experimental conditions. Significant peripheral arterial disease results in a fall in ankle pressure following exercise and the fall in ankle pressure is related to the severity of the disease [8].

The duration of exercise was originally taken as either the total walking time or a maximum of 5 minutes, but in the light of the findings described earlier, the possibility of reducing the workload to a more acceptable level was considered.

Preliminary observations with patients had indicated that even a short period of exercise was sufficient to result in a fall in ankle pressure after exercise, even if the patient remained symptom free. In order to examine the effects of different work loads a standard test of one minute at 4 km/hr at a 10% slope was compared with other, more strenuous periods of exercise. The result for an individual patient is displayed in Figure 17.1. Further studies demonstrated that the fall in ankle pressure following exercise was the same whether the patient walked to the claudication time (Fig. 17.2) or for a maximum of 5 minutes (Fig. 17.3).

These results indicate that the ankle pressure response to exercise does not depend solely upon the severity of the disease but also varies with the workload. The ankle pressure fall is the same whether the patient walks for one minute or for longer, but the recovery time increases with increased

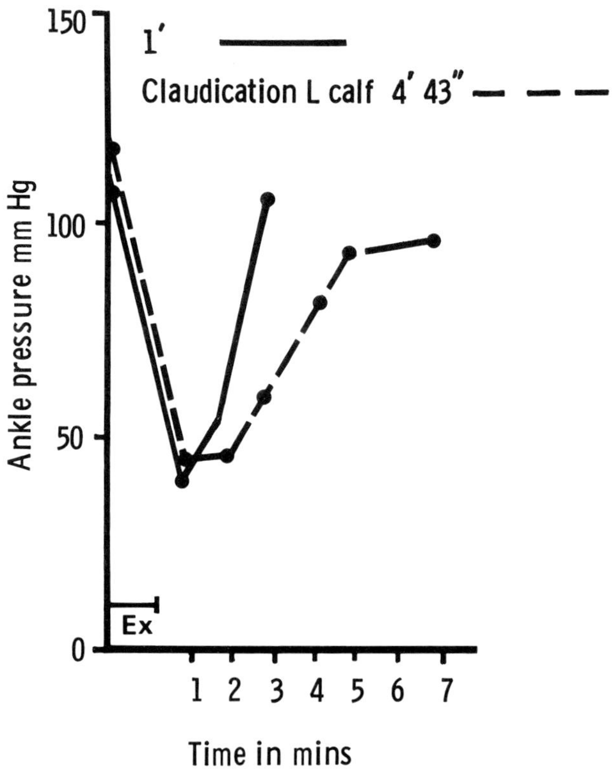

Figure 17.2. The ankle pressure response at the time of claudication (interrupted line) is compared with the response following exercise for one minute (continuous line).

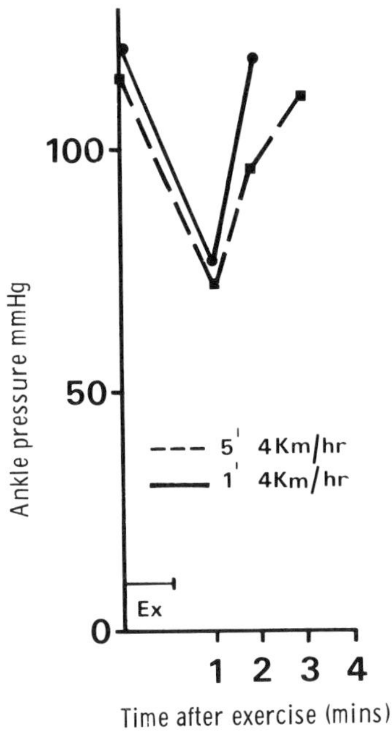

Figure 17.3. The ankle pressure response in a patient after exercise for 5 minutes and for one minute.

workload. This maximal fall in ankle pressure after comparatively short periods of exercise was first seen by Cappellen and Hall in 1960 [12] using direct intra-arterial measurements, and the findings described here were subsequently confirmed by Auckland and Hurlow in 1982 [13].

Ankle pressure measurements for peripheral arterial disease are therefore now performed before and after a standard one minute period of exercise (10% slope, 4 km/hr). The arm and ankle pressures are measured before exercise and one ankle pressure measurement is repeated 30–40 seconds after exercise and at one minute intervals thereafter. As the recovery time is likely to be fast with such a short period of exercise it is important that the post-exercise measurement be made quickly after exercise. For this reason the whole test is performed separately for each leg, the other ankle pressure being measured again following a five minute rest, before and after a second period of exercise. Severe disease will be manifest by a reduction in ankle pressure compared with the arm pressure even at rest, (ankle brachial pressure index – ABPI – less then 0.9) with a further fall in ankle pressure if the patient is exercised. Mild disease may be undetected at rest, the pressure index remaining normal, and a fall in ankle pressure only being detected after exercise (Figure 17.4). The sensitivity of the test to mild disease does

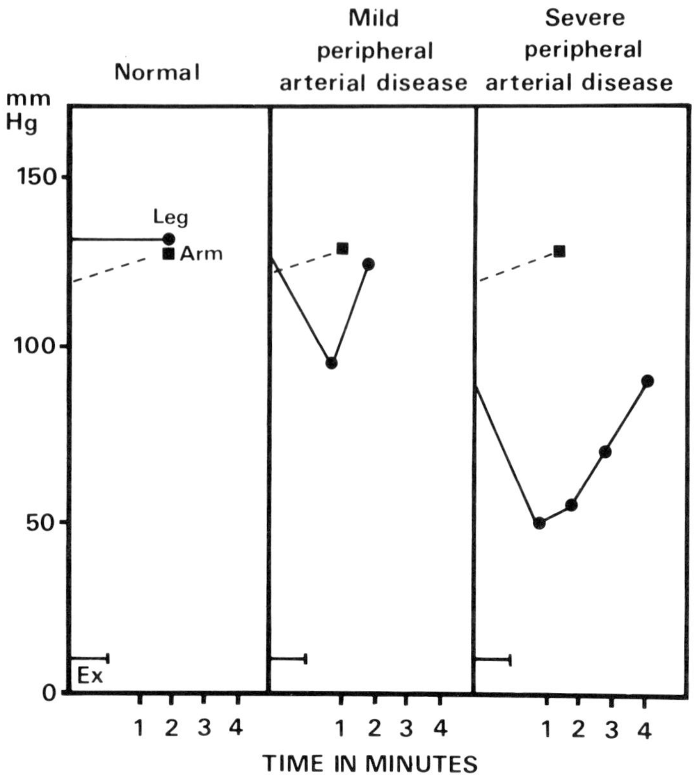

Figure 17.4. Comparison of the ankle pressure response to exercise between normal subjects, patients with mild peripheral arterial disease and patients with severe peripheral arterial disease. Note that the resting pressure is similar in normal subjects and in patients with mild peripheral arterial disease.

not appear to be diminished as a pressure fall of between 25–50 mm Hg after exercise cannot be increased if the patient walks further.

Further experiments with young controls were done to determine the level of pressure fall considered abnormal. Patients with mild disease do not undergo arteriography and there is therefore no 'gold standard' for comparison, and even if angiography had been possible, experimental work suggests that a stenosis seen at arteriography may not be functionally significant. The ankle pressure response to exercise in 100 legs of subjects under 35, (and thus considered unlikely to have early disease) were measured and the results for the first 50 legs are shown in Figure 17.5. A fall in ankle pressure of 30 mm Hg was subsequently taken to be indicative of functionally significant disease.

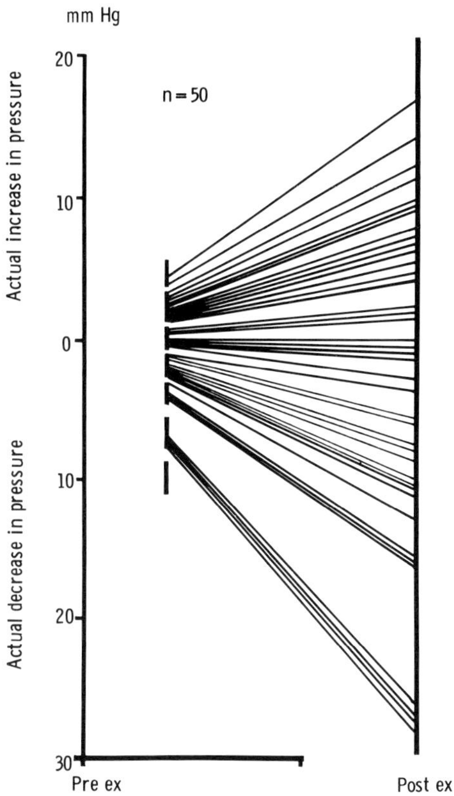

Figure 17.5. The change in ankle pressure following exercise is shown in 50 legs of 'normal' subjects. The post-exercise pressure is expressed as an increase or decrease compared with the pre-exercise pressure.

Patients with clinical evidence of peripheral arterial disease

A simple stress test can have an important part to play in the assessment of a patient with symptomatic peripheral arterial disease at every stage of the patient's management. Initially, a patient presenting with equivocal or mild symptoms may have the diagnosis supported by an abnormal ankle pressure response to exercise even if the resting ankle pressures are normal.

In patients with symptoms of intermittent claudication in one leg only, a stress test may determine the functional state of the asymptomatic leg. This is illustrated in Figures 17.6 and 17.7. Patients SH and SG both presented with intermittent claudication in the right calf, but had palpable pulses and a normal pressure index on the left. However, the left ankle pressure response

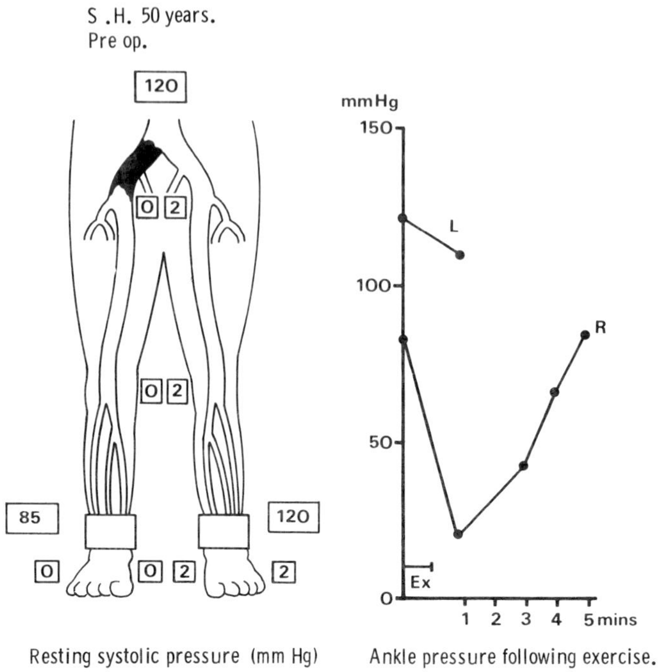

Figure 17.6. A normal pressure response in the left ankle (L) in the presence of intermittent claudication in the right calf (R).

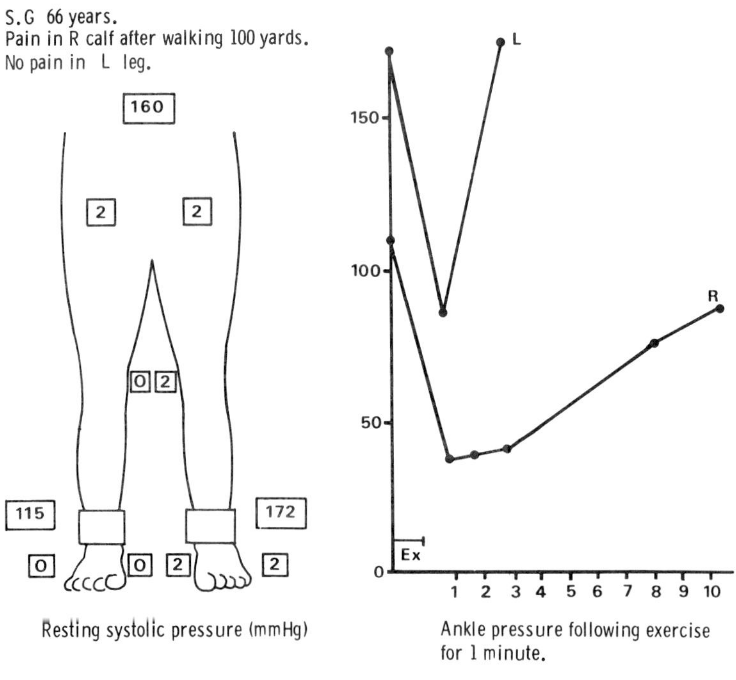

Figure 17.7. An abnormal pressure response in the left ankle (L) in the presence of intermittent claudication in the right calf (R).

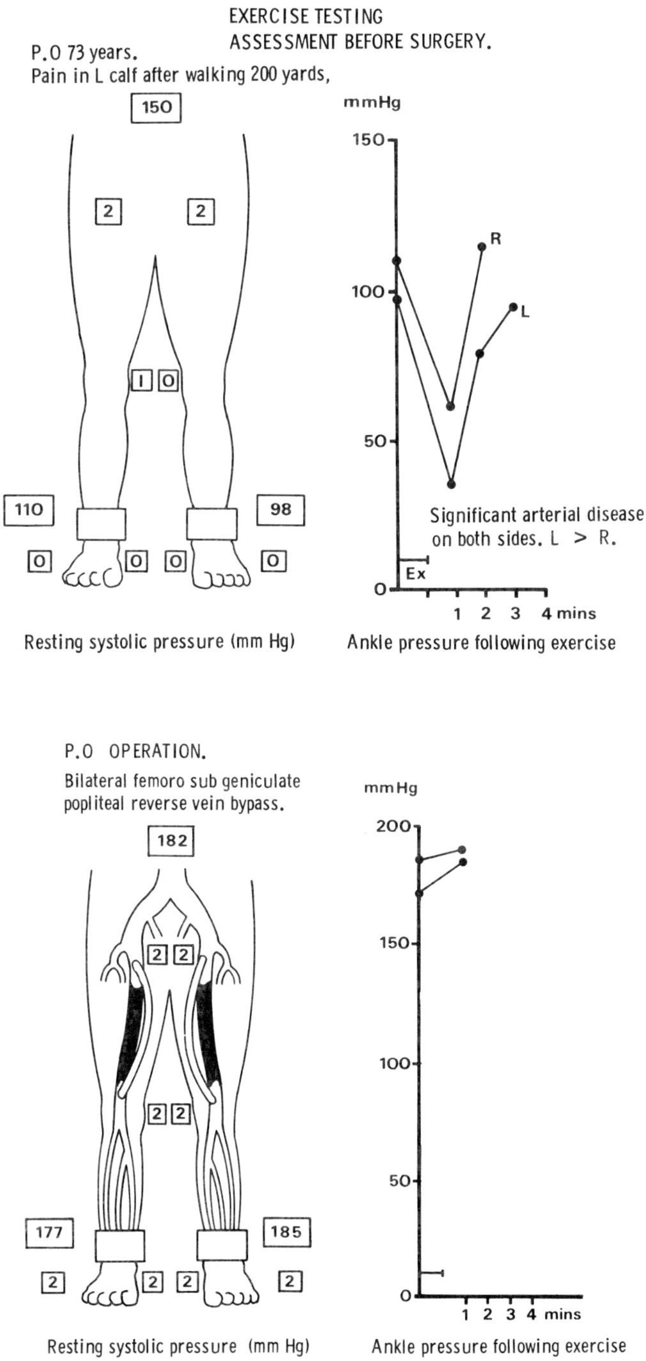

Figure 17.8. Ankle pressure both at rest and following one minute of exercise in patient P.O. before (top) and after (bottom) the operation of bilateral femoro popliteal grafting.

to one minute of exercise revealed two very different situations: patient SH was functionally normal, whereas patient SG had an abnormal response, suggesting that symptoms in the left leg were being 'masked' by symptoms in the right leg. In these situations surgery to one leg may simply unmask symptoms in the opposite leg. This situation may occur more frequently than is realised. In a consecutive series of 100 outpatients with symptoms of intermittent claudication in one leg only, 22 of the asymptomatic legs were shown to be abnormal on resting tests alone. Thirty-two of the remaining 78 asymptomatic legs had an abnormal ankle pressure response to exercise,

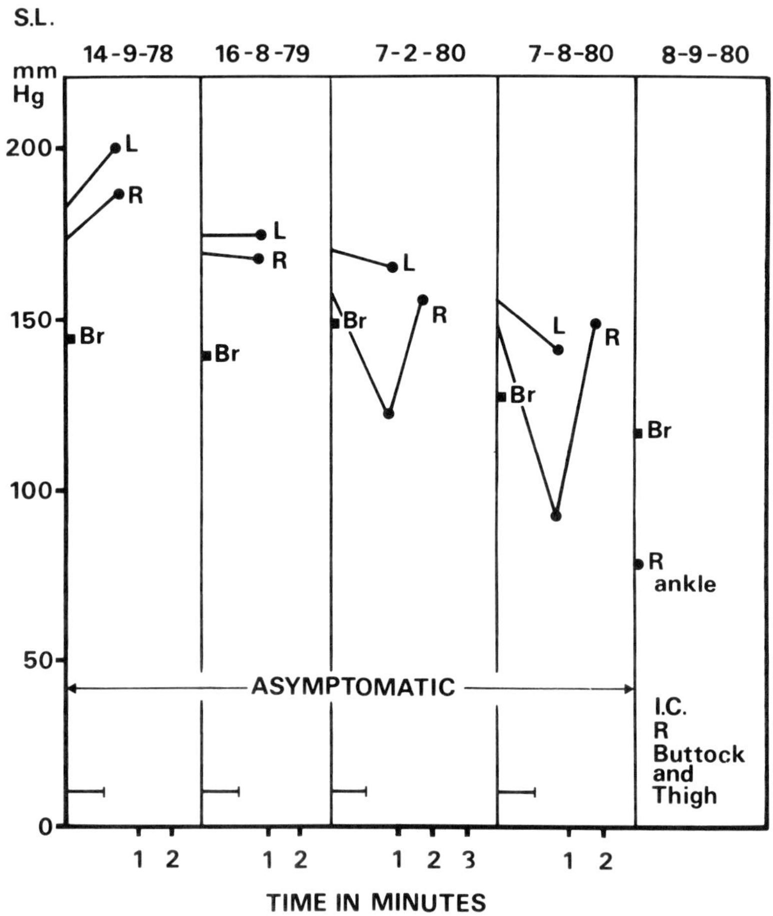

Figure 17.9. The ankle pressure response to exercise was initially normal in both legs following surgery. While he was still asymptomatic the patient developed an abnormal ankle pressure response to exercise on the right although the resting pressure index remained normal. Symptoms of intermittent claudication developed as the pressure worsened further.

whilst their resting pressures were normal. Asymptomatic peripheral arterial disease was thus detected in 54 of these patients using non-invasive tests. In only 16 of these patients was there any evidence of disease on clinical examination.

A stress test can also be used to assess the results of surgery. Patient PO presented with symptoms of claudication in the left leg, but had an abnormal ankle pressure on the right both at rest and in response to exercise (Fig. 17.8a). Following bilateral surgery both the resting and stress tests were normal (Fig. 17.8b).

One further important use of a simple stress test is in the follow-up of patients after surgery. Figures 17.9 and 17.10 illustrate this point. Both patients had a normal response to exercise following surgery but during subsequent years were shown to develop asymptomatic abnormalities before experiencing symptoms. Similarly, progression of disease in an asymptomatic leg can be demonstrated independently of disease in the symptomatic leg.

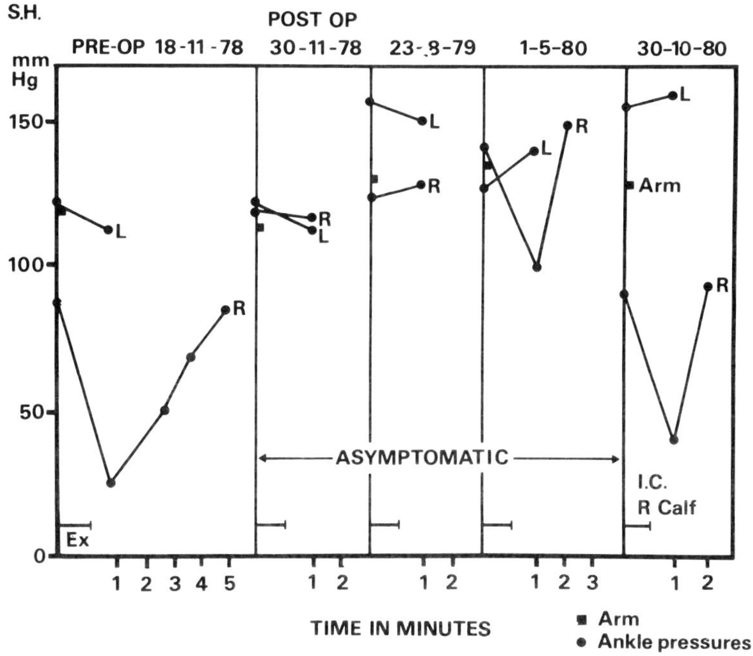

Figure 17.10. Following surgery the ankle pressure both at rest and in response to exercise was normal. Eighteen months later, while the patient was asymptomatic, he developed an abnormal ankle pressure response to exercise although the resting ankle pressure remained normal. Five months later he developed intermittent claudication in the right calf as the ankle pressure worsened further.

The one-minute exercise test in asymptomatic subjects

The previous clinical observations demonstrated that an abnormal exercise test was often the precursor of abnormal resting tests and symptoms. The scope of the test was then extended to the detection of occult peripheral arterial in asymptomatic subjects. Three consecutive groups were studied: patients admitted for hernia repair, patients admitted for coronary artery bypass grafts and diabetic outpatients over the age of 40 years. In addition to determining the prevalence of disease in each group we were concerned with the acceptability of the test and the value of an exercise test over and above measurements made at rest.

Table 17.1 depicts the total numbers in each group, the prevalence of symptoms and clinical signs of peripheral arterial disease, and the suitability of the remaining patients for the treadmill test.

Table 17.1. Suitability for treadmill testing

	Total no. assessed	Symptoms or signs of PAD[a]	No symptoms or signs of PAD	
			Suitable for treadmill	Unsuitable for treadmill
Hernia	165	8 (4.8%)	148	9
CABG	80	6 (7.5%)	65	9
Diabetic	219	31 (14.2%)	133	55

[a] PAD = Peripheral arterial disease

The prevalence of symptomatic peripheral arterial disease in the hernia group (4.8%) was similar to that expected for the same age group in the general population, whereas the prevalence in the other two groups appeared to be higher. It could also be seen that whereas only 6% of the asymptomatic hernia patients were unsuitable for treadmill testing, this figure was 29% in the diabetic group. In many this was due to other symptoms of cardiovascular disease (stroke or angina), the remainder were unsuitable for reasons such as blindness or severe shortness of breath.

Those patients with no symptoms of disease and suitable for treadmill exercise were invited to undergo testing for occult peripheral arterial disease. A resting pressure index of 0.9 or a fall in ankle pressure following exercise of 30 mmHg or more were considered abnormal. The results are shown in Table 17.2.

In each category it can be seen that many more abnormalities were detected using a more sensitive stress test than by resting tests alone, clearly demonstrating the value of a stress test.

One of the CABG patients died following surgery a week after these tests were performed. The aorto-iliac disease subsequently detected at post-

Table 17.2. Occult peripheral arterial disease

	number	Abnormal resting PI[a]	Abnormal exercise test	Total with occult PAD[b]
Hernia	100	1	9	10
CABG	50	1	18	19
Diabetic	100	3	27	30

[a] PI = ankle/brachial systolic blood pressure index
[b] PAD = Peripheral arterial disease

mortem had been reflected by an abnormal exercise test, as shown in Figure 17.11.

Very few other studies have used a stress test for the detection of occult disease, the majority confining their investigations to resting tests alone [14–17]. In each case it is postulated that the prevalence of occult disease would have been greater if a stress test had been used.

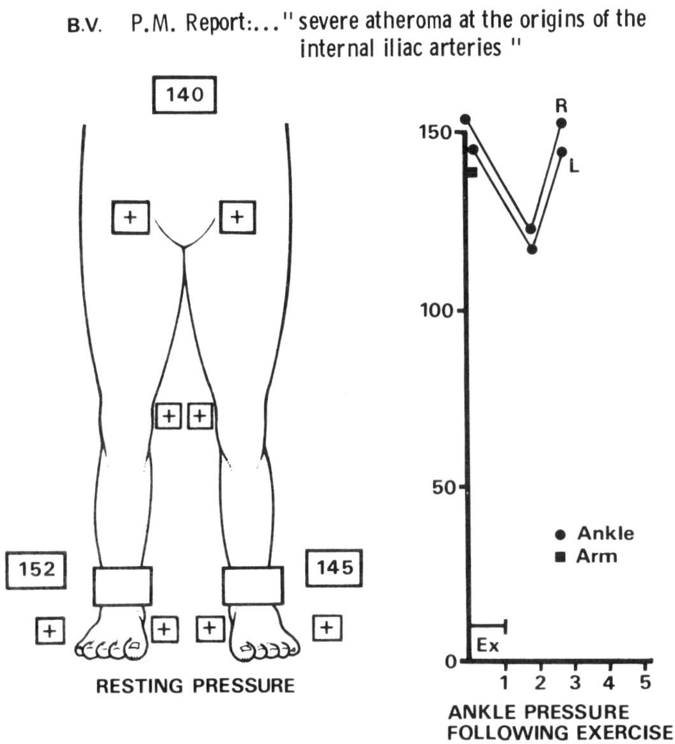

Figure 17.11. This patient had an abnormal ankle pressure response to exercise. One week later severe atheroma could be seen at post mortem.

Comparison of the treadmill test with other methods

Interest in occult peripheral arterial disease has developed only recently. Previously the use of non-invasive tests was confined to symptomatic patients and new methods have been aimed at matching, or even superceding arteriography. Investigations for use in a symptomatic patient, especially if done at rest, may be inadequate for an asymptomatic subject. Duplex colour Doppler for example, is excellent for imaging grafts, but less reliable for imaging the aorto-iliac segment and too time consuming for use in asymptomatic subjects. Pulse palpation, the use of a questionnaire and any tests which fail to incorporate a period of stress are also unlikely to be of much value in asymptomatic subjects. Simple stress tests are the most convenient and sensitive tool for epidemiological purposes.

Two types of stress test are used in this context – treadmill exercise and a post-occlusive reactive hyperaemia test. In the latter, the indirect ankle pressure or flow measurements are made following a period (usually 3–5 minutes) of calf or thigh occlusion. The hyperaemic blood-flow which follows a period of calf or thigh occlusion mimics the hyperaemic flow of exercise. The initial ankle pressure response appears to be the same in each case, although the recovery period is extended after treadmill exercise [18, 19].

Subject tolerance to the two tests will depend upon their age and disease status, and the discomfort of the reactive hyperaemic test must be offset against fitness for one minute of treadmill exercise. Sutton and co-workers [20] primarily used an exercise test in their study of elderly adults, reserving the reactive hyperaemia test for those unsuitable for the treadmill.

At present, therefore, these comparatively cheap and straightforward methods would appear to be the best means of detecting occult peripheral arterial disease. They may have restricted value in the evaluation of symptomatic patients, but are essential for asymptomatic subjects. Screening with resting tests alone will often fail to detect occult disease as disease of sufficient severity to result in abnormal pressures and flows at rest is often symptomatic. In every group of subjects that has been studied with the one-minute treadmill test, the stress test has provided considerably more information than the resting tests alone.

References

1. Bloor R. Natural history of arteriosclerosis of the lower extremities. Ann Roy Coll Surg Engl 1961; 28:36.
2. Kannel WB, Shurtleff D. The natural history of arteriosclerosis obliterans. Cardiovasc Clin 1971; 3:37.

3. Begg TB, Richards RL. The prognosis of intermittent claudication. Scot Med J 1962; 7:341.
4. Hughson WG, Mann JI, Tibbs DJ *et al.* Intermittent claudication: Factors determining outcome. BMJ 1978; 1:1377.
5. Hughson WG, Mann JI, Garrod A. Intermittent claudication: Prevalence and risk factors. BMJ 1978; 1:1379.
6. Criqui MH, Fronek A, Barrett Connor E *et al.* The prevalence of peripheral arterial disease in a defined population. Circulation 1985; 71 (3):510.
7. Hale WE, Marks RG, May FE *et al.* Epidemiology of intermittent claudication: evaluation of risk factors. Age and Ageing 1988; 17:57.
8. Yao JST. Haemodynamic studies in peripheral arterial disease: Br J Surg 1970; 57:761.
9. Boyd AB, Ratcliffe AH, Jepson RP *et al.* Intermittent claudication – a clinical study. J. Bone and Joint surgery 1949; 318:325.
10. May AG, Van de Berg L, De Weese JA *et al.* Critical arterial stenoses. Surgery 1963; 54:250.
11. Flanagan DP, Tullis JP, Streeter VL *et al.* Multiple sub-critical arterial stenoses: effect on post-stenotic pressure and flow. Ann Surg 1977; 186(5):663.
12. Cappelen C, Hall KV. The effect of obstructive arterial disease on the peripheral arterial blood pressure. Surgery 1960; 48:888.
13. Auckland A, Hurlow RA. Evaluation of a standard one minute walking test in patients with intermittent claudication. In: Non-invasive assessment of the cardiovascular system. Diagnostic principles and techniques. Dietrich EB (Ed.) 1982; John Wright PSG Inc.
14. Schroll M, Munck O. Estimation of peripheral arteriosclerotic disease by ankle blood pressure measurements in a population study of 60 year old men and women. J Chronic Disease 1981; 34:261.
15. Lamme S, Johansson BW, Lindell SE. Peripheral atherosclerosis in patients with myocardial infarction. Angiology 1984; 356:373.
16. Perphnieni V, Gylling H, Salmenkivi K. Peripheral atherosclerosis in familial hyperscholesterolaemia. J Intern Med 1989; 225:379.
17. Walsh JJ, Cofelice M, Lumpkin D *et al.* Is screening for vascular disease a valuable proposition? J Cardiovasc Surg 1988; 29(3):306.
18. Fox MJ, Tripolitis A, Kirby S *et al.* A comparison of a reactive hyperaemia test with a standard exercise test in the evaluation of peripheral vascular disease. Br J Surg 1977; 64:290.
19. Hummel BW, Hummel BA, Mowbray A *et al.* Reactive hyperaemia vs treadmill exercise testing in arterial disease. Arch Surg 1978; 113:95.
20. Sutton KC, Wolfson SK, Kuller LH. Carotid and lower extremity disease in elderly adults with isolated systolic hypertension. Stroke 1987; 18(5):817.

18. The management of occult atherosclerosis in arteries of the lower limbs

KENNETH A. MYERS, P. GEOFFREY MATTHEWS, MARK L. WAHLQVIST and CHE SAM LO

Most apparently normal adults have occult atherosclerotic disease in arteries to the lower limbs. Many older subjects have objective evidence of disease without being aware of disability. Even if disease is causing symptoms, the obvious stenosis or occlusion may be less important than occult disease in arteries above and below the lesion for planning the best treatment. Intervention to correct a stenosis or occlusion on one side may expose symptoms from occult disease on the other.

Most current knowledge about both the cause and natural history of atherosclerosis has come from epidemiological studies, and these have been a triumph for the modern scientific approach to evaluating disease. However, they have generally concentrated on coronary artery disease (CAD) rather than disease in arteries to the lower limbs. The Framingham study [1] has followed more than 5000 subjects now for over 40 years. The Multiple Risk Factor Intervention Trial (MRFIT) [2] screened more then 360,000 men to focus resources on some 12,000 who were in the top 10% for risk. At the other extreme, a Finnish study [3] and the Bogalusa study in the USA [4] are tracking children and adolescents.

The days of such enormous, prolonged, expensive trials must be numbered. Since clinical end-points are few and late in the evolution of disease, the trials need to follow large numbers over many years at enormous expense. They are being replaced or at least supplemented by studies that use objective techniques to detect early arterial disease, and these are well-suited to examine accessible peripheral arteries. They should require much smaller groups followed for a relatively short time at far less expense. Arteriography can detect early disease in arteries to the lower limbs and can measure disease progression with sufficient accuracy to relate progression to aetiological factors [5, 6]. However, it is probably not ethical to follow early arterial disease in asymptomatic subjects by this invasive technique. The thrust now is to study accessible arteries by non-invasive ultrasound techniques [7–14].

A.-M. Salmasi and A. N. Nicolaides (eds.), Occult Atherosclerotic Disease, 243–268.

Occult disease in arteries to the lower limbs in apparently normal subjects

The pathology of occult arterial disease

Rational treatment can be developed only if it is known how disease starts and progresses. These have been extensively reviewed by Ross [15] and by Schwartz *et al.* [16]. Atherosclerosis is considered to result from arterial injury on a background of inherited or acquired susceptibility. Changes start with fibrofatty thickening followed by accumulation of mononuclear inflammatory cells in the intima. These changes progress to smooth muscle proliferation and migration then thinning, fibrosis and necrosis in the media. In the later stages, there is extension of the inflammatory process into the adventitia. Thus, there are lipid-laden atheromas and associated fibrous sclerosis, and different methods of diagnosis and treatment may be required for each depending on the stage of evolution [17]. Presumably, the more advanced the changes through the wall, the more difficult it is to reverse the process, but it is not known whether it is ever too late to try.

Recent evidence suggests that active inflammatory processes may play an important role in development of plaques. In particular, recent studies by members of our unit examine the role that macrophages play as mediators of injury [18]. It appears that both macrophages and endothelial cells modify low density lipoprotein so that it can be taken up by scavenger receptors to form foam cells, macrophages may be activated to produce tissue factors which induce local thrombus formation, and modified low density lipoprotein may be an important stimulus for activating macrophages within the plaques.

Endothelial cells, smooth muscle cells (SMCs), macrophages derived from circulating monocytes, and cytotoxic T-lymphocytes all interact in the wall. SMCs replicate, migrate from the media to the intima, and change from functioning 'contractile' to lipid-containing 'synthetic' cells, but most lipid-rich foam cells at the edge of atheromas are macrophages, and SMCs may be more concerned with laying down the connective tissue matrix which develops in established lesions. Platelets adhere to the intima but probably contribute only to late phases of lesion progression. More needs to be known about cellular interaction to allow specific therapy to retard the changes.

The cells release attractant, suppresant, mitogenic and cytotoxic chemicals. Platelet chemo-attractants, notably platelet derived growth factor (PDGF), bring SMCs and monocytes to the region. Monocytes produce cytokinins which attract other cells, stimulate connective tissue matrix formation, carry in and oxidise LDL to release circulating tissue peroxides and produce free oxygen radicals which damage tissue. Endothelium produces growth factors and prostacyclins. Movement of SMCs from the media to intima may result from loss of normal inhibitory mechanisms. There is great untapped potential to develop drugs which influence these effects.

Risk factors for occult disease

Epidemiological studies have largely defined the factors responsible for atherosclerosis. Genetic predisposition has been shown by pedigree, twin and ethnic studies. The Framingham study showed innate susceptibility by a two-fold increased likelihood of coronary artery disease (CAD) if siblings had clinical CAD [1], and a 30% increased rate if parents died from CAD [19]. The added risk factors have been defined by cross-sectional, case-control and cohort studies. The Framingham study showed the personal characteristics and living habits which promote atherosclerosis, both endogenous (blood lipids, blood pressure, blood sugar, and fibrinogen) and exogenous (diet containing excess calories, fat and salt, sedentary habits, unrestrained weight gain and cigarette smoking, and perhaps 'Type A' behaviour and marital status) [1]. However, a WHO study to define the prevalence of risk factors in adults from 40 centres world-wide [20] showed wide disparity for prevalence and mortality rates and a poor correlation between the two in some centres, raising the possibility of other influences. Wahlqvist *et al.* [21] have reviewed the risk factors for lower limb arterial disease in diabetics. In general, risk factors become less active with advancing age and in females, there is debate as to whether they cause risk across their entire distribution or only above threshold levels, and it is not certain whether their effect is linear.

The diagnosis of occult disease in apparently normal subjects

Arteriographic studies

The difficulty has been to develop highly reproducible techniques. Brooks, Blankenhorn and colleagues [22] pioneered computer-controlled femoral arteriography to measure minor changes in wall thickness, and derived an index which they termed 'computer estimate of atherosclerosis' (CEA). In a preliminary study of 54 men, correlation between CEA and risk factors was significant at the first examination only for smoking and the diastolic blood pressure, and multivariate stepwise regression analysis for change between arteriograms showed that there was a significant correlation only with lipoprotein-a and maximum systolic blood pressure during exercise. The variance for CEA was low enough to predict that it should be possible to detect a 5% change in CEA over a 1-year trial with only about 130 subjects.

Ultrasound studies

Current interest is with techniques that show changes in the wall by ultrasound B-scans of carotid arteries and arteries to the lower limbs. Pignoli and colleagues [9, 10] performed *in vitro* studies of carotid arteries and the aorta and found two echo layers that correspond to the lumen/

intima and media/adventitia interfaces, the media appearing anechoic, and best definition of the inner surface was obtained from the far wall. They were able to measure thickness of the inner layer with an error less than 20%. Future *in vivo* studies are likely to confirm that the combined intima and media thickness relates to the degree of early fatty deposition, and when normal values have been defined, it should be possible to identify occult disease. If stereotactic techniques are then used to relocate the site of examination, it should be possible to track the progress of disease. We are using B-scans to measure common femoral arterial wall thickness and to relate the measurements to risk factors, and an example of a scan is shown in Figure 18.1.

Picano and colleagues [11, 12] used ultrasound backscattering to characterise arterial plaques in the aorta and found that peak amplitude and fast Fourier transform analysis of the reflected signal, particularly from the intima/media interface, were altered by collagen, cholesterol crystals and calcium, and this defined whether the segment was normal, fibrofatty or calcified. In the future, it may be possible to use this approach to relate the efficacy of treatment to the type of plaque.

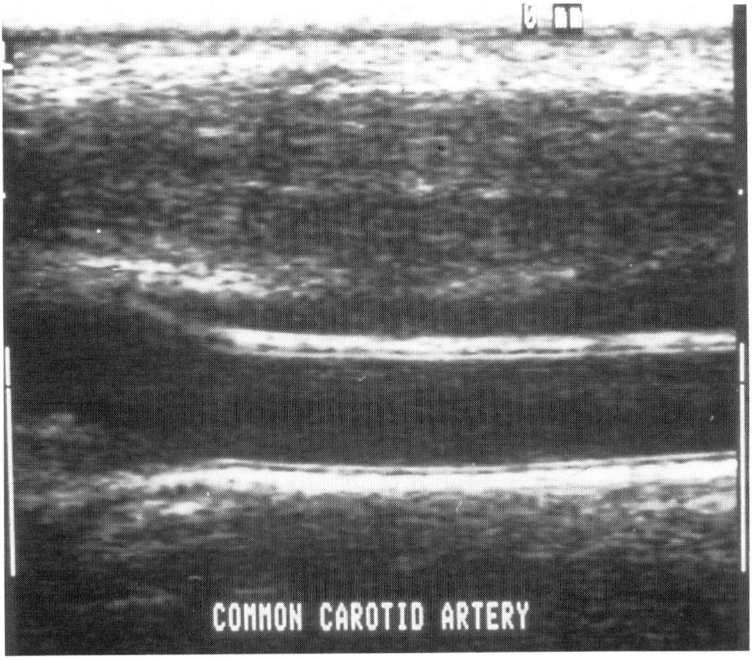

Figure 18.1. A high resolution ultrasound image of the artery in longitudinal section. The echogenic intima and echolucent media can be readily identified

Arterial wall rigidity relates to atherosclerosis and can be studied by further ultrasound techniques, although other changes such as glycosylation and calcification in the wall may cause confusion in the interpretation of findings. We studied subjects with no apparent clinical arterial disease by pulse wave transit times from the subclavian to common femoral arteries to calculate arterial wall compliance, and the Laplace Damping Factor (LDF) to measure pulsatility in the common femoral and posterior tibial arteries. Derivation of these measurements are described elsewhere [23]. There was a significant relation between compliance and advancing age, raised blood pressure, increased serum cholesterol and triglyceride levels, and reduced serum HDL levels. We found significant correlations between compliance and total cholesterol and HDL cholesterol even after partial correlation analyis to eliminate the effect of age and blood pressure [7]. In addition, there was significant decreased compliance and increased LDF in non-insulin dependant diabetic (NIDDM) men with no clinical evidence of arterial disease compared to normal controls [8]. Further, when the NIDDM subjects and normal controls were combined to provide as wide a range of blood glucose levels as possible, then after allowing for age, there were significant negative correlations between compliance and free fatty acid and insulin levels which were almost completely accounted for by differences in blood glucose levels, so that it was concluded that arterial compliance in the aortoiliac segment was best predicted in this part of the study by age and the area under the blood glucose curve [24, 25].

Current interest centres on the ability of ultrasound to measure arterial wall movement with each pulse, which should also be reduced as the wall becomes more rigid. This approach is used in the Bogalusa Heart Study of adolescents [4] to calculate the carotid pressure-strain elastic modulus (pulse pressure/fractional diameter increase during the pulse cycle); this was highly reproducible (r=0.84) and significantly higher in those with a high risk factor profile, particularly those with a positive parental history. Van Merode and colleagues [26] used the technique to show that carotid arteries are stiffer in hypertensives. Currently, we are measuring arterial wall movement by M-mode ultrasound techniques to calculate the arterial elastic modulus and to relate this to risk factors to confirm the earlier studies of arterial wall compliance. An example of the tracing used to obtain results is shown in Figure 18.2.

The natural history of occult disease in apparently normal subjects

The Atherosclerosis Risk in Communities (ARIC) Study [13] will use B-scan ultrasound measurement of wall thickness of the carotid and popliteal arteries on two occasions three years apart in some 16,000 subjects aged 45–64 years from four centres in the USA. Ultrasound findings will be

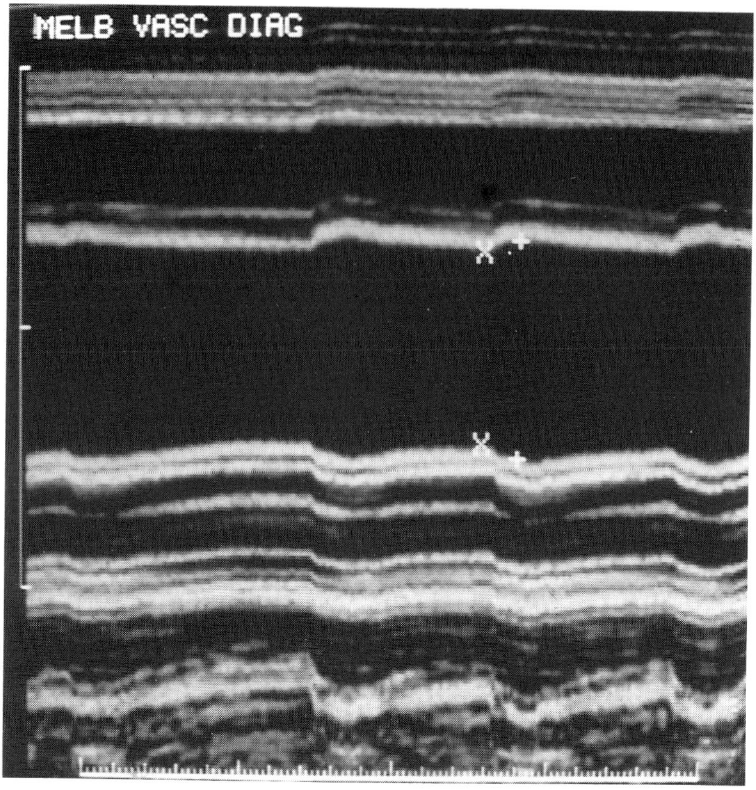

Figure 18.2. M-mode ultrasound imaging of the arterial wall showing the degree of wall movement through the pulse which allows calculation of the elastic modulus.

related to personal characteristics, blood analyses, and clinical events for CAD, stroke and intermittent claudication. Preliminary studies show that it should be possible to measure wall thickness to within 0.2 mm and to demonstrate a change in thickness of more than 0.3 mm. The aim is to investigate the aetiology, clinical sequelae, and variation in risk factors for atherosclerosis; it may be the first time that peripheral arteries will be examined in order to make indirect postulates about CAD, rather than the reverse. The same techniques will be used in the Multicenter Isradipine Diuretic Atherosclerosis Study (MIDAS) [27] to assess drugs intended to retard atherosclerosis in hypertensive patients. Expertise gained by the groups will then allow the techniques to be adapted to a wide range of studies.

Ultrasound measurements of arterial compliance and LDF can be used to study the course of pre-clinical disease. Campbell *et al.* [28] used LDF at the posterior tibial artery to follow 90 middle-aged men over 3 years, and found that 11 of 49 (22%) who had high values developed signs of lower limb arterial disease whereas only 2 of 41 (5%) with normal values developed signs of disease, but they were unable to accurately follow individual subjects with this technique.

Our longitudinal studies of the femoral and carotid arteries by measuring compliance, arterial wall thickness and arterial wall movement are designed to determine whether rates of progression vary in relation to risk factors and as part of randomised trials of drugs to lower lipid levels.

Treatment of occult disease in apparently normal subjects

Experiments in primates show that conservative treatment can inhibit progression of occult arterial disease or even cause regression [29–31] but it is not certain whether regression can occur in humans [32, 33]. However, since most subjects in 'western communities' have atherosclerosis, even from childhood, it is difficult to know how best to attempt to arrest the process. Rose [34, 35] distinguishes between 'sick individuals and sick populations' and compares the merits of the 'high-risk' and 'population' approaches for intervention to modify risk factors; at present, there is a combined approach of intensive treatment for those identified (usually by accident) as being at high risk and attempts at a community education programme. Since genetic predisposition may profoundly influence results in individuals but is generally lost in a heterogeneous population, it is far more difficult to predict the outcome in an individual subject than for a community.

There might seem to be benefit from concentrating on 'high risk' subjects but these could turn out to be the most difficult to motivate and the most refractory to treatment, while the 'high risk' approach is far more expensive [36]. The 'population' strategy to modify behaviour in the entire community is now preferred. The Australian National Heart Foundation Risk Factor Prevalence Surveys of 1980 and 1983 [37] provide typical evidence for the effects of educational programs. Changes between the two assessments were all in the appropriate direction and most achieved statistical significance, but the degree was encouraging rather than striking. Rose [34, 35] points out that 'a large number of people exposed to a low risk is likely to produce more cases than a small number of people exposed to a high risk' and suggests that 'hypertension clinics, lipid clinics, diabetic clinics . . . offer only a limited answer to the community problem', but he also points out that this means that many at low risk will be involved without benefit while those at high risk will be less well defined, eventually leading to the risk of both the community and doctors losing motivation. This may be the reason why recent critical reviews question the benefit from changing eating habits to attempt to reduce blood lipid levels, perhaps due to frustration at perceived regimentation, and a cynical attitude to commercial opportunities to promote costly aids to treatment.

Specific measures to modify risk factors
Since there is a direct relation between atherosclerosis and serum cholesterol, triglyceride, low density lipoprotein (LDL) and apoprotein-B levels, and an inverse relation with high density lipoprotein (HDL) and apoprotein-A levels, it seems reasonable to at least measure serum cholesterol, particularly if there is premature arterial disease or a strong family history of arterial disease or hyperlipidaemia [38]. The Australian National Heart Foundation recommend dietary treatment if the serum cholesterol is >5.5 mmol/1, the aim being to reduce saturated fatty acid and cholesterol intake by a low fat diet, to substitute oils and foods containing the omega-6 linoleic-acid, omega-3 polyunsaturated fatty acids and the monounsaturated oleic acid, and to avoid excess calories. However, even the best-motivated patients are unlikely to reduce their fat intake by more than 10% of energy intake. The Foundation also advise drug treatment if the serum cholesterol level is >6.5 mmol/1, and various drugs can reduce LDL to normal levels while most also increase HDL levels; it is not yet certain whether treatment to change the lipid status acts by causing a fall in LDL-cholesterol or an increase in HDL-cholesterol, and it is difficult to separate the effects of changing lipid levels from other biochemical changes.

A normal feedback mechanism to cell receptors stops continued LDL uptake when the cell is replete, but LDL altered by oxidation is taken up by alternate 'scavanger receptors' with no feedback inhibition. The largest cell mass is the hepatocyte population and if their lipid content rises due to increased ingestion of saturated fat, available LDL receptor numbers fall and plasma LDL levels rise. Thus, serum cholesterol may be reduced by not allowing it to get to hepatocytes, by diet or by drugs which bind bile-acids in the gut (bile-acid sequestrants). Alternatively, serum LDL may be reduced by agents which affect enzymes involved in uptake and synthesis in the cell, such as drugs which increase lipoprotein lipase activity (fibric-acid derivatives), or which compete with a rate-limiting coenzyme, 3-hydroxy-3-methylglutaryl coenzyme-A reductase (HMG CoA reductase inhibitors). Other drugs block LDL oxidation so as to reduce its uninhibited uptake. At present, the choice of the best drug is empirical and combinations such as a resin and nicotinic acid or a HMG CoA reductase inhibitor may be desirable. The overall reduction in disease progression must be weighed against side-effects for treatment over many years, so that it is not known at what age to start treatment, and whether less vigorous treatment should be chosen in the elderly.

Diet and exercise cause a fall in serum triglyceride and increase in HDL-cholesterol levels [39], but it is not known whether exercise and weight reduction result in benefit for pre-clinical lower limb arterial disease. Fish oil fatty acids (omega-3 acids) can have a beneficial effect [40], by acting through appropriate changes in lipids as well as reduced platelet aggregation and adhesion [41], but the precise role of these agents has yet to be defined.

The relation between diet and arterial disease is subtle but powerful and there is much yet to be learned. We showed that lower limb arterial wall indices of compliance and LDF in 31 apparently normal and 22 NIDDM patients without clinical evidence of arterial disease were significantly more likely to be within the normal range if the subjects had a wide variety of total food and plant food intake, and it was calculated that up to 20% of the variance in arterial wall indices was explained by food variety [42]. In addition, the same group were analysed to determine whether compliance and LDF were related to fish consumption, and it was found that compliance was significantly lower for 'non-fish eaters' in the healthy and NIDDM groups, and that LDF was significantly higher for 'non-fish eaters' for the healthy subjects and for both groups combined [43].

Stopping smoking should reduce lower limb arterial disease progression. Antihypertensive drugs have varying effects on serum lipid levels [44]. Rosenstock and colleagues [45] measured lipid levels at 6-month intervals in insulin-dependant diabetics and showed that they were significantly improved by 'intensive treatment' but not by 'conventional treatment' so that they postulated that intensive treatment should reduce the risk of future atherosclerosis. It is not certain whether benefit from treating these conditions is due simply to controlling associated risk factors or whether there is a direct effect [46]. Whether good control of hypertension or diabetes slows lower limb arterial disease progression is a further area for assessment by non-invasive ultrasound studies.

Clinical studies of risk factor modification

It is generally agreed that primary and secondary clinical intervention trials show that intensive modification of exogenous and endogenous risk factors result in a moderate reduction of cardiac events. It remains to be seen whether the same can be shown for disease in arteries to the lower limbs. Treatment to manipulate the biochemical environment can be achieved by removing exogenous influences, by diet, stopping smoking, and perhaps by avoiding stress, or by adding treatment, at a simple level by manipulating the diet or by exercise, or by drug treatment to reduce lipid levels, to reduce blood pressure, or to better control diabetes. The former is 'natural' and is unlikely to harm the subject, whereas the latter can lead to dangers.

The results of clinical trials relating to intervention have been extensively reviewed [47, 48]. Large primary prevention trials which reduced exogenous influences by diet, stopping smoking, etc. have shown a lower incidence of cardiac events, both in selected high risk groups (such as MRFIT and the

Oslo Trial) and in general community groups (such as the European Collaborative Trial and the North Karelia Study). The reduction in cardiac risk from drug treatment for high risk men has been shown in other large primary intervention trials (such as the WHO Cooperative Trial, Lipid Research Clinics Coronary Primary Prevention Trial, and Helsinki Heart Study) and secondary prevention trials after myocardial infarction (such as the Coronary Drug Project). It is not known whether early intervention in childhood would increase the benefit, whether it is ever too late to bother in older patients, and whether the results also apply to women and to subgroups such as diabetic or hypertensive patients. Unfortunately, results are often presented in such a way as to dramatise an effect which though significant may not be very striking [49]. The effect of such intervention on lower limb arterial disease has not yet been assessed by clinical trials.

Arteriographic studies of risk factor modification

Arteriography provides evidence that intervention can retard or perhaps even reverse occult arterial disease in humans. A review of small numbers of patients studied by coronary angiography to assess the effect of drug treatment [50] (such as the National Heart, Lung and Blood Institute Study, University of Helsinki Study and Cholesterol-Lowering Atherosclerosis Study) showed highly significantly reduced new lesion formation, delayed progression and even variable regression, associated with marked fall in serum lipids. Blankenhorn and colleagues [6] studied femoral arteries in 25 patients without clinical disease who were treated for hyperlipidaemia and they found that serial arteriograms at an average of 13 months apart showed that significant progression of disease correlated with triglyceride and cholesterol levels. However, Olsson [51] used femoral arteriograms performed 12 months apart to study 63 asymptomatic hyperlipidaemic patients randomised into a control group and a group treated with nicotinic acid to show that there were changes in atheroma size in only 25% and that there was no significant difference in the treated group. Two further separate femoral arteriographic studies from Sweden are in progress, with considerably larger numbers of patients.

Ultrasound studies of risk factor modification

The MIDAS trial [27] will compare isradipine and hydrochlorothiazide for their effectiveness in retarding progression of peripheral atherosclerosis in hypertensives. A number of other studies combining dietary and drug therapy to control cholesterol levels and associated risk factors such as hypertension are under way. In addition to clinical end-points, peripheral arteries will be studied by ultrasound techniques. While the difference in outcome is likely to be small so as to require relatively large numbers of patients followed for several years, with the consequent risk of type II errors, nevertheless we consider that this is the direction for the future.

Early clinical disease in arteries to the lower limbs

Pathology of early clinical disease

Widmer and colleagues [52] studied 6400 factory workers by oscillometry and found that about 5% had occlusive disease and that the distribution of occlusions was: superficial femoral arteries – 49%, crural arteries – 23%, iliac arteries – 14%, upper limb arteries – 12%, and the aorta – 2%. Atherosclerosis occurs particularly at vessel curves, angles and bifurcations, with predilection for disease at areas of low shear stress [53]. The aortic bifurcation angle appears to influence the risk of arterial disease. An autopsy study [54] showed that the normal angle is 35° (SD 11°) with no difference between males and females, although a wide range was quoted from other arteriographic studies. Sharp and colleagues [55] found that the average angle was 38° in the presence of occlusive disease and 52° in normal subjects or patients with aneurysms. The most common site for superficial femoral artery disease is at the adductor hiatus, but the mechanism for early changes at this site have not yet been adequately studied. Nor is there any clear explanation for the relatively high incidence of crural artery disease and low incidence of iliac disease in diabetics.

Risk factors for early clinical disease

Widmer and colleagues [52] found that the prevalence of occlusion in males was less than 1% under the age of 50 years, but that this rose to 5.2% at 55–59, and 7.5% at 60–64 years, with a male:female ratio of 1.6:1. The Framingham study [56] showed that 'women lagged behind men by 10 years', and that the incidence of claudication developing was about one-quarter of that for coronary artery disease. The relative effect of risk factors measured by regression coefficients differed at various sites [57]. For claudication, the association in descending order was with cigarette smoking, serum cholesterol, glucose intolerance and systolic blood pressure in men, and glucose intolerance, smoking, cholesterol and blood pressure in women, and these patterns were different to those for coronary and cerebrovascular disease. However, since claudication tends to present at a later age than CAD, the pattern of risk factors may appear to be different because the group is attenuated by death of patients due to myocardial infarction [58]. The prevalence of risk factors then determines their actual influence. In the Australian National Heart Foundation Risk Factor Prevalence Survey, a population study of 25–64-year-old males and females in 1983, the prevalence for each was: serum cholesterol >6.5 mmol/l – 20.9%; current smoking – 29.6%; hypertension – 29.6%; overweight or obesity – 34.7%. Fowkes [58, 59] reviewed the association between risk factors and lower limb arterial disease and concluded that smoking 'seems especially important' although clinical disease is more likely to be associated with smoking than early disease, perhaps because haemodynamic changes from smoking could bring more severe disease to attention, that hypertension is a risk factor, but that there is conflicting evidence for an association between glucose intolerance and disease in non-diabetics, and inconsistent results for an association with lipid abnormalities. Criqui and associates [60] used ultrasound techniques to relate disease to risk factors in 565 subjects aged 38–82 and found that 69 had lower limb arterial disease, that large vessel disease was related to age, smoking, systolic blood pressure, fasting plasma glucose and obesity in men, and age and systolic blood pressure in women, but that there was no significant relation between disease and any measured lipids in either sex. It may be that the distribution of obesity is of considerable importance.

There are at least 4 other confusing reports relating lower limb arterial disease to lipid abnormalities. A Dutch study of 37 young patients [61] showed a high incidence of abnormal cholesterol, triglyceride, LDL and HDL levels. A Danish study of 76 patients and 21 controls [62] showed significantly higher LDL and lower HDL in patients but no difference for cholesterol or triglycerides. A Norwegian study of 110 patients with lower limb arterial disease compared to 548 controls [63] showed that both cholesterol and triglyceride levels were significantly higher in the patients. A British study of 32 patients with peripheral arterial disease and 38 controls [64] showed that triglyceride levels were higher amongst male patients but that total cholesterol and HDL-cholesterol were not significantly different, although the ratio of HDL-chelesterol to total less HDL cholesterol was significantly reduced in both sexes, perhaps due to an association with smoking.

From Finland, Laakso and colleagues [65] studied over 2000 diabetics and controls aged 45–64 years and found that claudication was at least 4 times more likely in diabetics, and Siitonen and associates [66] showed that ankle pressure indices were reduced in 7.3% of NIDDM males compared to 2.3% of male controls, although there was no difference in females. Beach and colleagues [67] studied 258 NIDDM patients and 158 controls by ankle pressure indices at rest and after exercise and by Doppler waveform analyses of the femoral and tibial arteries, and found that the prevalence of lower limb arterial disease was 22% in NIDDM patients and 3% in controls, and that there was a 14% incidence of new disease and 87% likelihood of disease progression with NIDDM within 2 years; their patients had a higher incidence of elevated triglyceride, low HDL, hypertension and smoking, but diabetes was an independant risk factor.

Diagnosis of early clinical disease

Fowkes [68] has criticised the use of claudication as a marker for epidemiological studies, pointing out the difficulty in defining when an atheroma becomes a stenosis, what constitutes unequivical claudication, the inter-observer variability for assessing pulses and arteriograms, and the need for objective tests. Various non-invasive objective tests have been used to detect patients with stenosis or occlusion causing minimal or no disability. Widmer and colleagues [52] used oscillometry and Ulrich and associates [69–72] used plethysmography, but these are now outdated. Criqui and colleagues [73, 74] used strain gauges on the toes to measure segmental pressures down the legs and post-occlusion pulse reappearance half-time, and Doppler ultrasound to measure flow velocity and post-occlusion reactive hyperaemia patterns in the common femoral and posterior tibial arteries. Marinelli and colleagues [75] and Beach and associates [67] relied on Doppler ankle pressure indices at rest and after exercise and continuous-wave Doppler wave-forms from the common femoral and tibial arteries.

While early stenotic or occlusive disease is relatively common in arteries to the lower limbs, many subjects are asymptomatic or do not appreciate the significance of mild claudication. In Widmer's study [52] at least one-third of patients with occlusions were asymptomatic. Criqui and colleagues [73, 74] found that only about one-fifth of patients with abnormal ultrasound tests had claudication. In a study of 458 diabetic patients, Marinelli and colleagues [75] reported that 19% of diabetic patients who were thought to have a normal history and examination had abnormal non-invasive tests, and that 44% of those thought to have an abnormal history or examination had normal tests.

The natural history of early clinical disease

Dormandy and colleagues [76] reviewed the extensive evidence that the larger proportion of patients with claudication do not worsen, but that in part this is because many do not live for very long. Ulrich and associates [69–72] used plethysmography to follow 306 patients with intermittent claudication for an average of more than 3 years. There was a pattern characteristic of iliac occlusion in 49 legs, which remained unchanged in about 60% or converted to a pattern of femoro-popliteal disease in the other 40%, and about 40% showed gradually improving flow while none worsened. There was a pattern characteristic of femoro-popliteal disease in 271 legs, which remained unchanged in about 80% or converted to a pattern of iliac occlusive disease in some 10%, and most legs showed gradually worsening flow due to progression of distal disease while only about 10% improved. There were 153 contralateral limbs with a pattern of non-occlusive disease and follow-up showed that 12% improved to apparently become normal, about one-half remained unchanged, one-third worsened to develop a pattern of femoro-popliteal occlusion, and 2% worsened to develop a pattern of iliac occlusion; of those who apparently developed occlusions, only about one-third noted that symptoms became worse. Control legs in apparently normal subjects showed no change over a comparable period.

Treatment of early clinical disease

In general, conservative treatment to correct risk factors is all that is required, since there is no strong evidence to show that rapid disease progression is common and no means of predicting which patients are likely to be at future risk.

Duffield and colleagues [77] reported femoral arteriogram findings in 48 claudicants randomised to ‘drug treatment’ or ‘usual care’, and found that serum lipid levels became much lower in the drug-treated group and that lesion progression occurred in 10 of 144 segments in ‘drug-treated’ and 27 of 156 segments in ‘usual care’ patients, a 60% reduction in the rate of progression ($p<0.01$).

Objective studies measuring ankle pressures and walking distance have shown that stopping smoking significantly improves claudication [78]. However, a Norwegian study of 225 patients with claudication compared to a reference group of some 25,000 subjects in the community [79] showed the difficulties in persuading patients to stop smoking. The patients were evaluated by self-declaration and by serum thiocyanate measurements. Almost all males and 70% of females in the patient group stated that they were smokers or ex-smokers, but only 38% of smoking male patients compared to 77% of reference male smokers admitted smoking more than 10 per day, in spite of having higher thiocyanate levels. About 15% of patients who claimed to have stopped had raised thiocyanate levels.

Exercise has been shown to significantly improve walking distance [80]. The benefits claimed for more esoteric measures such as transcutaneous nerve stimulation, electrotherapy, external carbon dioxide, ultrasound, ultraviolet radiation, massage and external compression have yet to be evaluated [81].

Drug treatment may improve perfusion. Pentoxifilline reduces blood viscosity and improves walking distance in some claudicants [82]. Ketanserin, which inhibits platelet aggregation induced by serotonin, improves blood filtration and has an anti-hypertensive effect, has been studied in a randomised, placebo-controlled, double-blind trial of 3899 claudicants [83]; there were 17 major amputations in the treated group compared to 32 in the placebo group, but an adverse interaction between ketanserin and potassium-losing diuretics made it difficult to assess any real benefit from the drug.

Occult disease in patients with severe clinical disease in arteries to the lower limbs

Clinical peripheral arterial disease is usually focal so that treatment is possible by an operation to restore a circuit in the affected area. However, atherosclerosis is generalised so that further occult disease is likely to be present above and below the most affected segment on the affected side and on the other side. The severity and distribution of further disease may determine whether an operation relieves symptoms, how likely it is to succeed for a long time, and whether further symptoms will develop at another site. Thus, occult disease should be assessed before proceeding to any form of intervention, so as to allow a more accurate long-term prognosis.

Diagnosis of occult disease in patients with severe clinical disease

Clinical assessment
A careful history may disclose early claudication in the ipsilateral thigh or the contralateral calf at about the time that severe calf claudication stops the patient on the more affected side, but absence of symptoms does not exclude appreciable disease. Careful examination may raise the probability of pulse deficits, but we found that the ability of any of the members of our unit to agree as to whether femoral or popliteal pulses were normal or reduced in amplitude was little better than chance [84] so that it would be unwise to make a confident assessment of disease in proximal or contralateral arteries on the basis of palpating pulses.

Arteriography
If arteriography is required, it is our practice to show the full length of the arterial system on both sides from the renal arteries to the feet, in two planes if necessary. However, Slot and colleagues [85] found that arteriography is not very reliable; disease was classified into 4 grades by 11 observers and their agreement was not much better than expected from chance, particularly for the aorta, iliac and profunda femoris arteries. Even with biplanar arteriography, Theile and Strandness [86] could detect aorto-iliac disease with only 70% sensitivity and less than 80% specificity as judged by intra-arterial pressure measurements. Arteriographic scoring of runoff crural arteries can be calculated and has been compared to measured

resistance distal to femoral artery occlusions [87], with reasonably good correlation (r=0.64).

Invasive pressure measurements
Several authors have described the use of invasive common femoral artery pressures for diagnosis of occult aorto-iliac disease [88, 89] and others have described a combination of non-invasive tests with invasive pressure measurements in selected patients [90]. These can be performed well before intervention, seperately or at the time of arteriography, or in the operating theatre immediately before commencing surgery.

Non-invasive ultrasound techniques
In practice, we find that one of the most valuable investigations from the vascular laboratory is the measurement of pressure indices in each leg when the patient is first seen, for although these do not relate well to the severity of symptoms, they do show whether there is disease in the limb, and whether there is occult contralateral disease [91]. Laing and Greenhalgh [92] studied 100 asymptomatic contralateral legs in patients with claudication, and found that more than one-half had reduced ankle pressures but that less than one-third of these had abnormal physical signs.

Analysis of the common femoral artery Doppler ultrasound pulse wave can help to determine whether there is occult aorto-iliac disease. Several methods have been used including pulse rise time, pulsatility index (PI), the Laplace Damping Factor (LDF), and principal component analysis (PCA). Their derivation and relative merits have been reviewed elsewhere [23, 91] and there have been further recent reports. Bagi and colleagues [93] found an excellent correlation between common femoral pulse rise time and arteriographic assessment of disease, a pulse rise time >120 ms relating to stenosis >50% with a sensitivity and specificity of 95% and 97% respectively for aorto-iliac disease and 79% and 93% respectively for femoro-popliteal disease. However, Kitslaar and colleagues [94] compared pulse rise time and PI with arteriography and intra-arterial pressures to grade aorto-iliac disease and found that the correlation was poor, though it was best for the pulse rise time. Baker and associates [95] up-dated their experience with common femoral LDF compared to aorto-iliac arteriography in 98 legs and showed that LDF detected stenosis >50% with a sensitivity of 92% and specificity of 93%, independant of whether the superficial femoral artery was patent or occluded. Goss and colleagues [96] showed that a computer-generated diagnosis including PCA more accurately predicted the clinical outcome than did clinical judgment alone.

Various ultrasound tests have been used to assess stenosis in the femoro-popliteal segment. Baker and colleagues [97] studied transit times, pulse damping and an index of peripheral resistance derived by Laplace transform, but none showed good correlation with arteriographic measurement of stenosis.

There is now considerable interest in whether the duplex ultrasound scan can supplement or even replace arteriography for diagnosing the presence and severity of stenotic disease in arteries to the lower limbs [98]. Because the examination is extensive, it is really only feasible for regular practice using colour-Doppler scanning. Undoubtedly there is scope to more accurately define criteria for grading disease. At present, we follow criteria described by Cossman and colleagues [99] who rely on peak systolic velocity ratios and absolute velocities to define diameter stenoses as:

	Velocity Ratio	*Peak Velocity*
Minimal or no stenosis	—	<150 cm/sec;
30–49% stenosis	1.5–2:1	150–200 cm/sec;
50–75% stenosis	2–4:1	200–400 cm/sec;
More than 75% stenosis	>4:1	>400 cm/sec.

Cossman and colleagues [99] used these criteria to study arteries distal to the common femorals, with arteriography as the standard of reference, and found that they could grade >30% stenosis with a sensitivity of 83% and specificity of 96%, the highest accuracy being for the distal superficial femoral and popliteal arteries. Legemate and associates [100] found that >150% increase in peak systolic velocity predicted >50% stenosis on arteriography with sensitivity and specificity of 92% and 98% respectively for aorto-iliac disease and 88% and 98% respectively for femoro-popliteal disease, although the accuracy was less when compared to intra-arterial pressures, and they also found that an end-diastolic velocity >40 cm/sec accurately predicted that the diameter stenosis was >75%. Langsfeld and colleagues [101] calculated pressure gradients by the modified Bernoulli equation (pressure gradient = 4 × maximum velocity^2) to define significant aorto-iliac stenoses with a sensitivity of 82% and specificity of 93% as compared with arteriography, and showed an excellent correlation with pull-through intra-arterial pressures (r=0.9). The degree of turbulence shown by spectral analysis expressed as a power-frequency analysis should relate to the degree of stenosis [102]. Disagreement between duplex scans and arteriography appears to be more likely with minimal disease.

Treatment of occult disease in patients with severe clinical disease

Patients with severe ischaemia are likely to have disease at multiple levels, each contributing in different degree to restricted perfusion of the limb. One segment may stand out as being obviously affected but this does not mean that it is the only site that needs to be treated. Even although relief of rest pain or healing of necrotic sites is the prime goal, the traumas from intervention will be doubly rewarded if a procedure also leaves the patient with no claudication.

Occult disease above a symptomatic occlusion

It is probable that long-term patency after any form of intervention is less likely if there is low velocity and volume of blood flow through the segment. Flow could be restricted by occult disease in 'inflow arteries' above the operation, for example unrecognised iliac artery disease above a femoro-distal bypass [103].

A common problem is how to predict whether treating proximal stenotic disease by aorto-femoral bypass in a patient with a superficial femoral artery occlusion will improve symptoms. Faris and colleagues [104] measured intra-arterial common femoral and arm pressures to determine an aorto-femoral pressure gradient index and multiplied the pre-operative ankle or toe pressures by this index to predict the post-operative pressures. If the predicted post-operative ankle pressure index was >0.60, then claudication was relieved and if it was <0.56 it was not; if the predicted toe pressure was >40 mm Hg, it was likely that a conservative amputation for gangrene would heal.

Occult disease below a symptomatic occlusion

Again, it would seem likely that patency rates for bypass grafts and endo-vascular procedures might be adversely affected by disease in 'outflow arteries' below the operation site, but the evidence is inconclusive.

For aorto-femoral bypass, Harris and colleagues [105] found that late patency rates were significantly lower if there was associated superficial femoral artery occlusion than if the femoral outflow was patent, to the point where they advocate combined aortic and femoral artery bypass, but we found no difference between the two groups, perhaps because of a high proportion of distal anastomoses to the profunda femoris artery [106].

The influence of tibial artery and pedal arch disease have been studied after femoro-distal bypass. Early occlusion seems to be more likely if there is a high outflow resistance measured at operation [107] or if arteriography shows occlusion of the pedal arch [108]. However, late patency does not appear to be influenced by arteriographic grading of tibial artery outflow [109] or the state of the pedal arch [110], although Ascer and colleagues [111, 112] found that outflow resistance measurements predicted late patency rates for femoro-crural but not for femoro-popliteal grafts, and that foot-salvage rates in patients with critical ischaemia were well predicted by outflow resistance for all grafts.

There are varying opinions as to where to best place the distal anastomosis for a femoro-distal bypass. At one extreme, there is some enthusiasm for using the above-knee popliteal artery if possible, to keep the bypass short and to allow selection of a synthetic graft if preferred so as to spare the long saphenous vein for later use if needed [113], for the results of above-knee synthetic grafts may be little worse than those for vein [114], and best results from this approach may rely on being able to treat occult disease in the popliteal artery by endovascular procedures. There may be a place for taking a vein bypass to an 'isolated popliteal segment' below the knee, relying on collateral outflow to relieve symptoms and ensure long-term patency, and there is evidence that this may give as good results as more distal bypass [115]. However, there is now more enthusiasm for avoiding adverse effects from occult distal disease by taking autogenous vein down to a crural or pedal artery if the popliteal artery is not satisfactory, and there is no evidence that this gives worse long-term patency rates than for femoro-popliteal bypass. Andros and colleagues have shown that improved results can be obtained by taking bypass grafts down to below outflow occlusions by making the distal anastomosis to a tarsal artery [116]. There is also a push to perform multiple distal anastomoses if there is more than one patent crural artery, the proposition being that it is not possible to tell which has the best outflow and which is likely to give the best long-term results, so that there may be 'safety in numbers' [117], but there is no evidence yet to show that this is associated with improved results. There is not yet enough information to show whether these considerations also hold for endovascular procedures.

Occult contralateral disease

Frequently, arterial disease is bilateral but assymetrical. Claudication in the worst affected leg is likely to stop the patient from walking far enough for pain to develop in the contralateral leg. If claudication is relieved by operation in the worse leg, symptoms may then become manifest in the second leg. Predicting this may influence management, for a patient might wish to have one operation but not two operations to gain relief. A patient with critical ischaemia is not likely to complain of lesser contralateral symptoms, and critical ischaemia demands treatment to the worst affected leg, but residual claudication in the second leg after treatment is likely to lead to fear of future deterioration that may not be warranted. An least the patient should be warned if there is a possibility of staged bilateral surgery.

Management of occult contralateral disease is not always rational. It has long been conventional practice to treat serious aorto-iliac disease by aorto-bifemoral bypass, irrespective of whether disease is predominantly unilateral or bilateral. In a review of 57 aorto-bifemoral grafts [88], we found that the bypass on the 'second side' did not increase ankle pressure indices measured 4 weeks after operation in about three-quarters of the legs and indeed many had normal ankle pressure indices (>0.9) before operation. Because of this, it became our practice to treat apparently unilateral iliac disease by an extraperitoneal unilateral ilio-femoral/profunda synthetic bypass rather than by transperitoneal aorto-bifemoral bypass, and in 110 consecutive operations, we found that only 4 patients later required proximal surgery for contralateral iliac artery disease [118].

There is an increasing tendency to treat iliac disease by endovascular balloon dilatation, atherectomy or laser angioplasty, alone or in combination with femoral artery surgery. This allows a more selective approach to each side independently. The possible combinations of treatment are now considerable, with staged or simultaneous treatment of bilateral disease by endovascular surgery, or by balloon dilatation for the less affected side at the same time or separate from a unilateral ilio-femoral or femoro-femoral cross-over bypass. In our unit, aorto-bifemoral bypass is reserved now for patients with extensive aortic and bilateral iliac disease.

Conclusion

Detection and treatment of occult disease is becoming the prime focus for clinical research and practical management. Many people in the community are likely to develop lower limb ischaemia. Identifying subjects at risk when disease is still occult should allow appropriate modification of risk factors, hopefully to reduce and delay disease progression and defer or avoid expensive, traumatic surgical intervention. Surveillance will identify rapid progression and the need for early conservative treatment. Although a new era of proliferating non-invasive investigations should facilitate the process, how best to seek out subjects at risk with the greatest cost-benefit to the community has still to be determined. In the past, major arterial reconstruction tended to be reserved for foot-salvage in patients with advanced disease. However, claudication is a very disabling symptom and does not always follow a benign course. The next few years are likely to see greatly expanded indications for more early intervention by better bypass techniques and by endovascular surgery, as well as improved pharmacological management. Sophisticated non-invasive diagnostic techniques will be used to diagnose disease at an increasingly early stage, and more accurate mapping of disease will allow the most rational techniques for intervention.

References

1. Kannel WB. Contributions of the Framingham study to the conquest of coronary artery disease. Amer J Cardiol 1988; 62:1109.
2. Stamler J, Wentworth D, Neaton JD. Is relationship between serum cholesterol and risk

of premature death from coronary heart disease continuous and graded? JAMA 1986; 256:2823.
3. Akerblom H K, Viikari J, Uhari M *et al.* Atherosclerosis precursors in Finnish children and adolescents. I. General description of the cross-sectional study of 1980, and an account of the children's and families' state of health. Acta Paediatr Scand 1985; Suppl 318:49.
4. Riley W A, Freedman D S, Higgs N A *et al.* Decreased arterial elasticity associated with cardiovascular disease risk factors in the young: Bogalusa heart study. Arterioscleriosis 1986; 6:378.
5. Crawford D W, Brooks S H, Selzer R H *et al.* Computer densitometry for angiographic assessment of arterial cholesterol content and gross pathology in human atherosclerosis. J Lab Clin Med 1977; 89:378.
6. Blankenhorn D H, Brooks S H, Selzer R H, Barndt R. The rate of athrosclerosis change during treatment of hyperlipoproteinemia. Circulation 1978; 57:355.
7. Relf I R N, Lo C S, Myers K A, Wahlqvist M L. Risk factors for changes in aorto-iliac arterial compliance in healthy men. Arteriosclerosis 1986; 6:105.
8. Lo C S, Relf I R N, Myers K A, Wahlqvist M L. Doppler ultrasound recognition of preclinical changes in diabetic subjects: compliance and pulse-wave damping. Diabetes Care 1986; 9:1.
9. Pignoli P, Tremoli E, Poli A *et al.* Intimal plus medial thickness of the arterial wall: a direct measurement with ultrasound imaging. Circulation 1986; 74:1399.
10. Pignoli P, Longo T. Evaluation of atherosclerosis with B-mode ultrasound imaging. J Nuclear Med Allied Sci 1988; 32:166.
11. Picano E, Landini L, Lattanzi F *et al.* Time domain echo pattern evaluations from normal and atherosclerotic arterial walls: a study in vitro. Circulation 1988; 77:654.
12. Picano E, Landini L, Lattanzi F *et al.* Ultrasonic tissue characterization of atherosclerosis: state of the art 1988. J Nuclear Med Allied Sci 1988; 32:174.
13. Szkolo M, Barnes R, Folsom A *et al.* The ARIC investigators. The atherosclerosis risk in communities (ARIC) study: design and objectives. Amer J Epidemiol 1989; 129:687.
14. Bond M G, Wilmont S K, Enevold G L, Strickland H L. Detection and monitoring of asymptomatic atherosclerosis in clinical trials. Am J Med. 1989; 86 (Suppl. 4A):33.
15. Ross R. The pathogenesis of atherosclerosis – an update. New Engl J Med 1986; 314:488.
16. Schwartz S M, Campbell G R, Campbell J H. Replication of smooth muscle cells in vascular disease. Circulation Res 1986; 58:427.
17. Blankenhorn D H, Kramsch D M. Reversal of atherosclerosis and sclerosis. The two components of atherosclerosis. Circulation 1989; 79:1.
18. Tipping P G, Malliaros J, Holdsworth S R. Procoagulant activity expression by macrophages from atheromatous vascular plaques. Atherosclerosis 1989; 79:237.
19. Schildkraut J M, Myers R H, Cupples L A *et al.* Coronary risk associated with age and sex of parental heart disease in the Framingham study. Amer J Cardiol 1989; 64:555.
20. Dobson A J, Alexander H M, Leeder S R *et al.* Risk-factor levels and mortality of ischaemic heart disease in three Australasian centres. Med J Aust 1988; 48:61.
21. Wahlqvist M L, Relf I R N, Myers K A, Lo C S. Diabetes and macrovascular disease: Risk factors for atherogenesis and non-invasive investigation of arterial disease. Human Nutrition: Clinical Nutrition 1984; 38C:175.
22. Brooks S H, Blankenhorn D H, Chin H P *et al.* Design of human atherosclerosis studies by serial angiography. J Chron Dis 1980; 33:347.
23. Myers K A, Williams M A, Nicolaides A N. The use of Doppler ultrasound to assess disease in arteries to the lower limb. In Cardiovascular applications of Doppler ultrasound. Ed by A-M Salmasi and A N Nicolaides. Churchill Livingstone, Edinburgh. 1989; 289.
24. Wahlqvist M L, Lo C S, Myers K A, Simpson R W. Plasma insulin and free fatty acids as

risk factors for arterial compliance in type-2 diabetes. Recent Advances in Clinical Nutrition. 1986; 2:330.
25. Wahlqvist M L, Lo C S, Myers K A *et al.* Putative determinants of arterial wall compliance in NIDDM. Diabetes Care 1988; 11:787.
26. Van Merode T, Hick P J J, Hoeks A P G *et al.* Carotid artery wall properties in normotensive and borderline hypertensive subjects of various ages. Ultrasound Med Biol 1988; 14:563.
27. Furberg C D, Byington R P, Borhani N A. Multicenter isradipine diuretic atherosclerosis study (MIDAS): design features. Am J Med. 1989; 86 (Suppl. 4A):37.
28. Campbell W B, Skidmore R, Woodcock J P, Baird R N. Detection of early arterial disease: a study using Doppler waveform analysis. Cardiovasc Res 1985; 19:206.
29. Farrar D J, Green H D, Bond M G *et al.* Aortic pulse wave velocity, elasticity and composition in a nonhuman primate model of atherosclerosis. Circulation Res 1978; 43:52.
30. Farrar D J, Green H D, Wagner W D, Bond M G. Reduction in pulse wave velocity and improvement of aortic distensibility accompanying regression of atherosclerosis in the rhesus monkey. Circulation Res 1980; 47:425.
31. Malinow M R. Atherosclerosis: regression in non human primates. Circulation Res 1980; 46:311.
32. Graham G A. Is atherosclerosis a reversible lesion? Atherosclerosis 1976; 34:37.
33. Malinow M R. Regression of atherosclerosis in humans: fact or myth? Circulation 1981; 64:1.
34. Rose G. Strategy of prevention: lessons from cardiovascular disease. Br Med J 1981; 282:1847.
35. Rose G, Sick individuals and sick populations. Int J Epidemiol 1985; 14:32.
36. Hall J P, Heller R F, Dobson A J *et al.* A cost-effectiveness analysis of alternative strategies for the prevention of heart disease. Med J Aust 1988; 148:273.
37. Jamrozik K, Hockey R. Trends in risk factors for vascular disease in Australia. Med J Aust 1989; 150:14.
38. Nestel P J. Managing hyperlipidaemia. Med J Aust 1988; 148:29.
39. Wood P D, Stefanick M L, Dreon D M *et al.* Changes in plasma lipids and lipoproteins in overweight men during weight loss through dieting as compared to exercise. New Engl J Med 1988; 319:1322.
40. Vandongen R. Fish oils and cardiovascular disease. Med J Aust 1987; 146:236.
41. Gibson R A. The effects of diets containing fish and fish oils on disease risk factor in humans. Aust NZ J Med 1988; 18:713.
42. Wahlqvist M L, Lo C S, Myers K A. Food variety is associated with less macrovascular disease in those with type II diabetes and their healthy controls. J Amer Coll Nutrition 1989; 8:515.
43. Wahlqvist M L, Lo C S, Myers K A. Fish intake and arterial wall characteristics in healthy people and diabetic patients. Lancet 1989; 2:944.
44. Krone W, Nagele H. Effects of antihypertensives on plasma lipids and lipoprotein metabolism. Amer Heart J 1988; 116:1729.
45. Rosenstock J, Strowig S, Cercone S, Raskin P. Reduction in cardiovascular risk factors with intensive diabetes treatment in insulin-dependent diabetes mellitus. Diabetes Care 1987; 10:729.
46. Dollery C T. Risk predictors, risk indicators, and benefit factors in hypertension. Amer J Med 1987; 82:2.
47. Levy R I, Blankenhorn D, Davis C E *et al.* Intervention studies. Circulation 1989; 80:739.
48. Tyroler H A. Review of lipid-lowering clinical trials in relation to observational epidemiological studies. Circulation 1987; 76:515.

49. Brett A S. Treating Hypercholesterolaemia. How should practicing physicians interpret the published data for patients? New Engl J Med 1989; 321:676.
50. Bilheimer D W. Therapeutic control of hyperlipidemia in the prevention of coronary atherosclerosis: a review of results from recent clinical trials. Amer J Cardiol 1988; 62:1J.
51. Olsson A G. Review of angiographic studies of treatment of atherosclerotic vascular disease. Amer Heart J 1987; 113:609.
52. Widmer L K, Grensher A, Kanner W B. Occlusion of peripheral arteries. A study of 6400 working subjects. Circulation 1964; 30:836.
53. LoGerfo F W, Crawshaw H M, Nowak M *et al.* Effect of flow split on separation and stagnation in a model vascular bifurcation. Stroke 1981; 12:660.
54. Bargeron C B, Hutchins G M, Moore G W *et al.* Distribution of the geometric parameters of human aortic bifurcations. Arteriosclerosis 1986; 6:109.
55. Sharp W V, Donovan D L, Teague P C, Mosteller R D. Arterial occlusive disease: a function of vessel bifurcation angle. Surgery 1982; 91:680.
56. Kannel W B, Skinner J J, Schwartz M J, Shurtleff D. Intermittent claudication: incidence in the Framingham Study. Circulation 1970; 61:875.
57. Kannel W B, McGee D, Gordon T. A general cardiovascular risk profile: the Framingham study. Amer J Cardiol 1976; 38:46.
58. Fowkes F G R. Aetiology of peripheral atherosclerosis. Br Med J 1989; 298:405.
59. Fowkes F G R. Epidemiology of atherosclerotic arterial disease in the lower limbs. Europ J Vasc Surg 1988; 2:283.
60. Criqui M H, Browner D, Fronek A *et al.* Peripheral arterial disease in large vessels is epidemiologically distinct from small vessel disease. An analysis of risk factors. Amer J Epidemiol 1989; 129:1110.
61. Aronson D C, Ruys T H, Van Bockel J H *et al.* A prospective survey of risk factors in young adults with peripheral arterial occlusive disease. Europ J Vasc Surg 1989; 3:227.
62. Horby J, Grande P, Vestergaard A, Grauholt A M. High density lipoprotein cholesterol and arteriography in intermittent claudication. Europ J Vasc Surg 1989; 3:333.
63. Skrede S, Kvarstein B. Hyperlipidemia in peripheral atherosclerotic arterial disease. Acta Chir Scand 1975; 141:333.
64. Trayner I M, Mannarino E, Clyne C A C, Thompson G R. Serum lipids and high density lipoprotein cholesterol in peripheral vascular disease. Br J Surg 1980; 67:497.
65. Laakso M, Ronnemaa T, Pyorala K *et al.* Atherosclerotic vascular disease and its risk factors in non-insulin-dependent diabetic and nondiabetic subjects in Finland. Diabetes Care 1988; 11:449.
66. Siitonen O, Uusitupa M, Pyorala K *et al.* Peripheral arterial disease and its relationship to cardiovascular risk factors and coronary heart disease in newly diagnosed non-insulin-dependent diabetics. Acta Med Scand 1986; 220:205.
67. Beach K W, Bedford G R, Bergelin R O *et al.* Progression of lower-extremity arterial occlusive disease in type II diabetes mellitus. Diabetes Care 1988; 11:464.
68. Fowkes F G R. The measurement of atherosclerotic peripheral arterial disease in epidemiological studies. Int J Epidemiol 1988; 17:248.
69. Ulrich J, Engell H C. The natural history of arteriosclerosis in the lower extremities. I: a plethysmographic study of non-affected limb in unilateral disease. Danish Med Bull 1975; 22:129.
70. Ulrich J, Siggaard-Anderson J. The natural history of arteriosclerosis in the lower extremities. II: a plethysmographic study of non-occlusive arteriosclerotic disease in the lower limbs. Danish Med Bull 1975; 22:136.
71. Ulrich J. The natural history of arteriosclerosis in the lower extremities. III: a plethysmographic study of femoropopliteal occlusion. Danish Med Bull 1975; 22:141.
72. Ulrich J, Engell H C. The natural history of arteriosclerosis in the lower extremities. IV: a

plethysmographic study of occlusion in the aorto-iliac vessels. Danish Med Bull 1975; 22:147.

73. Criqui MH, Fronek A, Barrett-Connor E *et al.* The prevalence of peripheral arterial disease in a defined population. Circulation 1985; 71:510.
74. Criqui HH, Fronek A, Klauber MR *et al.* The sensitivity, specificity, and predictive value of traditional clinical evaluation of peripheral arterial disease: results from noninvasive testing in a defined population. Circulation 1985; 71:516.
75. Marinelli MR, Beach KW, Glass MJ *et al.* Noninvasive testing vs clinical evaluation of arterial disease. JAMA 1979; 241:2031.
76. Dormandy J, Mahir M, Ascady G *et al.* Fate of the patient with chronic leg ischaemia. J Cardiovasc Surg 1989; 30:50.
77. Duffield RGM, Lewis B, Miller NE *et al.* Treatment of hyperlipidaemia retards progression of symptomatic femoral atherosclerosis. Lancet 1983; 2:641.
78. Quick CRG, Cotton LT. The measured effect of stopping smoking on intermittent claudication. Br J Surg 1982; 69(Suppl): 24.
79. Vasli LR, Foss OP. Serum thiocyanate, smoking habits and smoking cessation trial in patients with peripheral atherosclerosis. Scand J Clin Lab Invest 1987; 47:399.
80. Larsen DA, Lassen NA. Effect of daily muscular exercise in patients with intermittent claudication. Lancet 1966; 2:1093.
81. Ernst E. Peripheral vascular disease: physical treatments may help. Br Med J 1989; 299:873.
82. Porter JM, Cutler BS, Lee BY *et al.* Pentoxifylline efficacy in the treatment of intermittent claudication: multicenter controlled double-blind trial with objective assessment of chronic occlusive arterial disease patients. Amer Heart J 1982; 104:66.
83. Verstraete M, Dormandy J, Bousser MG *et al.* Prevention of atherosclerotic complications: controlled trial of ketanserin. Br Med J 1989; 298:424.
84. Myers KA, Scott, DF, Devine TJ *et al.* Palpation of the femoral and popliteal pulses: a study of the accuracy as assessed by agreement between multiple observers. Europ J Vasc Surg 1987; 1:245.
85. Slot HB, Strijbosch L, Greep JM. Interobserver variability in single-plain aortography. Surgery 1981; 90:497.
86. Thiele BL, Strandness DE. Accuracy of angiographic quantification of peripheral atherosclerosis. Prog Cardiovasc Dis 1983; 26:223.
87. Peterkin GA, Manabe S, LaMorte WW, Menzoian JO. Evaluation of a proposed standard reporting system for preoperative angiograms in infrainguinal bypass procedures: angiographic correlates of measured runoff resistance. J Vasc Surg 1988; 7:379.
88. Flanigan DP, Williams LR, Schwartz JA *et al.* Hemodynamic evaluation of the aorto-iliac system based on pharmacologic vasodilation. Surgery 1983; 93:709.
89. Verhagen PF, van Vroonhoven TJMV. Criteria from intra-arterial femoral artery pressure measurements combined with reactive hyperaemia to assess the aorto-iliac segment; a prospective study. Br J Surg 1984; 71:707.
90. Thiele BL, Bandyk DF, Zierler GE *et al.* A systematic approach to the assessment of aortoiliac disease. Arch Surg 1983; 118:477.
91. Myers KA. Preoperative assessment of lower limb ischaemia. In Diagnostic techniques and assessment procedures in vascular surgery. Ed by RM Greenhalgh. Grune and Stratton, London. 1985; 217.
92. Laing S, Greenhalgh RM. The detection and progression of asymptomatic peripheral arterial disease. Br J Surg 1983; 70:628.
93. Bagi P, Sillesen H, Hansen HJB. Quantitative Doppler ultrasound evaluation of occlusive arterial disease in the lower limb. Europ J Vasc Surg 1988; 2:409.
94. Kitslaar PJEHM, Jorning PJG, Kohlen JPFM. Assessment of aortoiliac stenosis by

femoral artery pressure measurement and Doppler waveform analysis. Europ J Vasc Surg 1988; 2:35.

95. Baker J D, Skidmore R, Cole S E A. Laplace transform analysis of femoral artery Doppler signals: the state of the art. Ultrasound in Med Biol 1989; 15:13.
96. Goss D E, Simpson J, Roberts V C, Cotton L T. Evaluation of a computerised test for the assessment of peripheral arterial disease. Europ J Vasc Surg 1988; 2:333.
97. Baker A R, Prytherch D R, Evans D H, Bell P R F. Doppler ultrasound assessment of the femoro-popliteal segment: comparison of different methods using ROC curve analysis. Ultrasound in Med Biol 1986; 12:473.
98. Kohler T R, Nance D R, Cramer M M *et al.* Duplex scanning for diagnosis of aortoiliac and femoropopliteal disease: a prospective study. Circulation 1987; 76:1074.
99. Cossman D V, Ellison J E, Wagner W H *et al.* Comparison of contrast arteriography to arterial mapping with color-flow duplex imaging in the lower extremities. J Vasc Surg 1989; 1:522.
100. Legemate D A, Teeuwen C, Hoeneveld H *et al.* The potential of duplex scanning to replace aorto-iliac and femoro-popliteal angiography. Europ J Vasc Surg 1989; 3:49.
101. Langsfeld M, Nepute J, Hershey F B *et al.* The use of deep duplex scanning to predict hemodynamically significant aortoiliac stenoses. J Vasc Surg 1988; 7:395.
102. Harward T R S, Bernstein E F, Fronek A. The value of power frequency spectrum analysis in the identification of aortoiliac artery disease. J Vasc Surg 1987; 5:803.
103. Charlesworth D, Harris P L, Cave F D *et al.* Undetected aorto-iliac insufficiency. A reason for failure of saphenous bypass grafts for obstruction of the superficial femoral artery. Br J Surg 1975; 62:567.
104. Faris I, Tonnesen K H, Agerskov K *et al.* Femoral artery pressure measurement to predict the outcome of arterial surgery in patients with multilevel disease. Surgery 1982; 92:10.
105. Harris P L, Bigley D J C, McSweeney L. Aortofemoral bypass and the role of concomitant femorodistal reconstruction. Br J Surg 1985; 72:317.
106. King R B, Myers K A, Scott D F *et al.* The choice of operation in aortoiliac reconstructions for intermittent claudication. World J Surg 1983; 7:334.
107. Ascer E, Veith F J. Outflow resistance measurements in intrainguinal bypass operations by injecting saline and measuring the integral of pressure. In Diagnostic Techniques and Assessment Procedures in Vascular Surgery, Greenhalgh R M (Ed). London: Grune and Stratton. 1985; 269.
108. O'Mara C S, Flinn W R, Neiman H L *et al.* Correlation of foot arterial anatomy with early tibial bypass patency. Surgery 1981; 89:743.
109. Brewster D C, LaSalle A J, Robinson J G *et al.* Factors affecting patency of femoropopliteal bypass grafts. Surgery 1983; 157:437.
110. Ricco J-B, Flinn W R, McDaniel M D *et al.* Objective analysis of factors contributing to failure of tibial bypass grafts. World J Surg 1983; 7:347.
111. Ascer E, White S A, Veith F J *et al.* Outflow resistance measurement during infrainguinal arterial reconstructions: a reliable predictor of limb salvage. Amer J Surg 1987; 154:185.
112. Ascer E, Veith F J, White-Flores S A *et al.* Intraoperative outflow resistance as a predictor of late patency of femoropopliteal and infrapopliteal arterial bypasses. J Vasc Surg 1987; 5:820.
113. Rosenthal D, Levine K, Stanton P E *et al.* Femoropopliteal bypass: the preferred site for distal anastomosis. Surgery 1983; 93:1.
114. Veith F J, Gupta S K, Ascer E *et al.* Six-year prospective multicenter randomized comparison of autologous saphenous vein and expanded polytetrafluoroethylene grafts in infrainguinal arterial reconstructions. J Vasc Surg 1986; 3:104.
115. Brewster D C, Charlesworth P M, Monaham J E *et al.* Isolated popliteal segment v tibial bypass. Arch Surg 1984; 119:775.

116. Andros G, Harris RW, Salles-Cunha SX, Dulawa LB, Oblath RW. Lateral plantar artery bypass grafting: defining the limits of foot revascularization. J Vasc Surg 1989; 10:511.
117. Burdick JF, O'Mara C, Ricotta J *et al.* The multiple sequential distal bypass graft: improving nature's alternatives. Surgery 1981; 89:539.
118. Cham C, Myers KA, Scott DF *et al.* Extraperitoneal unilateral iliac artery bypass for chronic lower limb ischaemia. Aust NZ J Surg 1988; 58:859.

PART FIVE

Occult atherosclerotic disease of the renal and mesenteric arteries

19. Occult atherosclerotic involvement of the renal vasculature – pathophysiology, clinical manifestations and investigations contributing to management

CHRISTOPHER J. MATHIAS[1]

Atherosclerosis in the aorta increases in frequency from the arch downwards and may either directly affect the renal vessels or damage the kidney by thrombosis or thrombo-embolism. Hypertension and renal failure are major sequelae but they may not result in symptoms unless sufficiently severe. Involvement of other vessels, especially in the cerebral, coronary and peripheral circulation, are more likely to cause symptoms.

The relationship of atheromatous disease in the renal vasculature to hypertension and renal failure has long been recognised but it is not clear whether it is causal, resultant or coincidental. The high incidence of atheromatous plaques projecting into the renal arteries in patients with 'essential hypertension' was pointed out 50 years ago, by Blackman [1]. In a large multicentre study of 2242 hypertensives, angiography revealed renal vascular lesions in 20%, of which 63% were due to atherosclerosis [2]. Unfortunately however, the detection of atherosclerotic renal disease is often at a late stage, when substantial renal damage has already occurred and is irreversible. This chapter addresses the subject with a view to considering the pathological processes, the pathophysiological mechanisms in the genesis of renovascular hypertension, the clinical signs and symptoms, and those investigations which are of direct relevance, not only in confirming the presence of atheromatous involvement at an early stage, but in helping in clinical management, where the aims should be to prevent, and if possible reverse, renal damage.

1. Dr. Mathias is grateful to the Wellcome trust for their sustained support.

A.-M. Salmasi and A. N. Nicolaides (eds.), Occult Atherosclerotic Disease, 271–280.

Patho-physiological considerations

Anatomico-pathological processes

The renal vasculature can be involved in a number of ways (Fig 19.1). Atheromatous plaques in the aorta may encroach on the origins of the renal vessels causing ostial stenosis. There may be atheromatous changes involving the entire diameter of the vessel (circular or concentric form, which causes an hourglass appearance) or only part of the lumen (eccentric form).

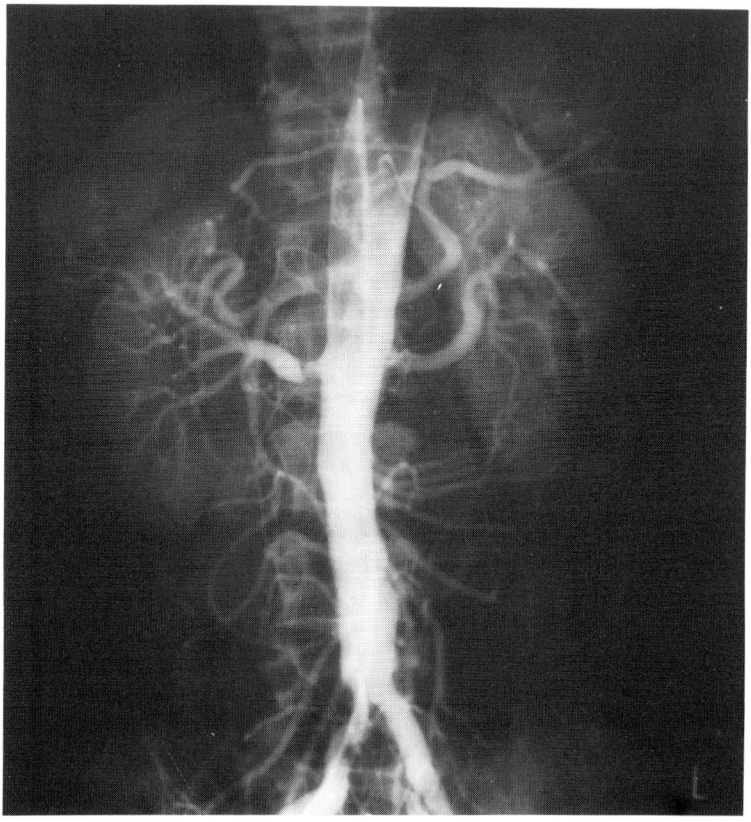

Figure 19.1. Intra-arterial flush aortogram, showing the branches of the aorta including the renal arteries. The right renal artery is stenosed just beyond its origin, with poststenotic dilatation. The right kidney is smaller than the left kidney. Above the renal arteries are the branches of the coeliac axis, with the splenic artery on the left and the common hepatic artery on the right. There is extensive atheroma in the lower part of the aorta and the iliac arteries, as indicated by the irregularity of the lumen. The catheter is placed in the right iliac artery and the tip is seen on level with the top of the left kidney. [from Mathias *et al.*, 1984(3)].

The main renal arteries or larger subdivisions are usually affected with relative sparing of the smaller vessels. These differences presumably result from the relationship between the deposition of cholesterol, the flow characteristics and shear forces in different blood vessels. The ensuing ischaemia may cause a small, shrunken kidney, although the formation of collateral vessels, especially through lumbar and other associated vessels, including ureteral arteries, may help to perfuse the kidney and maintain size and function.

The kidney also may be damaged by thrombotic or thrombo-embolic processes, originating either within the renal vessels, or more proximally from atheromatous ulcers or plaques in the aorta. This may result in segmental renal infarction or, if there is occlusion of the main vessel, infarction of the kidney and an autonephrectomy. A similar end-result may occur if there is dissection around an atherosclerotic plaque involving the ostia, or following aortic dissection which extends to the renal arteries.

Mechanisms contributing to hypertension

The concept that renal ischaemia stimulates the renin-angiotensin system which is instrumental in causing and maintaining hypertension, is attractive and commonly accepted. When considered in the context of clinical and experimental observations however, this does not stand up to rigorous analysis [3]. Experimental studies using models analagous to those seen clinically, (with a clip over the renal artery to cause stenosis), have extended our understanding of patho-physiological mechanisms. In the 1 clip-2 kidney Goldblatt model which is similar to unilateral renal artery stenosis, hypertension is predominantly renin-dependent, especially in the early stages. In other models, such as the 2 clip-2 kidney or 1 clip-1 kidney, there is a severe reduction in renal function, and hypertension is mainly volume dependent.

In the 1 clip-2 kidney Goldblatt model there appear to be three phases in the evolution of the hypertensive process [4], (Table 19.1). Soon after renal artery clipping the blood pressure rises promptly, along with levels of renin and angiotensin-II (A-II) and the hypertension is abolished by acute antagonism of A-II or by inhibiting A-II production with angiotensin converting enzyme inhibitors. This is Phase I, which is clearly renin dependent. Following this, blood pressure remains elevated or may rise further, while levels of renin and A-II plateau or fall. This is Phase II, where acute antagonism of A-II or inhibition of A-II formation does not necessarily lower blood pressure, unless administration of drugs is prolonged. In both Phases I and II, renal ischaemia is responsible for the hypertension, as revascularisation (by clip removal) or nephrectomy restores the blood pressure to previous levels. This suggests that in Phase II, mechanisms working independently of, or in addition to, the direct vascular effects of A-II are involved in the maintain-

Table 19.1. Outline of the three phases of experimental 1 clip-2 kidney Goldblatt hypertension showing the relationship between blood pressure (BP), renin/A-II (angiotensin-II) levels, A-II antagonism by saralasin, A-II inhibition by captopril and clip removal (revascularization) or nephrectomy.

	Blood pressure	Renin/A-II levels	A-II antagonism or inhibition	Revascularization or nephrectomy
Phase I	Elevated	Elevated	BP reduced	BP reduced
Phase II	Elevated	Elevated or normal	BP unchanged or falls if drug administration is prolonged	BP reduced
Phase III	Elevated	Normal or decreased	BP unchanged	BP unchanged

ance of hypertension. These will be discussed later. Following Phase II the hypertension appears irreversible, (Phase III), as drugs, revascularisation or nephrectomy have no effect. Hypertrophy of blood vessels and the heart and/or damage to the contralateral kidney, are factors contributing to 'resistant' hypertension.

These phases in the experimental model may bear some relevance to the clinical situation [5]. In man however, it is often difficult or impossible to know the precise duration the renal stenotic lesion or the duration of hypertension, especially as the stenosis is likely to be progressive, unlike the experimentally induced lesion. A more acute onset may occur with occlusion of a renal artery, and this can cause a marked elevation of renin/A-II levels and severe hypertension, which is responsive to converting enzyme inhibitors as in the experimental Phase I of the 1 clip-2 kidney Goldblatt model [6]. The majority of clinical cases however appear similar to experimental Phase II, as levels of renin/A-II are either modestly elevated or normal, and converting enzyme inhibitors may be effective in lowering blood pressure. The role of other factors in the maintenance of hypertension in this phase continue to be debated; an unfavourable redistribution of sodium, a questionable 'slow pressor component' of A-II and an increase or inappropriate maintainance of central neurogenic pressor mechanisms are some of the factors incriminated. Reversal of renal ischaemia, as in the experimental models, is often successful in amelioration or cure of the hypertension [5, 6]. These considerations have practical importance in the investigation of renovascular hypertension, in determining the relationship between renal ischaemia and hypertension, and in making decisions on therapeutic intervention.

Clinical manifestations

There are usually no specific symptoms which indicate involvement of the renal vasculature. Symptoms may be related to hypertension (headaches, dizziness, nocturia), or may be due to accompanying renal failure, especially when there is severe uraemia. When thrombo-embolism occurs, there may be loin pain which signals renal infarction. For the most part, atheromatous renovascular involvement is indeed 'occult'. Most patients will present because of symptoms resulting from atherosclerosis in other vascular territories, such as transient ischaemic attacks or amaurosis fugax (cerebral), angina pectoris (coronary) or intermittent claudication (peripheral).

Certain groups are at a greater risk. These include patients with familial hypercholesterolaemia, and disorders where hyperlipidaemia is of frequent occurrence, such as diabetes mellitus and hypothyroidism. Patients with long standing essential hypertension, even without elevated cholesterol levels, are at risk. Suspicion of renal artery stenosis should be aroused when the blood pressure is more difficult to control, especially when associated with impaired or deteriorating renal function (see chapter 21).

A renal bruit is often thought to be indicative of renal artery stenosis, but is present in only 32% of proven cases [7]. An epigastric bruit may originate from other abdominal vessels, including the normal aorta in thin women with lordosis. The presence of a bruit is therefore of significance, but its absence does not exclude renal artery stenosis. Bruits and weak or absent pulses in the cerebral and peripheral circulation are often present in atherosclerotic disease along with other signs indicating ischaemia or damage to vital organs. In bilateral renal artery stenosis, or renal artery stenosis in a solitary kidney, patients may present with volume overload and cardiac failure [8].

Investigations

The routine investigations often provide important clues to renal involvement. Examination of the urine may reveal microscopic haematuria, which in the presence of loin pain is suggestive of renal infarction, especially if there is no evidence of urinary tract infection. The haemoglobin level may be low in renal failure, although polycythaemia is occasionally observed in renal artery stenosis. Eosinophilia, thrombocytopenia and hypocomplementemia, which may be mistaken for immune-complex mediated vasculitis, have been associated with atheromatous renal emboli [9]. The degree of renal impairment is determined from the plasma creatinine level; however even when within the normal range there may be substantial renal damage and a creatinine clearance should ideally be performed. A deterioration in renal function during treatment with angiotensin converting enzyme in-

(a) (b)

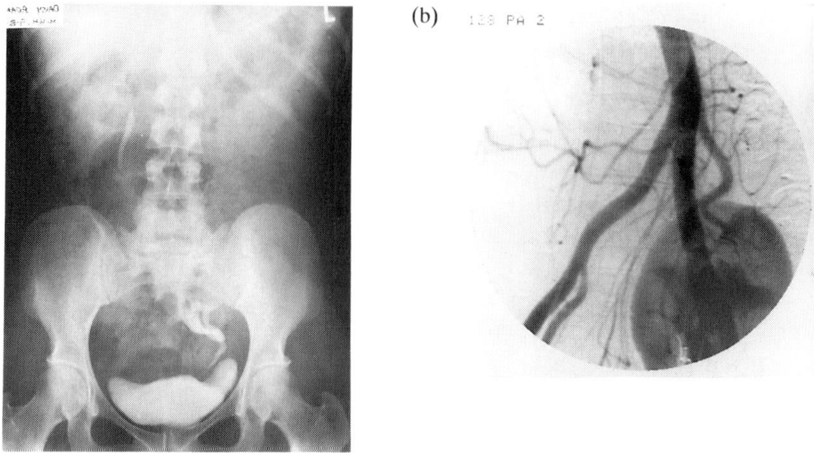

Figure 19.2a and b. Intravenous digital subtraction angiogram, which demonstrates the value of a post-angiography kidney-ureter-bladder film, in a woman undergoing investigation for hypertension. It was initially thought that there was only one kidney, on the right. The nephropyelogram indicates a pelvic kidney on the left (a). There was no evidence of stenosis of the left renal artery, as indicated in b and in views from other angles.

hibitors should draw attention to the likelihood of renal artery stenosis [10]. At an early stage one may proceed onto ultrasonography, to define rectifiable obstructive lesions, to determine the size of the kidneys, and in certain cases to exclude dissection of the aorta.

The definitive investigation however, is angiography [7]. With modern technology, intravenous digital subtraction angiography often clearly delineates the aorta, the ostia and the major renal arteries, which are the vessels usually involved in atherosclerotic renal disease. The investigation also provides information on the urinary outflow tract, and it is mandatory that a nephropyelogram is obtained at the end of the study (Fig 19.2). A denser nephrogram may help diagnose or confirm renal artery stenosis (Fig 19.3), especially if the vessels are not clearly visible because of overlapping bowel or other vessels. Occasionally ureteric notching is seen, because of hypertrophied ureteral arteries which help compensate for main vessel stenosis. The alternative, intra-arterial angiography has a number of advantages, including the ability to clearly define the lesion and also rectify it by dilatation angioplasty, or in select cases by therapeutic embolisation. It is imperative that a flush aortogram and selective renal angiograms are obtained. The former provides an overall view of the abdominal vasculature and importantly will enable assessment of other vessels in the coeliac axis, as the splenic or the hepatic artery may be used for revascularisation. Selective renal angiography provides views not only of the main, but also the smaller renal vessels. In atheromatous disease, care should be taken when cannulat-

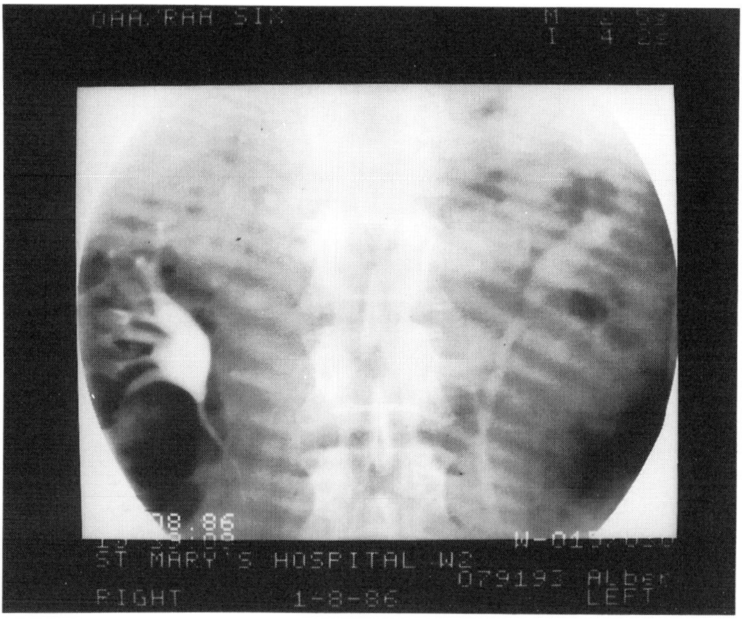

Figure 19.3. Nephropyelogram in a patient with hypertension and extensive atherosclerosis. There is a denser pyelogram on the right. Intra-arterial angiography confirmed right renal artery stenosis which was successfully dilated using balloon angioplasty.

ing the renal arteries to avoid dissection around an ostial plaque. In mild to moderate stenosis (<60%), it may be difficult to be certain of the degree of impaired perfusion and therefore measurement of the pressure gradient across the stenosis is of value. This also helps to determine the technical success of angioplasty.

Intra-arterial angiography has disadvantages which need to be considered. It is an invasive procedure which usually necessitates at least day admission into hospital. Although the incidence of serious side effects is extremely low in experienced hands, there is the potential for bruising, bleeding and peripheral embolisation. There is often a post-angiography elevation in blood urea and creatinine, which may be due to a variety of reasons. One cause may be the contrast medium [11], especially if large doses of high osmolarity agents are used. The risk however is small and nephrotoxicity is usually reversible. This may, of course, also occur with intravenous angiography. Other complications of the intra-arterial approach include dissection (which can further increase renal ischaemia), and thrombo-embolisation. Radionuclide studies are of particular value in assessment, as they provide comparative information quickly and non-invasively. We recommend 99mTC diethylene-triamine-penta-acetate (DTPA) scanning as a baseline

(a)

(b)

(c)

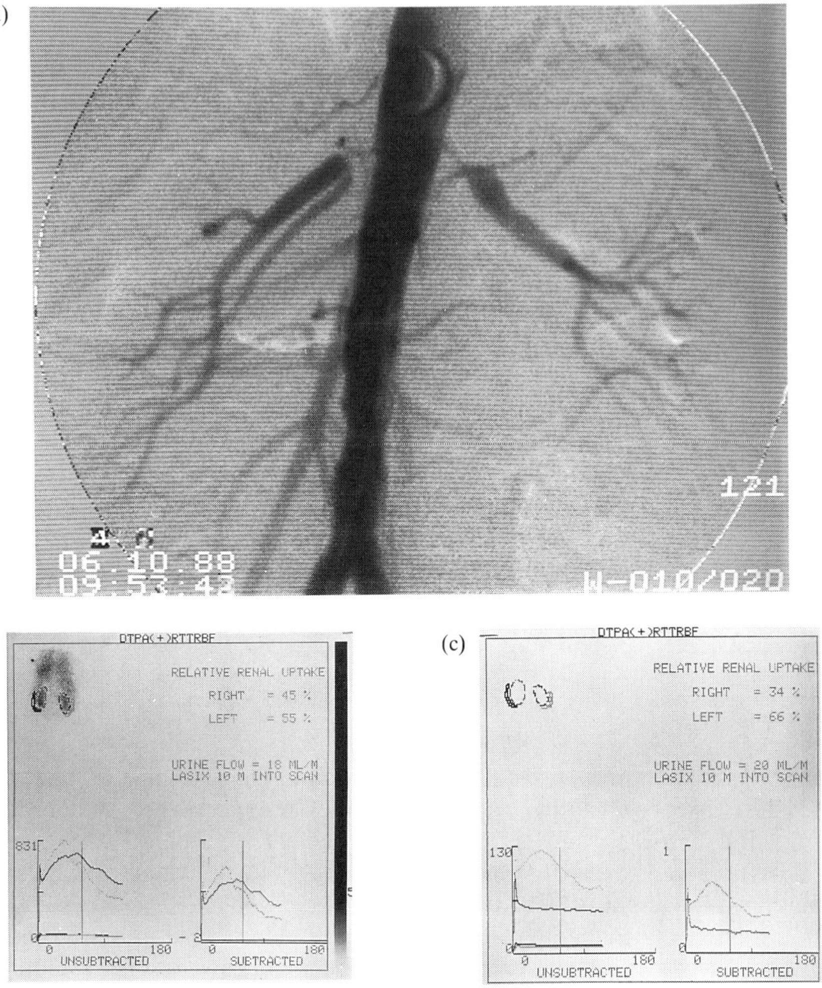

Figure 19.4a, b and c. Intra-arterial angiogram in a woman with widespread atherosclerosis (with involvement of the carotid and coronary circulation), demonstrating severe bilateral renal artery stenosis with an atheromatous lower aorta (a). The next two figures show 99mTc DTPA renograms before (b) and after the angiotensin converting inhibitor, Captopril (50 mg), (c). After captopril there is little change in the clearance of DTPA in the left kidney with virtually no clearance from the right kidney. The right kidney therefore is at considerably greater risk from ischaemic damage than the left. This study emphasises the potential danger of using angiotensin converting enzyme inhibitors in such patients.

investigation before angiography, especially where angioplasty is likely to be contemplated. It also provides the opportunity to measure renal function before and after the angiotensin converting enzye inhibitor, captopril (Fig 19.4a, b, c,). If there is a functionally significant stenosis, (where the post glomerular resistance is A-II dependent), there will be a deterioration of function after captopril which can be detected by renography.

Peripheral and divided renal vein renin measurements are less frequently used than previously. They help to assess the degree of renal ischaemia and determine if a small, poorly functioning kidney, for example, is hypersecreting renin. A number of factors influence renin levels [3] and people of African origin, for instance, normally have low levels of renin, which may not rise substantially despite significant renovascular involvement.

Management aims and options

The major aims are to improve the vascular supply to the kidneys so as to reverse or prevent further renal damage. If there is associated hypertension, as there often is, this may improve blood pressure control. In some situations, as with stenosis in a solitary kidney or bilateral stenosis, revascularisation is necessary to treat cardiac failure. The options consist of surgical intervention with revascularisation (using a range of procedures, or percutaneous transluminal angioplasty [3, 12]. The latter is of value especially in those unable to undergo major surgery. In some situations it may be better to watch and wait, especially if an adequate collateral circulation exists. Nephrectomy may be needed if the kidney is contributing minimally to overall renal function, but is a major factor in causing the hypertension. If the renal tissue mass is small, percutaneous embolisation should be considered.

The natural history of atherosclerotic renovascular disease often entails progressive ischaemia with either thrombosis or thrombo-embolic sequelae resulting in hypertension and/or renal failure with their attendant complications. The need to recognise the problem and intervene at an early stage is therefore of vital importance in preventing potential morbidity and mortality.

References

1. Blackman SS, Jr. Arteriosclerosis and partial obstruction of the main renal arteries in association with 'essential' hypertension in man. Bulletin of Johns Hopkins Hospital 1939; 65:353.
2. Foster J H, Maxwell A H, Franklin S S. Renovascular occlusive disease. Results of operative treatment. Journal of the American Medical Association 1975; 231:1043.
3. Mathias CJ, May CN, Taylor GN. The renin-angiotensin system and hypertension – basic and clinical aspects. In: Malcolm ADB (ed.), Molecular Medicine. Oxford: IRL Press, 1984; 1:178.
4. Brown JJ, Questa AV, Davies DL, Lever AL, Morton JJ, Padfield PL, Robertson JIS, Trust P, Bianchi G, and Schalekamp MAD. Mechanism of renal hypertension. Lancet 1976; 1,1219.
5. Mathias CJ, Kooner JS, Peart S. Do neurogenic mechanisms maintain hypertension in renal artery stenosis? In: Renovascular Hypertension. Pathophysiology, diagnosis, and

treatment. Glorioso N, Laragh J H, Rappelli A. (eds.) Raven Press, New York 1987; p. 173.

6. Mathias C J and Kooner J S. Neurogenic aspects of blood pressure control in man – with an emphasis on renovascular hypertension. In: Concepts in hypertension. Mathias C J and Sever P S (eds.), Steinkpoff Verlag, Darmstadt and Springer-Verlag, New York 1989; p. 67.
7. Carmichael D J S, Mathias C J, Snell M E and Peart S. Detection and investigation of renal artery stenosis. Lancet 1986; 1:667.
8. Pickering T G, Herman L, Devereux R B, Sotello J E, James G D, Sos T A, Silane M F and Laragh J H. Recurrent pulmonary oedema in hypertension due to bilateral renal artery stenosis: treatment by angioplasty or surgical revascularisation. Lancet 1988; 2:551.
9. Cosio F G, Zager R A, Sharma H M. Atheroembolic renal disease causes hypocomplementemia. Lancet 1985; 2:118.
10. Hricik D E, Browning P J, Kopelman R, Goorno W E, Madias N E, Dzau V J. Captopril-induced functional renal insufficiency in patients with bilateral renal artery stenosis or renal artery stenosis in a solitary kidney. New England Journal of Medicine 1983; 308:373.
11. Parfrey P S, Griffiths S M, Barrett P J, Paul M D, Genge M, Withers J, Farid N, McManamon P J. Contrast material-induced renal failure in patients with diabetes mellitus, renal insufficiency or both. A prospective controlled study. New England Journal of Medicine, 1989; 320:143.
12. Genest J, Cartier P, Roy P, Lefevre R, Kuchel O, Cantin M, Hamet P. Renovascular Hypertension. In: Hypertension. Genest J, Kuchel O, Hamet P, Cantin M. (eds.) 2nd. Edition. McGraw Hill, Montreal 1986; Chapter 63:1007.

20. Investigations of mesenteric and renal arteriosclerotic disease

PAUL S. VAN BEMMELEN and D. EUGENE STRANDNESS, JR.[1]

Disease of the mesenteric circulation can exist in three forms: (1) acute mesenteric occlusion with death of the small bowel; (2) chronic mesenteric angina; and (3) asymptomatic involvement. Acute ischaemia of the small bowel has a dramatic presentation dictating emergency measures for survival of the small bowel and the patient as well. Patients who are best subjects for non-invasive studies are those with symptoms suggestive of chronic mesenteric ischaemia.

A history of pain after eating with associated diarrhoea and weight loss is suggestive of the syndrome. A physical examination is of little help, but a bruit may be detected in the mid-epigastrium. It is this subset of patients who are ideal candidates for duplex scanning of the coeliac and mesenteric arteries.

In the past, aortography with lateral views was the only diagnostic method of any value. Because of the risks and high costs, this remained reserved only for those cases with a high suspicion of intestinal ischaemia. Duplex scanning has enabled a non-invasive functional assessment of the mesenteric circulation during postprandial stress conditions.

Methods and procedure

Preparation of the patient. In patients with abdominal symptoms the study is done after an overnight fast. The patient is placed supine and tilted 10–30 degrees feet down to displace the abdominal contents distally. For the examination of abdominal vessels, it is often necessary to use a low-frequency 3-MHz transducer to reach the vessels of interest.

1. The studies illustrated in Figures 20.1–5 were performed by Molly Zaccardi, RVT.

A.-M. Salmasi and A. N. Nicolaides (eds.), Occult Atherosclerotic Disease, 281–290.

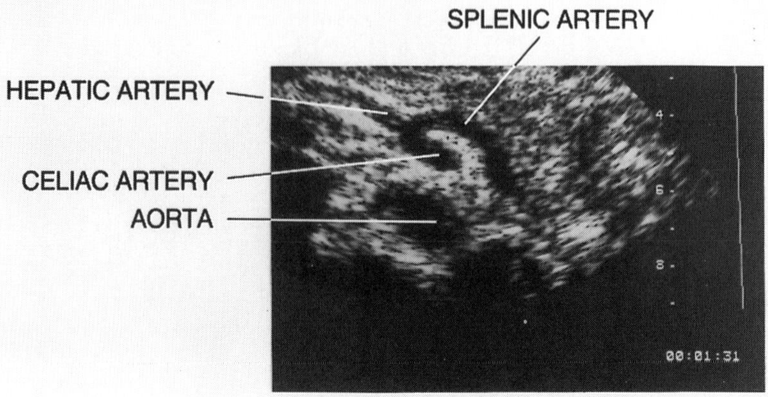

Figure 20.1. Cross-section showing the aorta, the celiac artery, hepatic artery, and splenic artery.

Once the baseline studies have been performed, postprandial values are obtained after a high caloric meal of 16 fl oz of Ensure[R] is given. This provides 710 calories with a distribution of protein 14.7% fat 32%, and carbohydrates 53.3%.

Imaging and identification

The coeliac artery can be identified by viewing in a cross-sectional plane through the proximal aorta. The bifurcation of the hepatic and splenic branches gives a characteristic image (Figure 20.1).

For the superior mesenteric artery, longitudinal views through the aorta will show the origin of the SMA with its acute angle to the aorta itself, Figure 20.2. It has been very difficult to routinely visualize the inferior mesenteric artery.

Characteristics of Doppler waveforms

The normal coeliac artery waveform in a fasting individual is notable for the absence of reverse-flow. Flow changes in the normal coeliac artery are minimal after eating, indicating that this vessel does not have a major supply function to the gut under normal conditions. The normal waveform from the superior mesenteric artery is characterized by reverse-flow after systole and low end-diastolic velocity in antegrade direction (Figure 20.2).

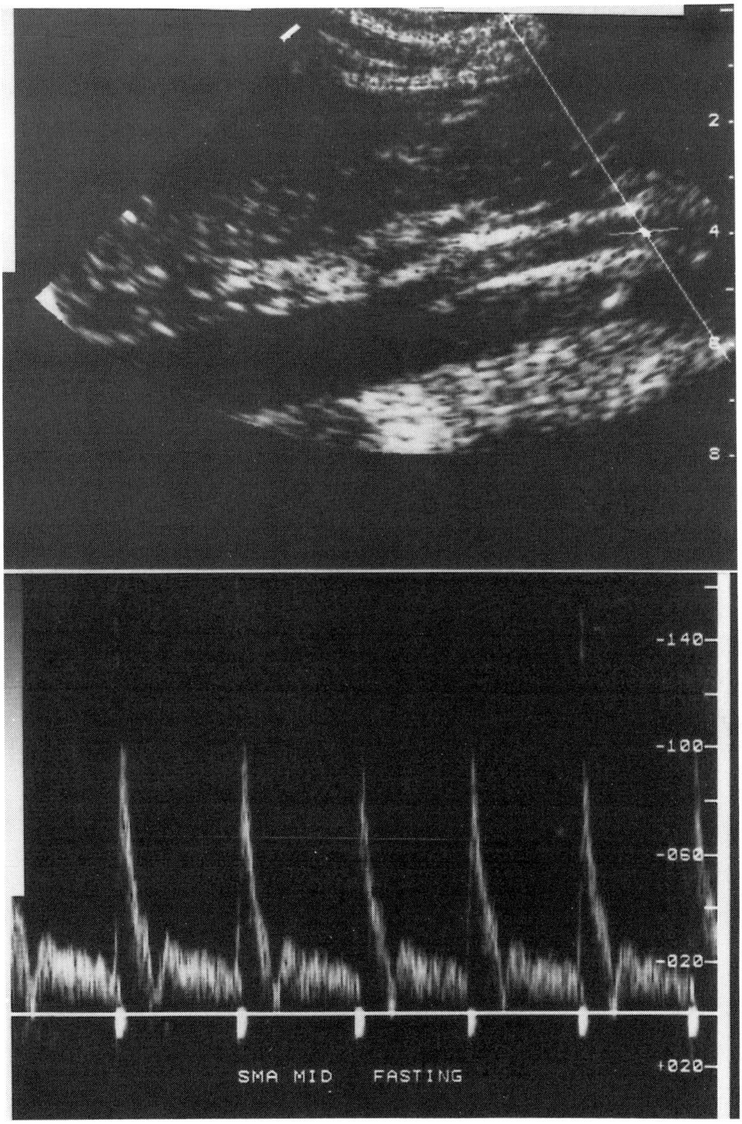

Figure 20.2. Normal superior mesenteric artery (SMA)-fasting. Acute angulation with aorta. Doppler waveform shows reverse flow in late diastole.

In coeliac artery stenosis, a significant increase in peak systolic velocity is found, followed by poststenotic flow patterns. The haemodynamic changes that occur in stenosis of the superior mesenteric artery are similar to those in

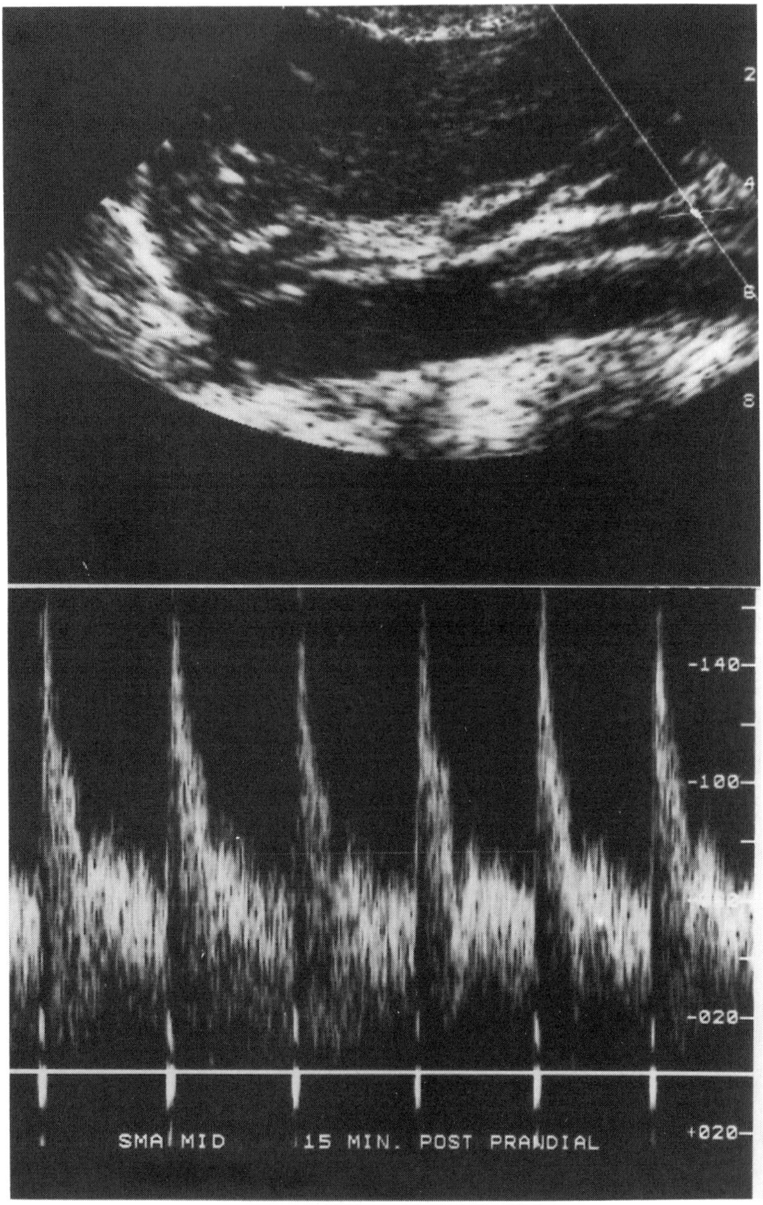

Figure 20.3. Normal SMA, 15 minutes postprandial. Increased diastolic forward flow velocity. Peak systolic velocity is 160 cm/sec.

peripheral arteries. The normal high-resistance outflow vessels decrease their resistance in order to maintain flow. As a result, the reverse component of diastolic flow disappears, and forward flow during the entire diastole is maintained at a higher level than in the normal high resistance situation [1, 2]. This is illustrated in Figure 20.3.

Normal values for duplex blood flow parameters for the coeliac artery and SMA in fasting individuals are given in Table 20.1.

Table 20.1. Normal fasting duplex blood flow parameters

	Peak systolic velocity	End-diastolic velocity
Celiac A	101 ± 3.5 cm/sec.	33 ± 1.4 cm/sec.
SMA	113 ± 3.9 cm/sec.	15 ± 1.1 cm/sec.

The postprandial changes in these parameters in normal individuals are given in Table 20.2.

Table 20.2. Normal postprandial duplex blood flow parameters. Maximal percentage increase over fasting values cm/sec

	Peak systolic velocity	End-diastolic velocity
Celiac A	20 ± 6	24 ± 9
SMA	42 ± 4	321 ± 100

In patients with intestinal angina, we have found that both the coeliac and superior mesenteric arteries have been involved with high grade stenoses. These lesions involve the ostia of the two vessels and lead to dramatic increases in the peak systolic and end-diastolic velocities [3, 4] (Figure 20.4).

Management of mesenteric arterial stenosis and chronic occlusion

Occult disease of the mesenteric circulation is difficult to manage, because very little is known about its natural history. Occult mesenteric arteriosclerosis does not include patients with a full-blown clinical syndrome of intestinal angina. Stenosis or occlusion of one or more mesenteric arteries is a common finding in routine autopsies. Due to the extensive collateral supply, there is no direct correlation between the anatomic cross-sectional lumen and clinical symptoms. Acute emboli usually lodge in a more distal area than the arteriosclerotic lesions near the orifice. Acute thrombosis occurs at the site of arteriosclerotic involvement and as a consequence leads to more extensive bowel ischaemia.

Physical signs in occult mesenteric arteriosclerosis are non-specific. Weight loss may occur from malabsorption but is usually related to fear of pain in symptomatic patients. Changes in bowel habits may occur. A systolic bruit

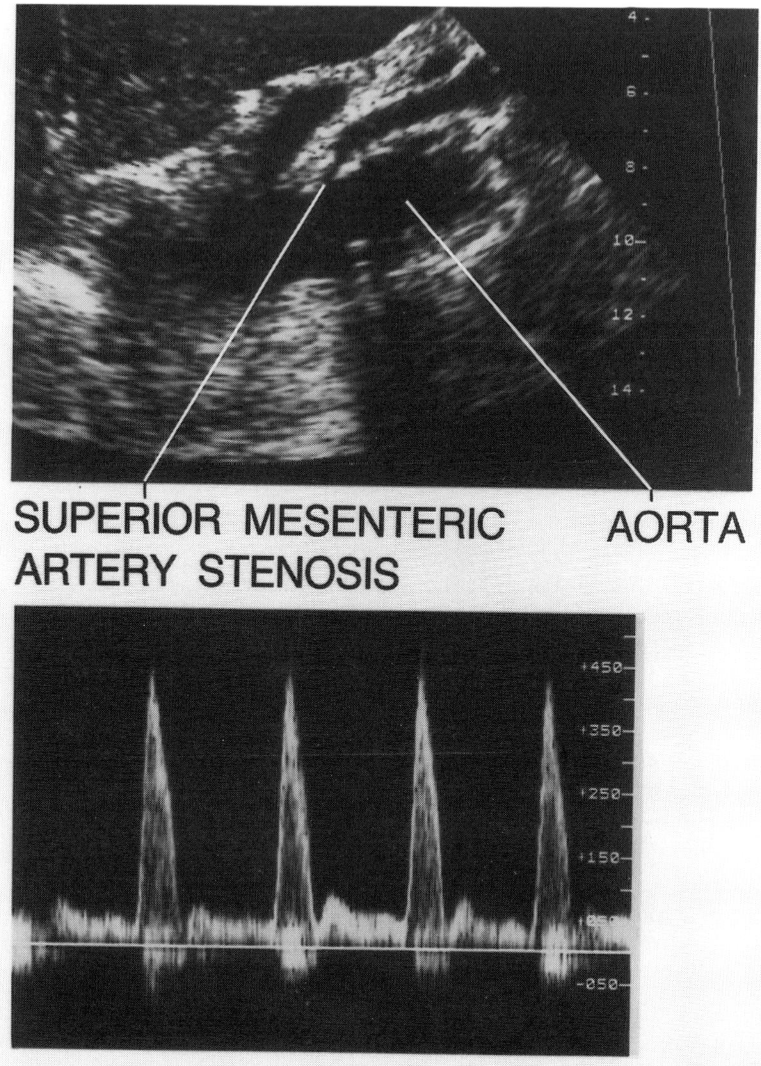

Figure 20.4. Stenosis of the SMA-fasting. The peak systolic velocity in the stenosis is 450 cm/sec.

near the umbilicus is not a specific symptom of mesenteric stenosis and may also be absent.

When mesenteric ischaemia is suspected in a patient with 'low flow,' it is wise to avoid medication with known vasoconstrictive effects on the splanchnic circulation such as digitalis. An elemental diet is reported to protect the intestinal mucosa. In particular, if the large bowel is suffering from limited ischaemia it is important to protect against bacterial toxin induced by antibiotics.

Arteriosclerotic renal artery disease

Measurement of the arterial blood pressure is one of the basic parts of any physical examination; therefore renovascular hypertension is a symptomatic form of renal arterial disease. On the other hand, mild hypertension is so common in the population that it is not prudent to perform angiography to discover renal artery lesions.

There are subsets of the population in whom non-invasive screening with duplex is worthwhile. These include:

1. Patients with severe hypertension.
2. Age group under five years old, or over 60 years old, with hypertension.
3. Lack of a family history of hypertension.
4. Presence of an abdominal bruit and hypertension.
5. Patients with malignant hypertension.

A major obstacle to the evaluation of patients suspected of having renal artery disease was the absence of a reliable non-invasive method to detect stenotic lesions in these arteries. Selective angiography was used only for those patients whose blood pressure was difficult to control. Duplex evaluation of the renal arteries is a good screening test for patients with suspected renovascular disease, which may be the cause of severe hypertension and/or renal failure.

Technique of renal artery duplex scanning

A bowel prep can be useful to improve visualization of the arteries of interest; the Dulcolax^R Bowel Prep Kit is used for preparing the patient. A non-fat lunch is recommended the day before the exam, followed by the ingestion of several glasses of water during the day. Supper consists of clear soup and juice. In the evening, four Bisacodyl^R tablets (5 mg) are taken. If patients have to be studied without the preceding preparations, a Bisacodyl^R suppository (10 mg) is used at 7.00 a.m., the morning of the study.

Bowel gas can be a major obstacle for the visualization; therefore 0.6 ml of Simethicon (Mylecon^R drops) is given orally immediately before the examination to diminish bowel gas.

The patients are studied in the supine position and from both flanks. The 3 MHz scanhead is used because of the distance of these vessels from the skin. The aorta is scanned longitudinally, and flow velocities are recorded at the level of the renal arteries. The scanhead is then turned transversely to identify the left renal vein and renal arteries. The renal arteries normally arise just distal to the origin of the SMA and at or just above the level of the left renal vein. The renal arteries can be identified by their characteristic waveform. Flow is always above zero with a high end-diastolic velocity. The arteries can be traced from their origin to the renal hilum and into the parenchyma. The kidney itself is imaged from the flank or back and measured in its maximal upper to lower pole dimension during inspiration.

Since the sample volume is large compared to the vessel, spectral broadening cannot be used in the diagnosis because it is often present in normal renal arteries. A renal artery stenosis of more than 60% diameter reduction can be identified by a localized velocity increase, poststenotic turbulence and a renal to aortic ratio of more than 3.5. [5–7], Figure 20.5. The renal aortic ratio (RAR) is the ratio of the highest peak systolic velocity in the renal artery to the peak systolic velocity in the adjacent aorta. Because aortic velocities are abnormally low in aneurysmal dilatation of the aorta, this ratio cannot be used when the aorta is dilated.

Distal renal waveforms are recorded 3–5 cm distal to the orifice in the main trunk. Medullary waveforms appear like mainstem vessel waveforms. They are obtained with the kidney viewed longitudinally and by increasing the size of the sample volume and placing it in the echogenic portion of the

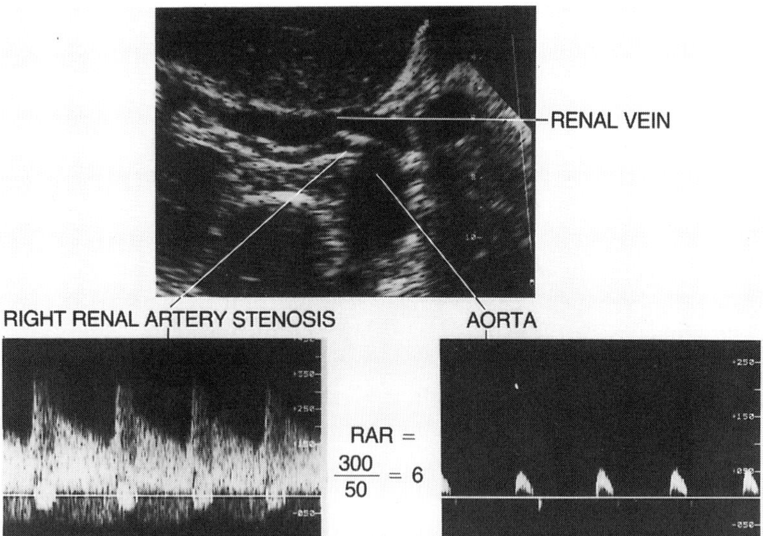

Figure 20.5. Stenosis of the renal artery. Peak systolic velocity in the right renal artery of 300 cm/sec; the peak velocity in the aorta is 50 cm/sec, therefore the renal; aortic ratio is 6.0

kidney. The arcuate vessels are found in the echofree cortical area of the kidney. Cortical waveforms are of a low amplitude.

An occluded renal artery is suggested by a low amplitude spectral waveform in the kidney and in kidneys less than 9 cm in length. Multiple renal arteries may be present and should be looked for.

The renovascular resistance can be estimated from the ratio of end diastolic to peak systolic velocity (EDR). The normal value (0.33) decreases with age and with parenchymal small artery disease. EDR's of below 0.2 represent increased renovascular resistance, which is seen in diabetic nephropathy and chronic renal failure.

Management of occult renal artery lesions

Studies on the natural history of renal artery stenosis have rendered conflicting data on the rate of disease progression. A non-invasive follow-up study from our laboratory [8] found a significant decrease in kidney size (−1 cm over a period of one year) associated with a 60–99% stenosis. None of the stenotic arteries progressed to occlusion during a mean follow-up of 13 months. Other studies that used serial angiography, however, found that 39% of arteriosclerotic arteries progressed to occlusion within 13 months and at an average rate of progression of 2% per month [9]. Wollenweber also found a high rate of progression (63%) in his angiographic follow-up study of 30 patients over 28 months.

At present, follow-up studies should consist of measurement of serum creatinine, measurement of kidney length and monitoring of the stenotic segment. In patients with associated aortic aneurysms, renal artery bypass may be done at the time of aneurysm resection. In these cases the added risk of the reconstruction has to be weighed against the likelihood that at a later time treatment of the renal artery lesion may become necessary.

Arteriosclerotic ostial lesions are the least amenable to dilatation and often require direct surgical repair. Fibromuscular hyperplasia can often be treated by balloon dilatation. The use of surgery or dilatation should be confined to those patients whose blood pressure is difficult to control and/or presence of early renal failure. Duplex scanning is ideal for following these patients in order to document the outcome and detect further problems that may require correction.

References

1. Jager K, Bollinger A, Valli C, Ammann R. Measurement of mesenteric blood flow by duplex scanning. J Vasc Surg 1986; 3:462.

2. Jager KA, Fortner GS, Thiele BL, Strandness DE. Non-invasive diagnosis of intestinal angina. J Clin Ultrasound 1984; 12:588.
3. Nicholls SC, Kohler TR, Martin RL, Strandness DE. Use of hemodynamic parameters in the diagnosis of mesenteric insufficiency. J Vasc Surg 1986; 3:507–510.
4. Moneta GL, Taylor DC, Helton WS, Mulholland MW, Strandness DE. Duplex ultrasound measurement of postprandial intestinal blood flow: Effect of meal composition. Gastroenterology 1988; 95:1294.
5. Kohler TR, Zierler RE, Martin RL, Nicholls SC, Bergelin RO, Kazmers A, Beach KW, Strandness DE. Non-invasive diagnosis of renal artery stenosis by ultrasound duplex scanning 1986; 4:450.
6. Taylor DC, Kettler MD, Moneta GL, Kohler TR, Kazmers A, Beach KW, Strandness DE. Duplex ultrasound scanning in the diagnosis of renal artery stenosis: A prospective evaluation. J Vasc Surg 1988; 7:363.
7. Taylor DC and Moneta GL. Duplex ultrasound scanning in the renal and mesenteric circulation. Seminars in Vascular Surgery 1988; 1:23.
8. Taylor DC, Moneta GL, Strandness DE. Follow-up of renal artery stenosis by duplex ultrasound. J Vasc Surg 1989; 9:410.
9. Wollenweber J, Sheps SG, Davis GD. Clinical course of atherosclerotic renovascular disease. Am J Cardiol 1968; 21:60.

PART SIX

New techniques, combined lesions and prevention

21. Use of DNA technology in the diagnosis of occult atherosclerotic disease

RICHARD S. HOULSTON and STEVE E. HUMPHRIES[1]

Cardiovascular disease (CVD) is a major contributor to mortality in western industrialised countries [1]. Its principle cause is atherosclerosis, with clinical effects only becoming apparant after years of asymptomatic development. Epidemiological studies have identified primary risk factors which are involved in atherosclerosis development, including hyperlipidaemia, hypertension and cigarette smoking. In addition, evidence from a number of studies examining coronary heart disease in first degree relatives of affected probands and twin studies, indicates a definite role of genetic factors in the aetiology of atherosclerotic disease.

Cardiovascular disease may initially appear unlikely to have a substantial genetic basis since any reduction in reproductive fitness even of late onset, would be expected to cause significant selection against such predisposing genetic defects. However, CVD has only become a frequent cause of early death in the later part of this century and over recent evolutionary history, previously with a vastly different socio/economic environment, different selection pressures may have operated.

The techniques of molecular genetics have made considerable impact in examining the metabolic variants involved in atherosclerosis development. It is to be hoped that future use of this information may identify individuals at risk of CVD at a young age. Subsequent risk of disease could then be modified by appropriate management.

Lipoprotein and apolipoprotein levels of individuals in the general population are influenced by both genetic and environmental factors. Extensive studies suggest that approximately 50% of the variability in normal plasma cholesterol levels in the general population is attributable to genetic differ-

1. The work in the authors laboratory is funded by the British Heart Foundation, the MRC and the Sunley Research Centre Trust. We wish to thank Fenella Holmes for her careful assistance in preparing this manuscript.

A.-M. Salmasi and A. N. Nicolaides (eds.), Occult Atherosclerotic Disease, 293–308.

ences among individuals [2–4]. Estimates for heritability of low density lipoprotein (LDL) cholesterol, high density lipoprotein cholesterol (HDL), apolipoprotein (apo) AI and apo B have yielded similar results [5, 6]. Additionally, studies suggest that responses of lipoprotein levels to dietary changes may be determined by variation at both the apo E and LDL receptor gene loci [7, 8].

Candidate genes

All genes involved in lipoprotein metabolism may be contributing to the determination of an individuals plasma lipoproteins and represent candidate genes for study; most have been cloned and sequenced (Table 21.1). In addition, many common polymorphisms of these genes have been documented, and represent the essential tools for delineating what fraction of variability in normal lipoprotein levels is attributable to each loci. Knowledge of this has considerable implications for understanding the genetic susceptibility to hyperlipidaemia and thence atherosclerosis. This chapter will address this area with examples of rare and common variants to illustrate the use of molecular biological techniques; for fuller reviews see references 9–11.

Table 21.1. Candidate genes involved in lipoprotein metabolism

Gene	Chromosome Localisation	Polymorphisms Documented
1 Apoproteins		
AI-CIII-AIV	11q	+
AII	1p	+
B	2p	+
E-CI-CII	19p	+
apo(a)	6q	+
2 Enzymes		
Lipoprotein Lipase	8p	+
Hepatic Lipase	15q	+
HMGCoA Reductase	5q	+
LCAT	16q	+
ACAT	?	–
CETP	16q	+
3 Receptors		
LDL-(B-E)	19p	+
Remnant (E)	12	–
HDL	?	–

The initial problem is which of these candidate loci to study first and how to assess which are making a significant contribution to atherosclerotic

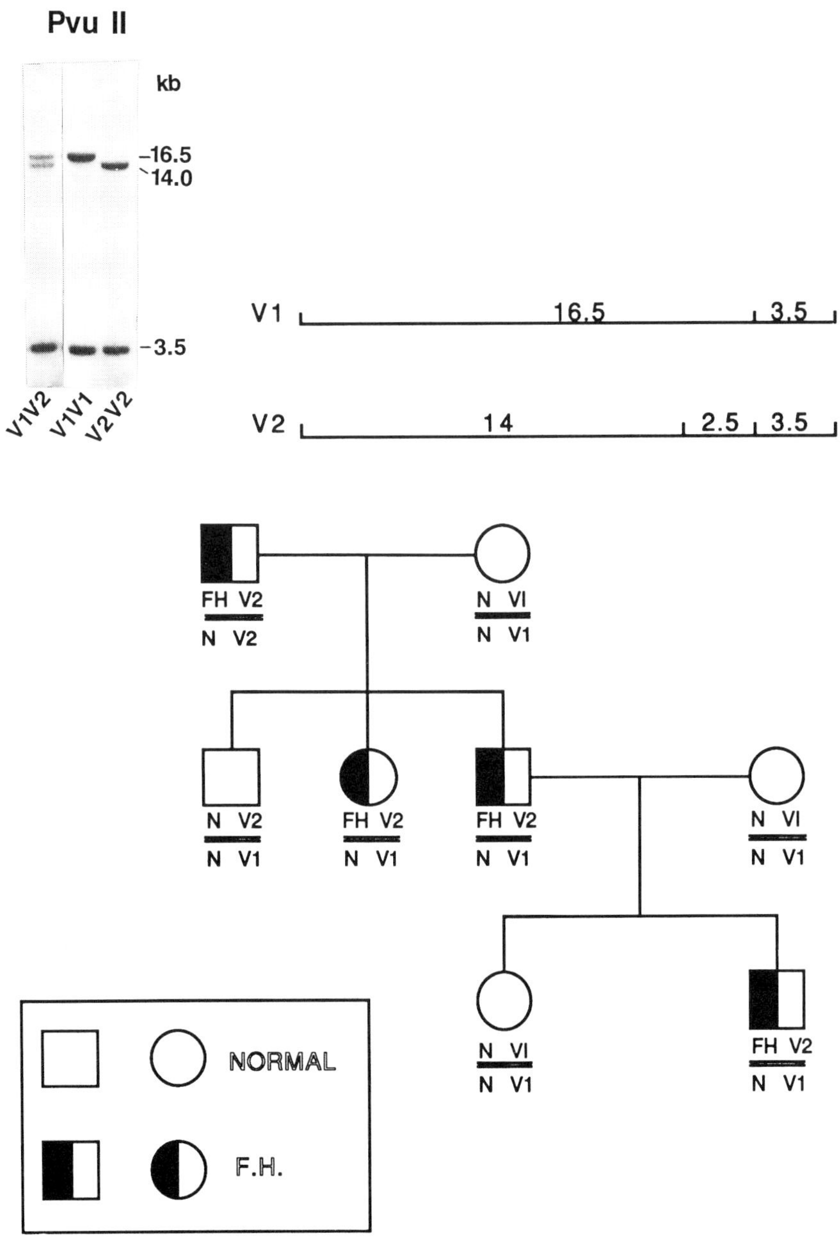

Figure 21.1. (a) Pvu II DNA polymorphism detected with the LDL-receptor gene probe. Southern blot analysis of hybridisation pattern obtained from a PvuII digest of DNA from three individuals. (b) Diagram of cutting sites for PvuII within LDL-R gene. (c) Segregation of familial hypercholesterolaemia and LDL-receptor gene polymorphism.

disease development either by quantitative or qualitative effects on circulating lipoprotein. This may be approached by examining either end of the reductionist tree; firstly by the study of rare inborn errors of lipid metabolism and secondly by use of DNA polymorphic markers to assess the relative contribution of each loci to normal variability in lipoprotein levels or to clinical end points such as myocardial infarction. These two approaches complement one another.

Candidate genes: rare variants

Familial hypercholesterolaemia

About one in 20 individuals suffering from premature heart attacks have a disorder called familial hypercholesterolaemia (FH), an inherited, autosomal dominant trait. Research by Brown, Goldstein and co-workers has demonstrated that FH is due to mutations in the low density lipoprotein (LDL) receptor gene [12]. This receptor, located on the cell surface, binds and internalises LDL particles. A reduction in the number of functional receptors is responsible for elevated levels of LDL and the subsequent increase in atherosclerotic risk. The availability of cDNA and genomic clones of the LDL-receptor gene [13, 14] has enabled these mutations to be characterised at the DNA level. In the UK approximately 5% of patients with FH possess a detectable deletion of part of the LDL-receptor gene [15] and direct diagnosis may therefore be carried out. At least 10 different deletions have now been characterised in the gene [14, 16], and in some populations, e.g. French Canadians [17] or Finnish [18], a high proportion of patients have a common deletion due to a founder effect. However, for other patients diagnosis requires family studies and the use of Restriction Fragment Length Polymorphisms RFLP(s). There are now 12 RFLPs of the LDL-receptor gene and using four of these roughly 80% of families are potentially informative for co-segregation studies [19] (see Figure 21.2 for illustrative family). The study of the naturally occurring defects leading to FH as well as those generated *in vitro* has enabled receptor function to be examined and shows that the receptor gene is important in lipid metabolism. However, it is possible that as well as the mutations with major effects that cause FH, there may be sequence changes in the gene that have a moderate effect on receptor function and thus on lipid levels. If such sequence changes are common they could be inherited, which in combination with variations in other genes could lead to hyperlipidaemia and atherosclerosis. The identification of individuals with both of these types of defects would be useful in the study of occult atherosclerotic disease.

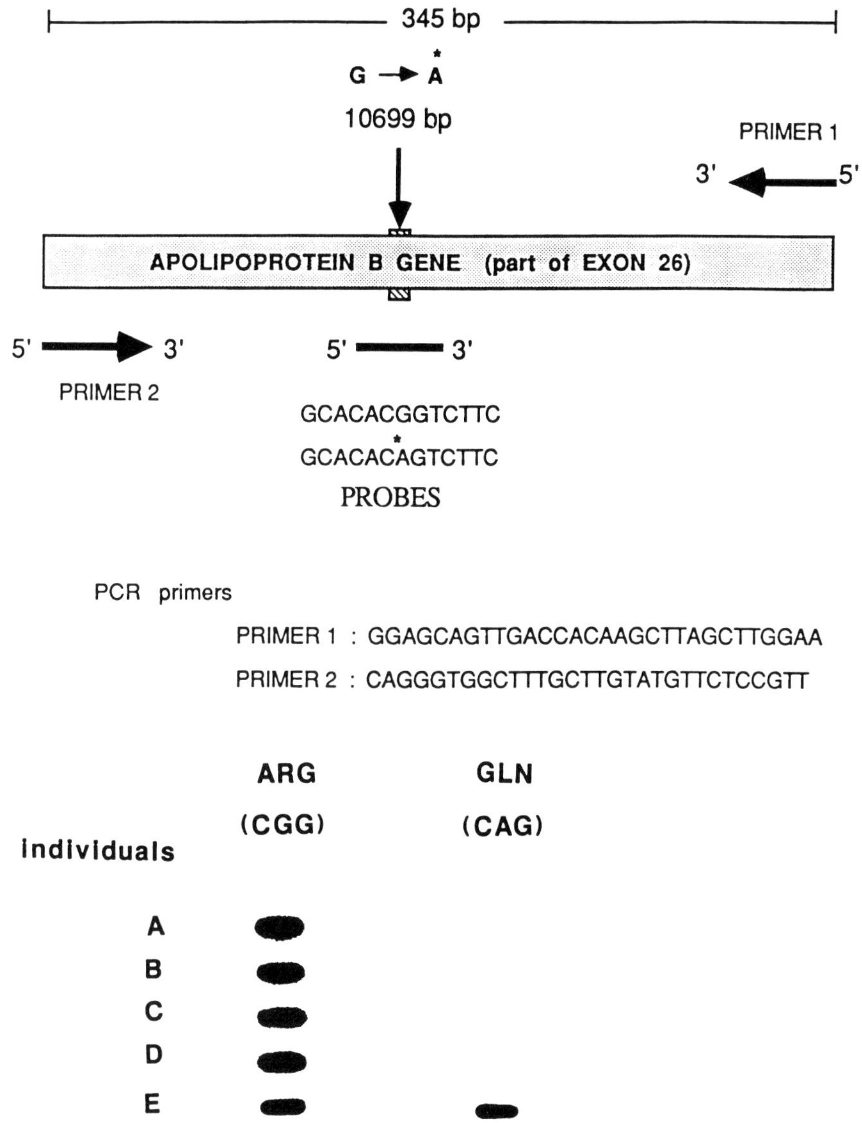

Figure 21.2. Two priming oligonucleotides are used to amplify a 345 bp region of apolipoprotein B containing 3500 (Arg → Gln) mutation by successive cycles of denaturation, annealling and extension. Allele specific oligonucleotides of 13 bases detect under appropriate hybridisation conditions the G to A substitution.

Apolipoprotein B 3500 mutation

Apoproteins AI, AII, B, CI-CIII and E are a family of genes evolutionarily related by random duplication as evidenced by their sequence and intron-exon structure [20]. The genes are dispersed over four chromosomes. Apolipoprotein B is the largest, and although showing certain common features, is structurally distinct from the other apoproteins. It is a protein of 4536 amino acids with a molecular weight of 513KD. As the principal protein component of LDL, it has a central role in the metabolism of this lipoprotein as the ligand for its cellular uptake through the B/E receptors and subsequent degradation [12, 21].

Recent work demonstrated that in some individuals with moderate hypercholesterolaemia there is a reduction in fractional catabolic rate of heterologous LDL and autologous LDL [22] which suggested that variation in apo B itself was affecting the catabolic rate of LDL. Further studies have demonstrated the defect is due to a single base change in the codon for amino acid 3500 (CGC $\rightarrow$ CAG) causing arginine to be substituted for glutamic acid [23]. The defective LDL displays reduced binding to the LDL-receptor and hypercholesterolaemia results from its accumulation. By use of the polymerase chain reaction (PCR) [24] to amplify a region of DNA spanning this defect, allows allele specific oligonucleotide (ASO) probes to be used to screen for this atherogenic disorder, and at-risk individuals to be identified (Figure 21.2). Such individuals have been identified by this technique both in the UK and in Denmark [25]. Furthermore this defect may represent approximately 5% of those previously diagnosed as having FH solely on clinical criteria. Clinical differences between this disorder and that of FH in respect of response to drug treatment and outcome remain to be established. However whilst this mutation is clearly rare it is the first mutation in apo B described, that leads to hyperlipidaemia and atherosclerosis, and the technology is already available to screen asymptomatic individuals for early identification.

Candidate genes: common polymorphisms

Within the genetic melieu there are a small number of loci exerting comparatively large effects on an individual's cholesterol and lipoprotein levels such as in familial hypercholesterolaemia, but because defects in these genes are relatively rare they have a small effect on cholesterol levels in the population as a whole. By contrast there are several gene loci each of which have a small effect on an individuals lipoprotein level, but in total, variation at these loci has a much larger effect on the determination of cholesterol concentrations in the population (Figure 21.3) and hence atherosclerotic disease development.

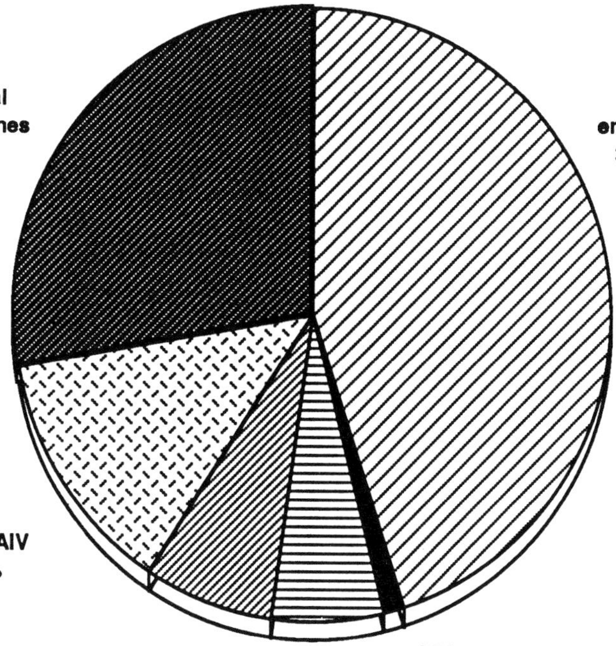

Figure 21.3. Relative contribution of gene loci to phenotypic variance in cholesterol levels.

Apolipoprotein E

Apo E is a 299 amino acid protein, the product of a single gene, and is present in very low density lipoproteins (VLDL), HDL and chylomicron remnants. Its primary function is a ligand for both the LDL-receptor and the hepatic E receptor [reviewed in reference 26] and it occupies a pivitol position in determining the metabolic fate of circulating lipoproteins. Three isoforms of apo E, E2, E3 and E4 are commonly observed in the general population. Isoform E2 differs from the most common isoform E3 by substitution of an ARG with a CYS at position 158 of the amino acid sequence and E4 differs from E3 by replacement of CYS with ARG at position 112. These amino acid changes result from single base changes of T to C or vice versa at the relevant coding position within the gene [27]. Over the past years a number of rare mutants have been identified some of which are associated with development of hyperlipidaemic states. Amplification of DNA spanning these base changes by the technique of PCR in conjunction with allele specific oligonucleotide probes has permitted a method of detecting these apo E variants [28–30].

Allelic variation of this gene locus has been studied by many workers with similar results [reviewed in reference 31]. Individuals possessing the E2 allele tend to have lower levels of plasma cholesterol than those with the E3 allele and those with possession of the E4 allele have amongst the highest levels. The genotype means rank E2E3 < E3E3 < E3E4 in all population samples studied, suggesting the effect of apo E genotype on the individuals levels of cholesterol is independent of the population mean, and that ecological and genetic differences among populations have little influence on the role of the apo E polymorphism in determining individual differences in circulating cholesterol. Variation at the apo E gene locus has been estimated to account for up to 8% of the total phenotypic variance in cholesterol levels in the general population [32–34].

The mechanism underlying such an association has been postulated to result from differences in catabolism of apo E2 and apo E4 carrying lipoproteins. Chylomicrons and VLDL possessing apo E4 are catabolised more efficiently and those with apo E2 less efficiently. Enhanced uptake by the hepatic lipoprotein receptors of apo E4 particles supplies the liver with more cholesterol, leading to a reduction in LDL receptor activity, thus elevating LDL levels. Conversely, lipoprotein particles carrying apo E2 are removed slowly by the liver, leading to up-regulation of the LDL-receptor and lower levels of LDL-cholesterol in the plasma.

Such a mechanism is thought to underly the development of type III hyperlipidaemia [35, 36], which is characterised by an accumulation of lipoprotein remnants in plasma, xanthomatosis and accelerated atherosclerosis, especially peripheral vascular disease. Whilst 90% of cases of hyperlipidaemia have the E2E2 phenotype, fewer than 5% of individuals of E2E2 phenotype exhibit type III. It would appear that a secondary disorder such as diabetes, hypothyroidism, obesity or drug effect is required for the disease to be manifest.

The importance of the apo E polymorphism in determining CVD risk within the general population has been addressed by a number of workers, however there is not universal agreement [31]. Projecting from the influence of apo E on circulating lipid levels to CVD risk, it has been estimated that the isoform of apo E may explain roughly 2.8% of the population CVD risk [31]. Thus this locus represents a gene where screening may be useful in identifying individuals at risk. Such screening could be carried out by either isoelectric focusing or by genotyping using PCR and ASOs.

Apoprotein (a)

A number of studies have shown levels of lipoprotein (a) (Lp(a)) to be a risk factor for CVD development with relative risks attributable ranging from 1.6–3.6 [37]. Furthermore it is a risk factor independent of the lipoproteins and may explain a large part of the risk associated with family history [38]. Plasma levels in individuals vary considerably from barely detectable to approximately 100 mg/dl [39] and are minimally affected by environmental influences. Lipoprotein (a) possesses many similarities to LDL in its physical and chemical properties. The major protein constituent of both lipoproteins is apolipoprotein B100 (apo B100) however, Lp(a) is unique in that it contains a highly glycosylated protein responsible for the apo(a) epitope. This apo(a) is attached to the apo B100 by disulphide bridges. In spite of close structural and kinetic resemblance the two lipoproteins appear to be under separate metabolic control. Furthermore, apo(a) exhibits both inter and intra variability in molecular size. At least 6 isoforms have been documented [40, 41], these variants being associated with quantitative variations in Lp(a). It would appear that the same gene locus is involved in determining Lp(a) glycoprotein phenotypes and Lp(a) concentrations [41], with a series of autosomal alleles operating at a single locus. These isoforms appear to result from variation in the number of Kringle repeats of the apo(a) gene as a result of intragenic recombination within repeated sequences [42, 43]. Striking homology between Lp(a) and that of plasminogen [42, 44] has been reported. The Kringle domains of plasminogen have been implicated in fibrin binding to endothelial cells and similar protease activity. It is thus conceivable that apo(a) could direct Lp(a) particles to sites of fibrin deposition (i.e. vascular injury) and thus provide a concentrated substrate for the acetyl LDL receptors of macrophages. An alternative hypothesis for Lp(a)s role in atherosclerosis development is via reduced fibrinolysis. Competition between plasminogen and Lp(a) for endothelial cell binding leads to reduced plasmin generation and fibrinolysis, so favouring thrombosis [45, 46].

Lp(a) levels of >30 mg/dl represent a considerably increased risk for atherosclerosis development [47] both in normolipidaemic and hyperlipidaemic individuals [48]. This together with the ease of measuring levels of Lp(a) by commercial, immunological techniques both allows and suggests that it should be routinely measured in order to assess potential risk for occult atherosclerotic disease development.

Apolipoprotein B

Epidemiological studies have demonstrated the approximately linear relationship between apo B levels and CVD risk. Furthermore case control studies have shown that levels discriminate well between those patients with and without clinical atherosclerotic disease [49, 50]. Clearly the apo B gene represents a good candidate for study in order to delineate common variants determining apo B levels within the general population, in a similar fashion to the apo E polymorphisms previously described. The XbaI RFLP of the

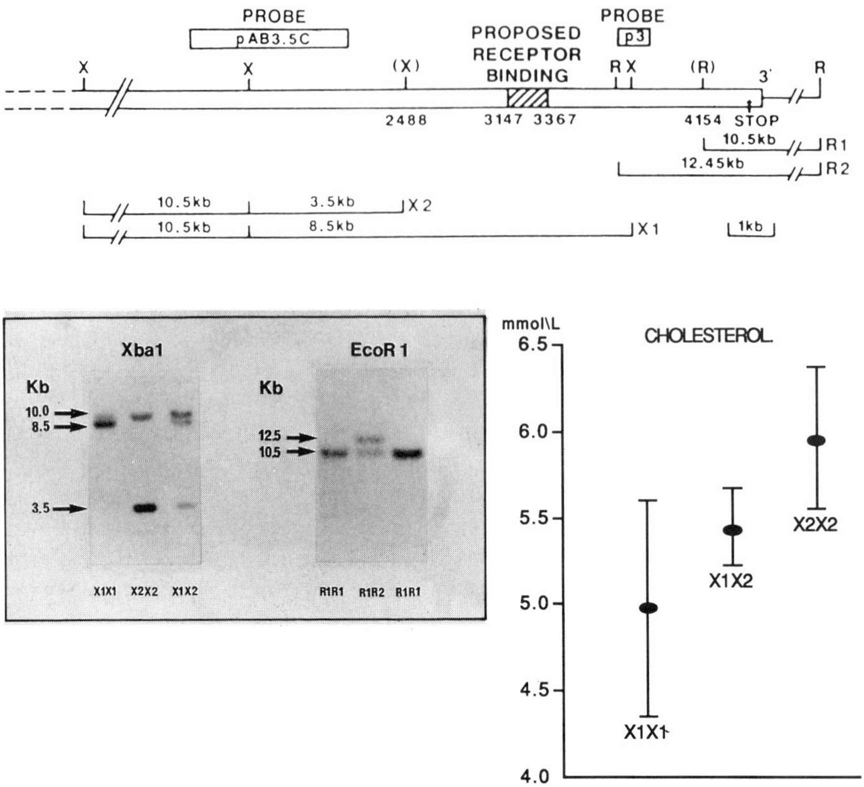

Figure 21.4. (a) Map of the relative positions of the XbaI and EcoRI variable sites in the apo B gene and the position of the region of the gene proposed to code for the amino acids that interact with LDL-receptor X – XbaI site, R – EcoRI site (*x*) and (*R*), variable sites. Positions of sites relative to the amino acids of apo B protein given. (b) Southern blot of Xbal and EcoRo polymorphism of apo B gene. 5µg of DNA from individuals with different genotypes are shown. Sizes of fragments are given in Kb. Individuals with both chromosomes lacking the variable cutting site for XbaI have the genotype *X1X1*, those with both chromosomes with the cutting site have the genotype *X2X2*. Individuals who have inherited one chromosome with and one without the variable site have the genotype *X1X2*. (c) Analysis of variance of serum cholesterol levels (mean ± SD) in individuals with different apo B XbaI genotype.

apo B gene has been shown in a number of independent studies to be associated with determination of lipid levels [51–54). Individuals may be divided by genotype into three classes (*X1X1*, *X1X2* and *X2X2*) and mean lipid levels estimated for each group (Figure 21.4) Individuals with the *X2X2* genotype (3.5Kb fragment) exhibit the highest levels of total cholesterol and LDL. In some, but not all studies heterozygotes, i.e. *X1X2*, have intermediate levels and those with the *X1X1* genotype the lowest levels. Similar influence on levels of triglyceride and apo B has been reported [51].

It has been estimated that the XbaI RFLP accounts for between 4–10% of the total phenotypic variance in cholesterol levels in individuals from the general population [53, 55], a result comparable to apo E. The XbaI RFLP is therefore detecting genetic variation in or around the apo B gene involved in the determination of cholesterol levels. The sequence change responsible for the XbaI RFLP has been shown to occur within the coding region of the gene but is in the third (Wobble) position of codon threonine 2488 and thus does not result in any amino acid substitution [56]. Therefore associations with this RFLP are acting through some other change in the apo B gene.

The reason that an RFLP such as XbaI is associated with lipoprotein levels is due to linkage disequilibrium based on evolutionary history. In the original population there were two chromosomes both with and without the cutting site, designated *X1* and *X2*. In one individual a mutation occurred in the gene leading to a functional change in expression and thus an altered phenotype such as high cholesterol. By chance, this occurred on the chromosome with the *X2* allele. In the population there were then three types of chromosome *X1*-normal, *X2*-normal and *X2*-mutant. When this population is examined many generations later, many individuals with high cholesterol will have the *X2* allele. Individuals with the *X1* allele will also be found with hyperlipidaemia as a result of independent mutational events or recombination at meiosis. The extent to which this is observed will be a function largely of the physical distance between the two sites, for sites within a few thousand base pairs of each other such loss of association will occur only after several hundred generations.

Amino acids 3147–3157 and 3357–3367 [57] of apolipoprotein B have been proposed to be the regions of interaction with the LDL-receptor. Amino acid changes in this region may therefore affect the rate of removal of LDL by altering the affinity of the LDL particle for the LDL receptor. This will lead to alteration of the rate of catabolism of LDL and so influence circulating cholesterol levels. Turnover studies of LDL indicate that variation in apo B itself is affecting the rate of LDL clearance; individuals with the *X2X2* genotype having the lowest clearance of LDL [58, 59]. Evidence from fibroblast cell studies has supported this hypothesis [60] with *X1*-LDL being degradated faster than *X2*-LDL via the LDL-receptor. This mechanism would appear to explain a proportion of the effect on serum lipid levels associated with the XbaI RFLP and illustrates the use of RFLPs to delineate the genetic factors involved in determination of lipid levels.

The frequency of apo B RFLPs has been studied in groups of patients with atherosclerosis by a number of workers [61–65]. The most consistent observation appearing to be an increased frequency of the EcoRI RFLP rare allele, both in coronary and in peripheral vessel disease when compared to

Table 21.2. Reported associations between atherosclerotic disease and RFLPs of the apo B gene

RFLP	Sample Origin	Sample No. Patients/ controls	Association	Rare allele (absence of Cultin sites) frequency patients/ controls	Reference
XbaI	Boston	84/ 84	+	0.64/0.50	[61]
	Seattle	117/102	–	0.50/0.54	[62]
				X1 allele (8.5kb)	
	London	124/186	–	0.53/0.48	[63]
	Austria	106/118	–	0.55/0.52	[64]
EcoRI	Boston	84/ 84	+	0.21/0.11	[61]
	Seattle	108/123	–	0.19/0.14	[62]
	London	124/186	+	0.21/0.15	[63]
	Austria	106/118	+	0.24/0.14	[64]
	London	200/115	+	0.20/0.14	[65]

control individuals (Table 21.2). The EcoRI RFLP results from a DNA base change in codon 4154 changing glutamine for lysine and is responsible for the t and z epitopes of the Ag antigens of LDL [66, 67]. However, the functional significance of this change is at present unknown although the finding of increased frequency in patients with CVD (Table 21.2) is suggestive that the LDL lysine may be more atherogenic.

Observations to date on the apo B gene suggest that variation at this locus is involved in differential lipoprotein metabolism and CHD risk, with further studies being required to define the precise mutations responsible for documented associations. Once identified they will be useful in the identification of individuals predisposed to occult atherosclerotic disease development.

Conclusions and future perspectives

The goal of this research is to examine how genetic variations are involved in determining quantitative and qualitative differences in lipoprotein metabolism and their contribution to CVD risk.

Current data suggests certain of the genes involved in lipoprotein metabolism exert considerable influence on the determination of lipoprotein concentrations, as well as the alterations responsible for different lipoprotein phenotypes and CVD. In the majority of patients diagnosis of occult atherosclerotic disease is not yet feasible by DNA technology. There are, however, notable exceptions, exemplified by the rare apo B 3500 mutation. The transition from research using imprecise polymorphisms to the availability of specific tests such as the polymerase chain reaction in conjunction with ASO probes to detect specific mutations will be likely in the near future. Using a number of such tests, detection of predisposition to occult atherosclerotic disease through variation in many gene loci may then be a reality.

References

1. NIH Consensus Development Conference Statement. Lowering blood cholesterol to prevent heart disease. JAMA 1985; 253:2080.
2. Sing CF, Chamberlain MA, Block WD, Feiler S. Analysis of genetic and environmental sources of variation in serum cholesterol in Tecumseh Michigan T. Analysis of the frequency distribution for evidence of genetic polymorphisms. Am J Hum Genet 1975; 27:333.
3. Sing CF, Orr JD. Analysis of genetic and environmental sources of variation in serum cholesterol in Tecumseh, Michigan, IV. Separation of polygene from environmental effects. Am J Hum Genet 1978; 30:491.
4. Moll PP, Powsner R, Sing CF. Analysis of genetic and environmental source of variation in serum cholesterol in Techumseh Michigan, V. Variance components estimated from pedigrees. Ann Hum Genet 1979; 42:343.
5. Berg K. Genetics of coronary heart disease. In: Progress in medical genetics, Volume V. AG Steinberg, AG Bearn, AG Motulsky, Childs (eds) Saunders Company Philadelphia 1983; p. 35.
6. Hamsten A, Tselius T, Dahlen D, de Faire U. Genetic and cultural inheritance of serum lipids, low density and high density lipoprotein cholesterol and serum lipoproteins AI, AII and B. Atherosclerosis 1986; 60:199.
7. Weintraub MS, Eisenberg S, Brewlow J. Dietary fat clearance in normal subjects is regulated by genetic variation in apolipoprotein E. J Clin Invest 1987; 80:1571.
8. Weight M, Cortesse Sule U, Miller NE, Lewis B. Heritability of low density lipoprotein receptor activity of human blood mononuclear cells: studies in normolipidaemic adult male twins. Clin Sci 1982; 62:397.
9. Goldbourt U, Neufeld HN. Genetic aspects of Arteriosclerosis. Arteriosclerosis 1986; 64:357.
10. Lusis A. Genetic factors affecting blood lipoproteins: the candidate gene approach. J Lipid Res 1988; 29:397.
11. Humphries SE. DNA polymorphsms of the apolipoprotein genes – their use in the investigation of the genetic component of hyperlipidaemia and atherosclerosis. Atherosclerosis 1988; 72:89.
12. Brown MS, Goldstein JL. How LDL receptors influence cholesterol and atherosclerosis. Scientific American 1984; 251:52.
13. Yamamoto T, Davis LG, Brown MS, Schneider WJ, Casey ML, Goldstein JL and Russell DW. The human LDL receptor: a cystein-rich protein with multiple Alu sequences in its mRNA. Cell 1984; 39:27.
14. Lehrmann MA, Goldstein JL, Brown MS, Russell DW, Schneider WJ. Internalization-defective LDL receptors produced b genes with nonsense and frameshift mutations that truncate the cytoplasmic domain. Cell 1985; 47:735.
15. Horsthemke B, Beisiegel U, Dunning A, Havinga JR, Williamson R, Humphries SE. Unequal crossing-over between two alu-repetitive DNA sequences in the LDL receptor

gene: A possible mechanism for the defect in a patient with familial hypercholesterolaemia. Eur J Biochem 1987; 164:77.

16. Horsthemke B, Dunning A, Humphries SE. Identification of deletions in the human, low-density lipoprotein receptor gene. J Med Genet 1987; 24:144.
17. Hobbs HH, Brown MS, Russell PW, Davignon J, Goldstein JL. Deletion in LDL receptor gene occurs in majority of French Canadians with FH. N Engl J Med 1987; 317:734.
18. Aalta-Setälä K, Gylling H, Meittinen T, Kontula K. Identification of a deletion in the LDL-receptor gene. FEBS. LETT. 1988; 230 1, 2, 31.
19. Humphries SE, Taylor R, Jeenah M, Seed M. The use of recombinant DNA techniques for the diagnosis of familial hypercholesterolaemia. J Inher Metab Dis II Suppl. 1988b; 1:33.
20. Luo CC, Li WH, Moore MM and Chan L. Structure and evolution of the apolipoprotein multigene family. J Mol Biol 1986; 187:325.
21. Sparks JD, Sparks CF. Apolipoprotein B and lipoprotein metabolism. Ad Lipid Res 1985; 21:1.
22. Vega GI, Grundy SM. *In vivo* evidence for reduced binding of low density lipoproteins to receptors as a cause of primary moderate hypercholseterolaemia. J Clin Invest 1986; 78:1410.
23. Soria LF, Ludwig FH, Clarke HRG, Vega GL, Grundy SM, McCarthy BJ. Association between a specific apolipoprotein B mutation and familial defective apolipoprotein B100. Proc Natl Acad Sci USA 1989; 86:587.
24. Saiki RK, Bugawan TL, Horn GT, Mullis KB, Erlich HA. Analysis of enzymatically amplified B-globin and HLA DQα DNA with allele specific oligonucleotide probes. Nature 1986; 324:163.
25. Tybjærg-Hansen A, Gallagher J, Vincent J, Houlston R, Talmud P, Dunning AM, Seed M, Hamsten A, Humphries SE, Myant NB. Familial defective apolipoprotein B100. Detection in the United Kingdom and Scandinavia and clinical characteristics of ten cases. Atherosclerosis; 80:235.
26. Mahley RW. Apolipoprotein E: Cholesterol transport protein with expanding role in cell biology. Science, 1988; 240:622.
27. Wallis SC, Rogne G, Gill L, Markham A, Edge M, Woods D, Williamson R, Humphries SE. The isolation of cDNA clones for human apolipoprotein E and detection of apo E RNA in hepatic and extrahepatic tissues. EMBO J 1983; 12:2369.
28. Smeets HJM, Poddighe J, Stuyf PMJ, Stalenhoef AFH, Ropes HH, Wieringa B. Identification of apolipoprotein E polymorphism by using synthetic oligonucleotides. J Lipid Res 1988; 29:1231.
29. Weisgraber KH, Newhouse YM, Mahley RW. Apolipoprotein E genotyping using polymerase chain reaction and allele specific oligonucleotide probes. Biochem Biophys Res Comm 1988; 157:3, 1212.
30. Houlston RS, Snowden C, Green F, Alberti G, Humphries SE. Apolipoprotein (apo) E genotypes by polymerase chain reaction and allele specific oligonucleotide probes: no detectable linkage disequilibrium between apo E and apo CII. Hum Genet 1989; 83:364.
31. Davignon J, Gregg E. Sing CF. Apolipoprotein E polymorphism and atherosclerosis. Arteriosclerosis 1988; 8:1.
32. Sing CF and Davignon J. Role of apolipoprotein E polymorphism in determining normal plasma lipid and lipoprotein variation. Am J Hum Genet 1985; 37:268.
33. Boerwinkle E, Utermann G. Simultaneous effects of the apolipoprotein E polymorphism on apolipoprotein E, apolipoprotein B and cholesterol metabolism. Am J Hum Genet 1988; 42:104.
34. Smit M, Kniff P, Rosseneu M, Burg J, Klasen F, Frants R, Havekes L. Apolipoprotein E

polymorphism in the Netherlands and its effect on plasma lipid and apolipoprotein levels Hum Genet 1988; 80:287.

35. Utermann G, Hess M, Steinmetz A. Polymorphism of apolipoprotein E and occurrance of dysbetalipoproteinaemia in man. Nature 1977; 269:604.
36. Zannis V I and Breslow J L. Characterisation of the unique human apolipoprotein E variant associated with type III hyperlipoproteinaemia. J Biol Chem 1980; 1759.
37. Rhoads G G, Dahlen G, Berg K, Morton N E, Dunnenberg A L. Lp(a) lipoprotein is a risk factor for myocardial infarction. JAMA 1986; 256:18, 2540.
38. Durrington P N, Tshola M, Hunt L, Arnol S, Bhatnager D. Apolipoproteins (a) AI and B and Parental History in men with early onset ischaemic heart disease. Lancet 1988; 1070.
39. Albers J J, Adolphson J L, Hazzard U R. Radioimmunoassay of human plasma (Lp(a)) lipoprotein. J Lipid Res 1977; 18:331.
40. Fless G M, Zumthallen M F, Scanu A M. Physiochemical properties of apolipoprotein (a) and lipoprotein (a–) derived from the dissociation of human plasma lipoprotein (a). J Biol Chem 1986; 261:8712.
41. Utermann G, Menzel H J, Kraft H G, Duba H C, Kemmler H G, Seitz C. Lp(a) glycoprotein phenotypes: inheritance and relationship to Lp(a) – lipoprotein concentrations in plasma J Clin Invest 1987; 80:458.
42. McLean J N, Tomlinson J W, Kuang W J, Eaton D L, Chan E Y, Fless G M, Scanu A M, Laen R M. cDNA sequence of human apolipoprotein (a) is homologous to plasminogen. Nature 1987; 330:132.
43. Lindahl G, Gersdorf E, Menzel H, Seed M, Humphries S E, Utermann G. Variation in the size of human apolipoprotein (a) is due to a hypervariable region of the gene Hum Genet 1989; 81:149.
44. Eaton D L, Fless G M, Kohn W J, McLean J W, Xu Q T, Miller C D, Lawn R M, Scanu A M. Partial amino acid sequence of apolipoprotein (a) shows that it is homologous to plasminogen. Proc Natl Acad Sci USA 1987; 84:3224.
45. Miles L A, Fless G M, Levin E G, Scanu A M, Plow E F. A potential basis for the thrombotic risks associated with lipoprotein(a). Nature 1989; 339:301.
46. Hajjar K A, Gavish D, Breslow J L, Nachman R L. Lipoprotein (a) modulation of endothelial cell surface fibrinolysis and its potential role in atherosclerosis. Nature 1989; 339:303.
47. Kostner G M, Avogaro P, Cazzolato G, Marth E, Bittolo-Bon G, Quinnci G B. Lipoprotein Lp(a) and risk of myocardial infarction. Atherosclerosis 1981; 38:51.
48. Houlston R, Quiney J, Mount J, Watts G F, Lewis B. Lipoprotein (a) and coronary heart disease in Familial Hypercholesterolaemia. 1988; Lancet ii: 8606:405.
49. Whayne, T F, Alaupovic P, Curry M D, Lee M T, Anderson P S and Schecter E. Plasma apolipoprotein B and VLDL – LDL – and HDL-cholesterol as risk factors in the development of coronary arterial disease in male patients examined by angiography. Atherosclerosis. 1981; 39:411.
50. Durrington P N, Hunt L, Ishola M, Kanea J. Stephens, W P. Serum apolipoproteins AI and B and lipoproteins in middle aged men with and without previous myocardial infarction. Br Heart J 1986; 56:206.
51. Law A, Powell L M, Brunt H, Knott T J, Altmann D G, Rajput J, Wallis S C, Pease R J, Priestly L M, Scott J, Miller G J, Miller N F. Common DNA polymorphisms within coding sequence of apolipoprotein B gene associated with altered lipid levels. Lancet, 1986; i:1301.
52. Berg K. DNA polymorphism at the apolipoprotein B locus is associated with lipoprotein levels. Clin Genet 1986; 30:515.
53. Talmud P J, Barni N, Kessling A M *et al.* Apolipoprotein B gene variants are involved in the determination of serum cholesterol levels: a study in normo- and hyperlipidaemic individuals. Atherosclerosis 1986; 67:81.

54. Aalta-Setälä K, Tikkanen MJ, Taskinen MR, Nieminen M, Holmberg P. XbaI and c/g polymorphisms of the apolipoprotein B gene locus are associated with serum cholesterol and LDL-cholesterol levels in Finland. Atherosclerosis 1988; 74:47.
55. Talmud P, Houlston RS, Hutson JL *et al.* A comparison of the effect of genetic variation at the apolipoprotein (apo B) and apo E loci in the determination of plasma lipoprotein and apolipoprotein concentrations in the normal population. (in preparation)
56. Carlsson P, Darnfors C, Olofsson S, Bjursell G. Analysis of the human apolipoprotein B gene; complete structure of the B74 region. Gene 1986 49:29.
57. Knott TJ, Pease RJ, Powell *et al.* Human apolipoprotein B: complete cDNA sequence and identification of structural domains of the protein. Nature 1986; 323:734.
58. Demant T, Houlston RS, Caslake MJ *et al.* The catabolic rate of low density lipoprotein is influenced by variation in the apolipoprotein B gene J Clin Invest 1988; 82:797.
59. Houlston RS, Turner PR, Revill J, Lewis B, Humphries SF. The fractional catabolic rate of low density lipoprotein in normal individuals is influenced by variation in the apolipoprotein B gene: a Preliminary study. Atherosclerosis 1988; 71:81.
60. Series J, Cameron T, Caslake M, Gaifney D, Packard C, Shepherd J. The XbaI polymorphism of the apolipoprotein B gene influences the degradation of low density lipoprotein *in vitro*. BBA 1989; 1003:183.
61. Hegele RA, Huang L-S, Herbert *et al.* Apolipoprotein B-gene DNA polymorphisms associated with myocardial infarction. New Engl J Med 1986; 515:1509.
62. Deeb S, Failor A, Brown BG, Brunzell JD, Albers JJ Motulsky AG. Molecular genetics of apolipoproteins and coronary heart disease. Cold Spring Harbour Symp Quant Biol 1986; 51:403.
63. Myant NB, Gallagher J, Barbir M, Thompson GR, Wile D, Humphries SE. Restriction fragment length polymorphisms in the apo B gene in relation to coronary vessel disease. Atherosclerosis 1989; 77:193.
64. Paulweber B, Freidl W, Krempler F, Humphries SF, Sandhoefer F. Association of DNA polymorphism at the apo B gene locus with coronary heart disease and serum VLDL levels. Atherosclerosis 1990; 10:17.
65. Monsalve MV, Young R, Jobsis J *et al.* DNA polymorphisms of the gene for apolipoprotein B in patients with peripheral arterial disease. Atherosclerosis 1988; 70:13.
66. Ma YH, Schumaker V, Butler R, Sparkes R. Two DNA restriction fragment length polymorphisms associated with Ag(z) and Ag(cg) antigenic sites of human apolipoprotein B. Arteriosclerosis 1987; 71:301.
67. Dunning AM, Tikkanen MJ, Enholm CE, Bütler R, Humphries SE. Relationships between DNA and protein polymorphisms of apolipoprotein B. Hum. Genet 1986; 78:325.

22. Occult cardiovascular atherosclerotic disease in the diabetic

ROBERT S. ELKELES

Cardiovascular disease manifesting as coronary heart disease, cerebrovascular disease and peripheral vascular disease, is the most important cause of mortality and morbidity in people with diabetes mellitus [1]. The cause of this appears to be accelerated atheromatous formation.

The two major types of diabetes mellitus, insulin-dependent (Type 1), and non-insulin-dependent (Type 2), differ in many respects. There are differences in aetiology, genetic basis, pathophysiology and metabolic derangement. Yet in both types, cardiovascular disease, due to enhanced atherogenesis, is a major cause of premature morbility and mortality.

For all cardiovascular diseases, data from the Joslin Clinic [2] shows that mortality for male diabetics due to cardiovascular disease is 2.5 times that of the general population. The mortality rate for female diabetics for cardiovascular disease is even greater, at 3.5 times that of the general population. In the age group 15–44, the difference between diabetics and non-diabetics is particularly prominent. The mortality ratio for all cardiovascular diseases in diabetic males was 12.2 times that of the general population, and for females, 19.5 times that for the general population in this age group. Mortality rate for cerebrovascular disease in the diabetic is increased in both male and female by two-fold, compared with the general population. A follow-up study of 307 juvenile-onset diabetics, in whom the diagnosis of diabetes was made before 1933, and under the age of thirty-one, was carried out [3]. The patients were surveyed after forty years' duration of diabetes. Fifty-six percent of the diabetic population had died, whereas the expected mortality rate for the general population was only ten percent. In thirty-one percent the cause of death was uraemia, but in twenty-five percent the cause was coronary heart disease.

For non-insulin-dependent diabetics, coronary heart disease represents the most prominent cause of death. Panzram [4] has recently summarized the findings of twelve prospective population studies on coronary heart

A.-M. Salmasi and A. N. Nicolaides (eds.), Occult Atherosclerotic Disease, 309–318.

disease and mortality risk in predominantly middle-aged diabetic patients. These studies, from several countries, included those from the United States, Israel, Poland, Great Britain and Finland. These show that the age adjusted cause specific mortality ratio for coronary heart disease is 2–4 times higher in diabetic patients than in non-diabetic controls. A relatively greater risk for females is evident. The excess risk is due to a higher incidence of myocardial infarction, as well as increased acute case fatality and a less favourable long-term prognosis. Furthermore, there is good evidence that cardiac failure occurs more frequently in diabetics than non-diabetics. The second major cause of death in non-insulin-dependent diabetes is cerebrovascular disease and its close relationship to hypertension. Stroke accounted for about fifteen percent of all deaths in non-insulin-dependent diabetics in the World Health Organization Study Group Survey [5]. There appears to be a 2–4 fold excessive risk of death from cerebrovascular disease in non-insulin-dependent diabetics, compared to the general population [4].

For peripheral vascular disease, the Framingham Study [6] has shown that the average age adjusted incidence of intermittent claudication was 12.6/1000 for diabetic men, compared with 3.3/1000 for non-diabetic men. For women, the figure was 8.4/1000, compared with 1.3/1000 for non-diabetic women.

Thus, in comparison with the general population, diabetics have a markedly increased cardiovascular mortality in all age groups, but mostly before middle-age. In insulin-dependent diabetics, nephropathy is the predominant cause of death in the first thirty years, but with longer duration of disease, atherosclerotic changes are the main cause of mortality, especially coronary heart disease.

In diabetics with the onset of disease in middle-age or later cardiovascular disease, due to atherosclerosis, accounts for 70 to 75 percent of deaths, and there appears to be no relationship between this and duration of diabetes. The majority of deaths are due to coronary heart disease. In comparison with the general population, female diabetics show a larger excess of coronary heart disease and mortality than males, whereas the excess for cerebrovascular disease is equally distributed between the two sexes [1]. As cardiovascular disease has a long incubation period, it follows that occult disease must be common in the diabetic, both in the non-insulin-dependent and insulin-dependent types.

Coronary heart disease

The prevalence of coronary heart disease, left ventricular failure and hypertension was examined in 133 newly-diagnosed Type 2 diabetics – 70 males and 63 females – aged 45 to 64, and compared with that in 144 controls match for sex and age [9]. The prevalence of previous myocardial infarction, major Q/QS abnormalities on the resting ECG and/or hospital admissions for myocardial infarction increased 1.7-fold in male and 4.4-fold for female non-insulin-dependent diabetics, compared with controls. Chest pain and ECG abnormalities suggestive of ischaemia were approximately twice as frequent in non-insulin-dependent diabetics as in controls. The frequency of coronary heart disease defined by chest pain, ECG abnormalities, was 3.5 times higher in males and 3.1 times higher in female diabetics than in controls. The frequency of current digitalis therapy was 3.3 times higher in males and 3.9 times higher in females non-insulin diabetics than in controls, suggesting an increased frequency of congestive cardiac failure in the diabetics. The prevalence of hypertension, based on elevated blood pressure levels and the current use of antihypertensive drugs, was 1.6 to 1.7 times higher in the diabetics than in the controls.

Several studies have in dicated that coronary heart disease is frequently present at the time of diagnosis of non-insulin diabetes. In the Bedford Survey [7] a group of 104 previously undiagnosed diabetics were studies for the presence of arterial symptoms (angina or chest pain of cardiac origin) and ECG abnormalities. The presence of arterial symptoms was 1.4 times higher in diabetic men than in non-diabetic men, and 2.4 times higher in diabetic women than non-diabetic women. ECG abnormalities were 1.7 to 2.5 times higher in diabetic men than in non-diabetic men, and 1.2 to 2.0 times higher in diabetic women than in non-diabetic women. In a group of 90 newly diagnosed diabetic women, aged 35 to 70, the prevalance of major S-T segment depression was four times higher in diabetics than in non-diabetics. [8].

Coronary heart disease in insulin-dependent diabetes

It has recently been realized that there is also a high instance of coronary heart disease in insulin-dependent diabetes. The risk of premature coronary heart disease has been studied [10] in a cohort of 292 insulin-dependent diabetics followed for between 20 and 40 years. By the age of 55, the cumulative mortality rate due to coronary heart disease was 35 percent, compared to 8 percent of the non-diabetic control population in the Framingham Study. Angina and acute non-fatal myocardial infarction followed a similar pattern, as did asymptomatic coronary artery disease detected by a stress test, so that there was a combined prevalence rate of 33 percent in the age group, 45 to 59. Mortality due to coronary artery disease in the group was related to the prevalence of nephropathy. It was estimated that the age specific mortality rate due to coronary artery disease would be halved in the absence of nephropathy. Nevertheless, even in the absence of proteinuria, age specific mortality for coronary heart disease in insulin-dependent diabetes was still much higher than in non-diabetics.

The influence of nephropathy on the incidence of coronary heart disease in insulin-dependent diabetes has been further studied. In a case control study [11] fifty-nine insulin-dependent diabetics with nephropathy, and fifty-nine without, were followed for ten years, for five years before proteinuria developed and for five years after proteinuria developed. Within six years after the onset of proteinuria, the cumulative incidence of coronary heart disease in those with proteinuria was forty percent, compared with five percent in those without. Blood pressure was higher in those with nephropathy than in those without, and serum cholesterol was elevated from the time of onset of proteinuria.

Silent myocardial infarction

Several studies have pointed out the high frequency of painless and unrecognized myocardial infarction in diabetics. In one study chest pain was absent in twenty-four percent [12] of diabetics with myocardial infarction, whilst in another the frequency was forty-two percent [13]. In the Framingham Study an unrecognized myocardial infarction was found to occur twice as often in diabetics as in non-diabetics, although this difference was not statistically significant.

The detection of occult coronary heart disease

The detection of occult coronary heart disease in these patients is difficult. 116 insulin-dependent diabetics were followed prospectively [14] for one hundred months. During this time fourteen had clinical evidence of coronary heart disease, with myocardial infarction, sudden cardiac death or the onset of angina. A Treadmill ECG result that was either abnormal or inconclusive because of failure to achieve ninety percent of the predicted maximum heart rate identified each patient in whom evidence of coronary heart disease developed within fifty months after entry. (For further details on the use of stress ECG testing see Chapter 17.)

Cardiac failure

The Framingham Study found that diabetics had a considerably increased risk or congestive cardiac failure particularly in insulin-dependent diabetics [6]. This excessive risk has led to the concept of a specific diabetic heart muscle disease. The studies using non-invasive techniques for the assessment of left ventricular function, e.g. systolic time intervals, apex cardiography and echo-cardiography, have shown that subtle signs of impaired left ventricular function are often found in diabetic patients, even in the absence of clinically detectable congestive cardiac failure. No non-invasive techniques can absolutely distinguish functional abnormalities due to coronary and non-coronary disease. In a group of twenty-five diabetics without known complications, abnormal systolic time intervals were found [15]. However, other studies [16–18] have not confirmed these findings, and in complication-free patients, systolic time intervals were found to be normal. An increased pre-ejection period and left ventricular ejection time were found in diabetics with proliferative retinopathy and nephropathy. These abnormalities seemed to correlate with the extent of micro-angiopathy [17, 18]. It would appear, however, that although heart disease is common in diabetes, the evidence that there is a specific dilated form of cardiomyopathy is not yet firm [19].

Peripheral vascular disease

An extensive survey of occult peripheral vascular disease was carried out by Janka *et al.* [20]. 623 unselected diabetics from the Schwabing City Hospital were studied. Forty-five percent were receiving insulin, while, forty percent were receiving tablets and fifteen percent were on diet. Peripheral vascular disease was sought by ankle/brachial Doppler pressure measurements and oscillometry after one minute of exercise. Peripheral vascular disease was further classified into proximal (pelvic, femoral and popliteal) and peripheral (below the knee). The overall prevalence of peripheral vascular disease was 15.9 percent for the whole group, 14.4 percent for women and 18.0 percent for men. In those with peripheral vascular disease it was proximal in 32.4 percent and peripheral in 63.6 percent. Patients with proximal peripheral vascular disease were likely to have hypertension, smoke and have high serum cholesterol values, and a higher degree of cardiovascular risk factors than those without peripheral vascular disease. An influence on duration of diabetes was not seen in those with proximal peripheral vascular disease. The survey also did not show a greater prevalence of cardiovascular risk factors, in those with peripheral vascular disease, except for greater prevalence of severe hypertension. In this group there was a greater prevalence of patients on insulin, presumably insulin-dependent diabetes and there was a significant correlation between peripheral vascular disease and duration of diabetes.

A detailed prospective study of peripheral vascular disease in diabetes has been carried out by Beach *et al.* [21]. Peripheral vascular disease was ascertained by measuring ankle/brachial pressure ratio using Doppler ultrasound and examination of Doppler velocity wave forms. The prevalence of lower limb arterial disease in 252 Type 2 non-insulin-dependent diabetics was twenty-two percent, compared with three percent in controlled subjects. The progress of lower limb arterial disease was also studied. In non-insulin-dependent diabetics with no detectable peripheral vascular disease at initial testing, fourteen percent developed abnormalities during the two years of study. However, eighty-seven percent of patients with evidence of peripheral vascular disease at the onset of the study showed progression of disease during the study.

Carotid artery disease

There have been few studies of the prevalence of carotid artery disease comparing diabetics and non-diabetics. Chan *et al.* [22] examined 271 non-insulin-dependent diabetics and compared them with 135 non-diabetic controls. Carotid artery disease was studied by ultrasonic B-mode pulsed Doppler/real time spectrum analysis. Carotid artery stenosis was not found in any of the 46 diabetics or 6 controls under the age of fifty. In those over fifty, the prevalence of carotid artery stenosis was 9.6 percent in the diabetics, compared with 0.8 percent in controls. There was a significant association between the history of cigarette smoking and the prevalence of carotid artery disease.

Aetiology and prevention

Non-insulin dependent diabetes

In the general population abnormalities of serum lipids and lipoproteins are associated with the development of atherosclerosis. Lipid and lipoprotein abnormalities are common in non-insulin-dependent diabetes, and are likely to be important in the aetiology of the increased tendency to cardiovascular disease in these subjects. The most frequent abnormality in circulating lipids and lipoproteins in non-insulin-dependent diabetes is an increase in serum triglyceride [23] and a decrease in high density lipoprotein (HDL) cholesterol [24]. These changes are more marked in women than in men [24, 25]. Whether total or low density lipoprotein (LDL) cholesterol is altered in non-insulin-dependent diabetes is controversial. Total plasma cholesterol may be normal or slightly elevated. LDL cholesterol is usually normal, but very low density lipoprotein (VLDL) cholesterol is increased. This suggests that it is the increased circulating VLDL, which is responsible for the elevation of total cholesterol [26]. Nevertheless, kinetic studies have shown an increase in LDL turnover, although whether this is important in atherogenesis is not known. The increase in serum triglyceride and decrease in HDL cholesterol may be related to peripheral insulin resistance, which is a common feature of non-insulin-dependent diabetes. Insulin resistance occurs in the general population. Diabetes supervenes when the beta cells are not able to respond to the challenge by increase in insulin production. Hyperinsulinaemia resulting from insulin resistance is associated with hypertriglyceridaemia, low HDL cholesterol and impaired glucose tolerance [27]. Insulin resistance may also be implicated in the aetiology of essential hypertension.

The relationship between serum lipids and cardiovascular disease has been studied in a group of non-insulin-dependent diabetics [28]. In males those with macrovascular disease had higher levels of serum cholesterol and LDL cholesterol than those without. In females those with macrovascular disease had higher concentrations of serum triglyceride, cholesterol and LDL cholesterol, as well as lower HDL, HDL_2 and HDL_3 cholesterol and apoprotein A1 than in those without. On multivariate analysis LDL cholesterol was the most important association with macrovascular disease in males, and apoprotein A1 in females.

Insulin-dependent diabetes

In well controlled insulin-dependent (Type 1) diabetics, serum lipids and lipoproteins do not differ from those in non-diabetics. In insulin deficiency, when control is poor, there is elevation of VLDL, LDL and HDL triglycerides. However, in a group of 57 male insulin-dependent diabetic, lower levels of serum apolipoprotein B, with a concomitant increase in the cholesterol content of LDL, was found in comparison with eighty-one non-diabetic controls [29]. It was concluded that this could have resulted from a build up in intermediate density lipoprotein subclass of LDL, which is an atherogenic lipoprotein.

Proteinuria developing in insulin-dependent diabetes is an important predictor of cardiovascular disease. In a study from Steno Memorial Hospital in Denmark [30], in insulin-dependent diabetics, who developed proteinuria, the relative mortality from cardiovascular disease was thirty-seven times higher than in the general population. In those without proteinuria, it was only 4.2 times higher than in the general population.

In another group of insulin-dependent diabetics [31], the prevalence of macrovascular disease (coronary heart disease and peripheral vascular disease) was greater in those with proteinuria and normal renal function than in those without. Blood pressure was also higher in those with proteinuria, who also had decreased concentrations of HDL and HDL_2 cholesterol and a tendency to higher total serum cholesterol. The presence of proteinuria, even with normal renal function, is associated with changes in lipoproteins and an increased incidence of cardiovascular disease in insulin-dependent diabetes.

Other possible mechanisms for the increased tendency to cardiovascular disease in diabetes, such as abnormalities in serum fibrinogen, viscosity, haemostatic variables, platelet aggregation, hyperglycaemia itself, and abnormal glycation of lipoproteins, may be important, but are beyond the scope of this chapter. Insulin may act like a growth factor on the arterial wall promoting the infiltration of smooth muscle cells into the intima and their replication there [32].

Prevention

In non-insulin-dependent diabetes several epidemiological studies have failed to show a relationship between the control of blood glucose and the prevalence of cardiovascular disease. The treatment of hyperglycaemia in non-insulin-dependent diabetes has had little impact on the morbidity and mortality on coronary heart disease. Conventional therapy, by diet, oral hypoglycaemic drugs, or even insulin, may not reverse the lipoprotein abnormalities in these patients [33]. The use of lipid-modifying drugs, such as Bezafibrate has been suggested as a pharmacological way of restoring the lipoprotein pattern in these patients to normal, and reducing the incidence of cardiovascular disease [27]. This subject is reviewed elsewhere [33]. The avoidance of treating hypertension in these patients with drugs which adversely affect serum lipids and lipoproteins, such as thiazide diuretics and beta-adrenergic blockades may also be important [33]. In insulin-dependent diabetes insipient nephropathy with proteinuria seems to predispose the cardiovascular disease. There is evidence that the development of nephropathy is related to the quality of glycaemic control [34] and that good glycaemic control may delay the onset of micro-angiopathy in general. As the aetiology of the premature development of cardiovascular disease in insulin-dependent diabetes is much less well understood than in non-insulin-dependent diabetes, it is difficult to give sound advice on prevention. However, there is some evidence that cigarette smoking carries an even greater risk for cardiovascular disease in diabetics than in non-diabetics [35] and clearly smoking should be actively discouraged. Attention to other risk factors in cardiovascular disease, such as hyperlipidaemia and hypertension, which are important in the general population, are probably even more important in patients with insulin-dependent diabetes.

References

1. Pyorala K, Laasko M. Macrovascular disease in diabetes mellitus. In: Mann J I, Pyorala K, Teuscher A, (eds), Diabetes in Epidemiological Perspective. Churchill Livingstone, Edinburgh, 1983; p. 183.
2. Marks H H, Krall L P. Onset, Course, Prognosis and Mortality in Diabetes Mellitus. In: Marble A, White P, Bradley R F, Krall L, (eds). Joslin's Diabetes Mellitus. Philadelphia: Lea and Feabiger, 1971; p. 209.
3. Deckert T, Poulsen J E, Larsen M. Prognosis of diabetes with diabetes onset before the age of thirty-one. 1. Survival, causes of death and complications. Diabetologia, 1978; 14:363.
4. Panzram G. Mortality and survival in Type 2 (non-insulin dependent) diabetes mellitus. Diabetologia 1987; 30:123.
5. WHO Study Group on Diabetes Mellitus. World Health Organization Tech. Rep. Series 727. WHO Geneva. 1985.
6. Kannel W B, McGee, D L. Diabetes and Cardiovascular Disease: The Framingham Study. JAMA 1979; 241:2035.
7. Keen H, Rose G, Pyke D A, Boyns D, Chlouverakis C, Mistry S. Blood sugar and arterial disease. Lancet 1965; 2:505.
8. Weaver J A, Bhatia S K, Boyle D, Hadden D R, Montgomery D A D. Cardiovascular state of newly discovered diabetic women. Brit Med J 1970; 1:783.
9. Uusitupa M, Siitonen U, Aro A, Pyorala K. Prevalence of coronary heart disease, left ventricular failure and hypertension in middle-aged, newly diagnosed Type 2 (non-insulin-dependent) diabetic subjects. Diabetologia 1985; 28:22.
10. Krolewski A, Kosinski E J, Warram J H, Leland O S, Busick E J, Asmal A C, Rand L I, Christlieb A R, Bradley R F, Kahn C R. Magnitude and determinants of coronary artery disease in juvenile-onset, insulin-dependent diabetes mellitus. Am J Cardiol 1978; 59:750.
11. Jensen T, Borch-Johnsen K, Kofoed-Enevoldsen A, Deckert T. Coronary heart disease in young Type 1 (insulin-dependent) diabetic patients with and without diabetic nephropathy: incidence and risk factors. Diabetologia 1987; 30:144.
12. Partamian J O, Bradley R F. Acute myocardial infarction in 258 cases of diabetes. New Eng J Med 1965; 273:455.
13. Soler N G, Pentecost B L, Fitzgerald M G, Malins J M. Myocardial infarction in diabetics. Quart J Med 1975; 44:125.
14. Margolis J R, Kannel W B, Feinleib M, Dawber T R, McNamara P M. Clinical features of unrecognized myocardial infarction – silent and asymptomatic; eighteen year follow-up. The Framingham Study. Am J Cardiol 1973; 32:1.
15. Ahmed S S, Jaferi G A, Narang R M, Regan T J. The pre-clinical abnormality in left ventricular function in diabetes mellitus. Am Heart J 1975; 89:153.
16. Rubler S, Sajadi M R M, Arayoe M, Holford F D. Non-invasive estimation of myocardial performance in patients with diabetes. Diabetes 1978; 27:127.
17. Seneviratne B I B. Diabetic cardiomyopathy: the pre-clinical phase. Br Med J 1977; 1:1444.
18. Shapiro L M, Leatherdale B A, McKinnon J, Fletcher R F. Left ventricular function in diabetes mellitus: Relation between clinical features and left ventricular function. Brit Heart J 1981; 45:129.
19. Shapiro L M. Functional aspects of diabetic heart disease in diabetes and heart disease. Jarrett, R. J (Ed.) Elsevier, Amsterdam, New York, London. 1984; 81.
20. Janka H U, Standl L, Mehnert H. Peripheral vascular disease in diabetes mellitus and its relation to cardiovascular risk factors; screening with the Doppler ultrasonic technique. Diabetes Care 1980; 3:207.

21. Beach KW, Bedford GR, Bergelin RO, Martin DC, Vandenberghe N, Zaccardi M, Strandness DE. Progression of lower-extremity arterial occlusive disease in Type 2 diabetes mellitus. Diabetes Care 1988; 11:464.
22. Chan A, Beach KW, Martin DC, Strandness DE. Carotid artery disease in NIDDM diabetes. Diabetic Care 1983; 6:562.
23. Barrett-Connor E, Grundy SM. Holdbrook MJ. Plasma lipids and diabetes mellitus in an adult community. Am J Epidem 1982; 115:657.
24. Barrett-Connor E, Witztum JL, Holdbrook M. A community study of high density lipoproteins in adult non-insulin-dependent diabetics. Am J Epidem 1983; 117:186.
25. Walden CE, Knopp RH, Wahl PW, Beach KW, Strandness E. Sex differences in the effect of diabetes mellitus on lipoprotein triglyceride and cholesterol concentrations. N Eng J Med 1984; 311:953.
26. Reaven GM. Non-insulin-dependent diabetes mellitus, abnormal lipoprotein metabolism and atherosclerosis. Metabolism 1987; 36:2 (Suppl 1) 1.
27. Seviour PW, Teal T, Richmond W, Elkeles RS. Serum lipids, lipoproteins and macrovascular disease in non-insulin-dependent diabetics: a possible new approach to prevention. Diabetic Med 1988; 5:166.
28. Zavaroni I, Bonora E, Pagliara M, Dall'Aglio E, Luchetti L, Buonanno G, Bonati PA, Bergonzani M, Gnudi L, Passeri M, Reaven G. Risk factors for coronary artery disease in healthy persons with hyperinsulinaemia and normal glucose tolerance. N Eng J Med 1989; 320:702.
29. Winocour PH, Ishola M, Durrington PN, Anderson DC. Lipoprotein abnormalities in insulin-dependent diabetes mellitus. Lancet 1986; 1:1170.
30. Borch-Johnsen K, Kreiner S. Proteinuria: value as predictor of cardiovascular mortality in insulin-dependent diabetes mellitus. Brit Med J 1987; 294:1651.
31. Winocour PH, Durrington PN, Ishola M, Anderson D, Cohen H. Influence of proteinuria on vascular disease, blood pressure, and lipoproteins in insulin-dependent diabetes mellitus. Brit Med J 1987; 294:1648.
32. Nakao J, Ito H, Kanayasau T, Murota S-I. Stimulatory effect of insulin on aortic smooth muscle cell migration induced by 12 L-hydroxy-5, 18, 10, 14-eicosatetraenoic acid and its modulation by elevated extracellular glucose levels. Diabetes 1985; 34–185.
33. Baynes C, Feher MD, Elkeles RS. The effect of treatment of non-insulin-dependent diabetes mellitus (NIDDM) on serum lipids and lipoproteins. Quart J Med (1989) in press.
34. Sherwin RS, Tamborlance WV. Metabolic control and diabetic complications in diabetes mellitus: management and complications. Ed. Olefsky JM, and Sherwin RS. Churchill Livingstone, New York, Edinburgh, London and Melbourne, 1985; 1.
35. Suarez L, Barrett-Connor E, Interaction between cigarette smoking and diabetes mellitus in the prediction of death attributed to cardiovascular disease. Am J Epidem 1984; 120:670.

23. Who should be investigated for occult atherosclerotic disease?

SUSAN LAING, MARY ELLIS and ROGER M. GREENHALGH[1]

Atherosclerosis is a major cause of death and disability in the Western world. During the past few decades, vascular surgery has developed rapidly and alongside the surgical advances has been the development of invasive and non-invasive investigations. Initially, these tests were an adjunct to surgery: to confirm the diagnosis, to locate and quantify the severity of the disease and to provide a baseline measurement for post-operative assessment and follow-up. With the further development of these techniques, it has become possible to detect occult atherosclerosis. The detection of occult disease will not only enable a better understanding of the natural history of the disease, but also open the way for intervention at an earlier stage.

It is becoming increasingly apparent that atherosclerosis is a multi-site disease and that the prevalence of symptomatic disease represents only a fraction of the true prevalence of atheroma. This chapter will discuss the widespread nature of arterial disease in patients presenting with symptoms and also discuss the extent to which occult atherosclerotic disease can be detected in asymptomatic populations.

Atherosclerosis as a multi-site disease

The widespread nature of atherosclerosis has been recognised for a long time from both post mortem [1] and post-operative mortality studies. In 3 studies from the Cleveland Clinic, Hertzer and co-workers [2–4] reported the late post-operative deaths from myocardial infarction following vascular

1. We are grateful to the Nissan UK Arterial Research Foundation for supporting our research. The following people are employed through the foundation and are involved in the screening programme: Sharon Sykes (Programme Coordinator), Simon Hales, Michael O'Meara, Elizabeth Yea, Nicola Stubbing.

A.-M. Salmasi and A. N. Nicolaides (eds.), Occult Atherosclerotic Disease, 319–334.

surgery. Myocardial infarction was the principle cause of late post-operative death, accounting for 55% of deaths following lower extremity re-vascularisation, 38% of deaths following carotid endarterectomy and 37% of deaths following aortic aneurysm resection. Myocardial infarction is also responsible for many early post-operative deaths [5]. Stroke has been associated with the outcome of surgery, Kallero and co-workers [6] reported an increase in mortality and morbidity from both myocardial infarction and stroke after reconstructive surgery, although generally the risk from stroke appears to be low [7].

Those patients not undergoing surgery are also more likely to die of atherosclerosis than another disease although very few patients with peripheral arterial disease are likely to die as a direct result of this [8]. In his Hunterian Lecture in 1960 Bloor [9] described the follow-up of 1476 patients with intermittent claudication followed for 4–10 years. Of the 673 deaths during this period 401 (59.5%) were cardiac, 112 (16.6%) cerebral and 55 (8.1%) due to other forms of arterial disease such as a ruptured aortic aneurysm. Only 105 (15.5%) of the deaths were due to non-atherosclerotic causes. The Framingham study [10] demonstrated that survival rates in patients with intermittent claudication and no evidence of coronary or cerebrovascular disease were similar to those for the general population free from arterial disease. It is due to co-existent arterial disease that the mortality of patients with intermittent claudication is much higher than expected for the general population [11, 12].

Co-existence of symptomatic atherosclerosis

To determine the extent of co-existent symptomatic disease, we reviewed retrospectively two groups of vascular patients and noted symptoms related to carotid artery disease (amaurosis fugax, TIA's, strokes) and coronary artery disease (angina, myocardial infarction). Group I consisted of 1730 patients (1204 men, 526 women) with either symptoms of peripheral arterial disease or previous reconstructive surgery. Group II consisted of 265 patients

Table 23.1. Co-existent symptomatic disease

	n	Carotid Artery Disease	Coronary Artery Disease	Carotid and Coronary Artery Disease	No Symptomatic Disease Elsewhere
Group I PAD	1730	318 (18.4%)	707 (40.9%)	161 (9.3%)	866 (50.1%)
Group II AA	265	55 (20.8%)	96 (36.2%)	26 (9.8%)	140 (52.8%)

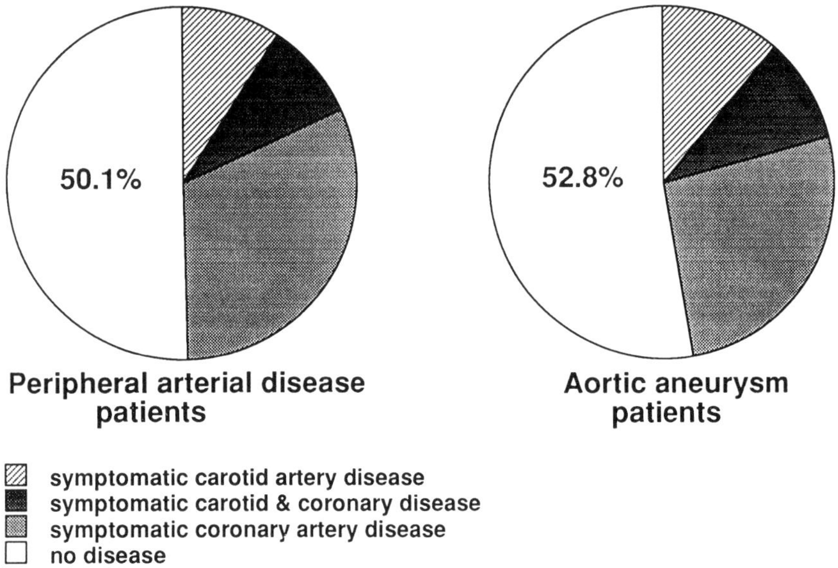

Figure 23.1. Co-existent symptomatic disease

(207 men, 58 women) who had previously undergone aortic aneurysm resection. The results are displayed in Table 23.1. The prevalence of symptomatic coronary artery disease is higher than carotid artery disease in both groups. A total of 49.9% patients in Group I and 47.2% patients in Group II had symptomatic disease in at least one other site and a significant number had symptomatic disease in both sites (Figure 23.1).

Many other studies also confirm this co-existence of symptomatic or clinically detectable disease. In a series reported by Ennix and co-workers [13], of 1238 patients undergoing consecutive carotid endarterectomies, a total of 608 (49%) had either angina or a history of myocardial infarction. In another large study by Hertzer and co-workers [14] of 1000 patients undergoing peripheral vascular surgery of all types, 198 had symptoms of angina and 221 a previous myocardial infarction. Symptomatic carotid artery disease is also frequently documented in these patients. In a study of 160 patients undergoing peripheral vascular surgery, Turnipseed, Berkoff and Belzer [7] reported 69 patients with a history of cerebrovascular disease.

There are fewer studies reporting the morbidity in co-existent disease, but clearly the presence of symptomatic atherosclerosis at any site in the arterial tree confers a poor prognosis elsewhere. Hughson and co-workers [15] showed that both cerebrovascular and coronary disease have an adverse effect on the outcome of intermittent claudication. Patients in the

Framingham study [16] with a previous stroke had a 4 times greater chance of a subsequent myocardial infarction than those who had not had a previous stroke and the rate of developing intermittent claudication was 7 times greater in subjects with angina pectoris than in those without.

The detection of occult atherosclerotic disease

It is almost entirely due to the recent developments in diagnostic techniques that has led to the current interest in occult atherosclerosis although, of course, not every method used in the investigation of symptoms is necessarily appropriate or sufficiently sensitive for the detection of occult disease.

Clinical examination, for example, the disappearance of pedal pulses after exercise, a carotid bruit or palpable aortic aneurysm, may suggest the presence of underlying disease, but this alone is unreliable [17, 18].

Methods for the detection of occult atherosclerosis will be discussed extensively in other chapters and will only be briefly mentioned here. An understanding of the method used and its limitations is essential for interpreting data regarding the prevalence or incidence of occult disease. Tests for diagnosing occult coronary artery disease are mainly, although not entirely, restricted to tests of function. These include both resting and exercise ECG recordings [19] (Chapter 7), thallium scanning [20] (Chapter 9) (both after exercise and dipyridamole induced stress) and measurement of exercise induced stroke volume changes by transcutaneous aorto velography [21] (Chapters 7 and 11). In other anatomical studies coronary arteriography has been used [14].

Carotid artery disease testing is also based on a mixture of anatomical and functional tests. Anatomical details are reflected by B-mode ultrasound images of the vessel wall [22], whereas Doppler ultrasound allows measurements of flow velocities within the vessels and thus gives an assessment of function [23, 24]. Duplex machines combine these functions [25–27]. Occasionally carotid arteriography is used [28].

Aortic aneurysm assessment is also invariably done using B-mode ultrasound [29, 30], whereas ultrasound imaging is used very little for the detection of occult peripheral arterial disease, and if it is used it is restricted to isolated areas such as the popliteal trifurcation. Many other techniques incorporating blood pressure and flow measurements are used for detection of peripheral arterial disease either at rest or following a period of stress [17, 31, 32]. Femoral angiography is used only rarely in asymptomatic patients [33].

Studies of the prevalence of occult atherosclerotic disease, to be discussed later, report widely varying yields. In many cases this is due to differences in the populations under investigation. However, a proportion of the discrepancies arise from both the variation in the method used and in the interpretation of the results. For example, a stress test will yield a greater number of subjects with occult peripheral arterial disease than will a resting test alone [34]. In other cases, the tests will be comparable but the authors will put a different emphasis on the findings, a carotid stenosis of 20% may be regarded as normal in one centre and abnormal in another [22, 35]. Finally, caution must be exercised when comparing the prevalence of occult atherosclerosis at different sites, occult carotid disease may be detected more readily by the techniques available than occult coronary artery disease. An imaging test will detect more minimal disease than a test of function.

Occult atherosclerosis in symptomatic arteriopaths

Despite the fact that patients are often classified according to the site of their initial symptoms, (thus becoming 'aneurysm patients' or 'heart patients') the evidence, not only from co-existing symptoms but from the post-mortem and mortality studies as well, suggests the general widespread nature of the disease. Symptomatic arteriopaths, therefore, are one group in whom we might expect to detect extensive occult atherosclerosis.

Coronary artery disease

As myocardial infarction is the predominant cause of both early and late mortality following vascular surgery many centres now routinely investigate their patients for occult coronary artery disease before surgery. The most extensive study of this kind has been done by Hertzer and co-workers [14]. They performed coronary angiograms on 263 patients prior to abdominal aortic resection, 295 patients prior to carotid endarterectomy and 381 patients prior to lower limb revascularisation with the aim of detecting severe and correctable coronary artery disease which could be operated upon first. Not surprisingly more coronary disease was found in those clinically suspected of it. However, normal coronary arteries were found in only 16 (6%) of the aneurysm patients, 27 (9%) of the cerebrovascular patients and 38 (10%) of the lower limb patients. Overall, severe correctable coronary disease was found in 31% of the aneurysm group, 26% of the cerebrovascular group and 21% of the lower limb group. More interestingly, occult coronary artery disease was often seen in patients with neither symptoms nor standard ECG evidence of disease. In these patients, severe and correctable coronary artery disease was seen in 18% of the aneurysm group, 17% of the cerebrovascular group and 8% of the lower limb group. The prevalence of advanced coronary artery disease which was either inoperable or which did not merit surgery was, of course, even higher.

For those patients not undergoing surgery, in whom coronary angiography may not be appropriate, the prevalence of occult coronary artery disease detected from ECGs alone is also high [17]. Vecht and co-workers [19] examined 100 consecutive patients with intermittent claudication only. Fifty six had an abnormal resting ECG, and during an exercise ECG a further 6 developed abnormalities not detected at rest. Using myocardial scintigraphy in a group of claudicants Stavenow and co-workers [36] confirmed clinical evidence of coronary disease in 36% and detected occult coronary disease in a further 38%. Despite the range of results and the variation in methodology these studies all suggest that occult coronary disease is often concomittant with symptomatic atherosclerosis elsewhere.

Carotid artery disease

Occult carotid disease has also been studied extensively in arteriopaths. Although the post-operative mortality and morbidity from stroke is low, cerebrovascular events play a significant part in the overall reduction of life expectancy in an arteriopath. Furthermore, the debilitating effect of a stroke renders the detection (with a view to correction) of occult carotid artery disease an attractive proposition.

The detection of a carotid bruit is not enough. In a series of patients with carotid bruits [17] it was shown that 52% of these patients had a carotid stenosis resulting in more than 50% reduction in diameter but that a further 13% of patients without bruits also had this extent of carotid disease.

In an early study using continuous-wave Doppler flow measurements Hennerici and co-workers [24] studied 375 patients with symptomatic peripheral arterial disease and 264 with symptomatic coronary disease. Carotid disease (greater than 50% stenosis) was demonstrated in 33% of the peripheral and 7% of the coronary patients. Later studies using Duplex ultrasound scanning report higher yields. In a small study by Stavenow and co-workers [36] of only 25 claudicants, only 2 had a history of cerebrovascular disease but 8 had carotid stenoses greater than 75% shown by the Duplex. Turnipseed, Berkoff and Belzer [7] in a larger study of 160 peripheral vascular patients reported a high prevalence of 69 with concomittant symptomatic cerebrovascular disease, but the Duplex demonstrated significant carotid artery disease in 83 patients (52%).

Our own studies confirm that Duplex scans will detect significant, previously unsuspected, disease. We reviewed 2 groups of patients and noted symptomatic evidence of cerebrovascular disease. Duplex scans were performed on all patients, and occult carotid artery disease greater than 25% was recorded. Group I was 2118 patients with a history of symptomatic peripheral arterial disease and Group II was 383 patients who had previously

Table 23.2. Symptomatic and occult carotid artery disease

	n	Symptomatic Carotid Artery Disease	Occult Carotid Artery Disease	Total Prevalence Carotid Artery Disease
Group I PAD	2118	386 (18.2%)	789 (37.3%)	1175 (55.5%)
Group II AA	383	68 (17.8%)	136 (35.5%)	204 (53.3%)

undergone resection of an abdominal aortic aneurysm. The results are shown in Table 23.2. In both groups of patients the prevalence of significant carotid artery disease was over 50%.

Aortic aneurysm

The interest in occult aortic aneurysm is much more recent (see chapter 16). Again, rupture of an aortic aneurysm does not contribute significantly to the post-operative mortality in arteriopaths, but as the mortality from rupture is probably greater than 80% and mortality from elective surgery less than 5% [37], it is not surprising that a number of centres are now turning their attention to aneurysms. Most of these have been general population studies, and only a few restricted to patients with established, symptomatic disease elsewhere in the arterial tree. Bengtsson and co-workers reported findings from 2 studies [38, 39] in which they looked for abdominal aortic dilatation in either patients operated upon for carotid artery stenosis or patients with intermittent claudication. In the carotid group followed for 2–13 years, 109 died and 96 had autopsies during this time. Aortic aneurysms were demonstrated in 13 (13.5%). Another 154 were screened by ultrasound and 17 (11%) had aortic dilatation. In the intermittent claudication group, 110 patients died and 8 had autopsies. Aortic aneurysms were found in 7 (8%). Another 183 patients were screened and 25 (13.7%) shown to have an aortic diameter greater than 3 cms. In both groups, the prevalence of aortic aneurysms was much higher in men than women.

A more detailed study of 100 peripheral arterial disease patients, compared with a control group, was done recently by Allardice and co-workers [30]. Aneurysms (minimum diameter 2.5 cm), or ectatic aortas (minimum diameter of 3 cm) were detected by ultrasound in 13 (20%) of 75 men and 3 (12%) of 25 women. Only 5 of the aneurysms were detected on clinical examination. In contrast, aneurysms were found in only 2% of the control group.

Peripheral arterial disease

Because peripheral arterial disease is rarely life-threatening much less attention has been paid to the prevalence of occult peripheral arterial disease.

We have used an abnormal Ankle/Brachial systolic blood Pressure Index (ABPI) of less than 0.9 or a fall in ankle pressure of 30 mmHg following a one minute period of exercise to indicate significant peripheral arterial disease [34]. Using this test we have examined the prevalence of occult peripheral arterial disease in 80 consecutive patients undergoing coronary artery bypass graft surgery (CABG). Six (7.5%) of these patients had intermittent claudication. We studied 50 of the remaining asymptomatic patients and compared the results with an age matched control group of 50 asymptomatic patients admitted for a hernia repair. The results are shown in Table 23.3. The prevalence of occult peripheral arterial disease in the CABG group (36%) was significantly higher than in the hernia group (8%) and in only one patient was occult disease detected using resting tests alone. The overall prevalence of peripheral arterial disease in CABG patients is thus well over 40%.

Table 23.3. Occult peripheral arterial disease in patients who underwent CABG[a]

	Peripheral arterial disease according to:				
	Clinical Examination	Resting PI	Exercise Test	Total	
50 CABG Patients	0	1	18	19	(36%)
50 Hernia Patients	0	0	4	4	(8%) $p<0.001$

[a]CABG = Coronary artery bypass grafting

Occult atherosclerosis in asymptomatic high risk groups

The high prevalence of occult atherosclerosis in established arteriopaths confirms the generalised nature of the disease. However, the previous studies (with the very few exceptions of those with controls) give no indication as to whether this high level of occult disease would be found throughout the population or is confined to established symptomatic patients. To provide a comparison we must examine the prevalence of occult atherosclerosis in patients without symptoms of arterial disease.

However, even in asymptomatic subjects the prevalence will vary according to the population chosen. Hypertension, hyperlipidaemia, diabetes, and a strong family history are all known risk factors and there is some evidence that the prevalence of occult disease is higher in these groups.

Hypertension

A number of studies have looked for occult carotid artery disease in hypertensive patients [26]. Lewis and co-workers [40] using Doppler flow measurements to detect severe carotid stenoses demonstrated occult disease in 14% of an elderly hypertensive group, and none in an age matched normotensive group. Looking for less severe disease Lusiani and co-workers [41] showed carotid atheroma in 24.5% of a group of asymptomatic hypertensives compared with 10.2% in a group of age-matched normotensive controls.

Hypertensive patients have also been screened for aortic aneurysms. Lederle, Walker and Reinke [29] demonstrated 18 aneurysms (9%) in a group of 201 men between 60–75 years with either hypertension or heart disease, and Allen and co-workers [42] screening 168 patients over 65 years with hypertension found 9 aneurysms (5.3%). However, Lindholm and co-workers [43] in the Dalby study screened 245 elderly hypertensive patients and found only one aneurysm.

Hyperlipidaemia

Premature coronary artery disease is a well recognised symptom of familial hypercholesterolaemia [44], but peripheral arterial disease was previously thought to be rare in this group. Perphoniemi and co-workers [32] measured the ankle/brachial systolic blood pressure index in 20 asymptomatic patients with hypercholesterolaemia and 20 normolipid controls. An abnormal ABPI (<0.97) was found in 13 (65%) of the study group and in one of the controls. Ruhn and co-workers [33] subjected 65 asymptomatic men with hyperlipidaemia to arteriography and demonstrated femoral atherosclerosis in 45.

Diabetes

Many reports have already shown the high prevalence of coronary artery disease in diabetics [45, 46], and occult peripheral arterial disease has also been demonstrated in diabetics [47].

We have studied a consecutive group of 219 diabetic patients. Twenty-four had symptoms of peripheral arterial disease. A further 7 had significant abnormalities on clinical examination giving a total of 14.2% with symptoms or signs of disease.

One hundred of the remaining group were studied again using ankle pressure measurements at rest and after exercise. The results were compared with a control group of 100 age matched hernia patients. The results are shown in Table 23.4. The prevalence of asymptomatic disease in the diabetic group (30%) was significantly higher than in the control group (10%). The

Table 23.4. Occult peripheral arterial disease in diabetic patients

	Peripheral arterial disease according to:			
	Clinical Examination	Resting PI	Exercise PI	Total
100 Diabetic Patients	0	3	27	30
100 Hernia Patients	0	1	9	10 p<0.001

severity of the peripheral arterial disease was also related to both age and the duration of diabetes (Figure 23.2).

Family history

A particularly strong association with family history has been shown in aortic aneurysm patients. Johansen and Koepsell [48] in 1986 screened the families of 250 patients with aortic aneurysms and a further 250 control families. First degree relatives with an aneurysm were found in 48 (19.2%) of the patients' families and in only 6 (2.4%) of the control families. Bengtsson and co-workers [49] have studied 36 brothers and 52 sisters of aortic aneurysm patients. Ten (29%) of the brothers and 3 (6%) of the sisters also had an aneurysm greater than 3 cm in diameter.

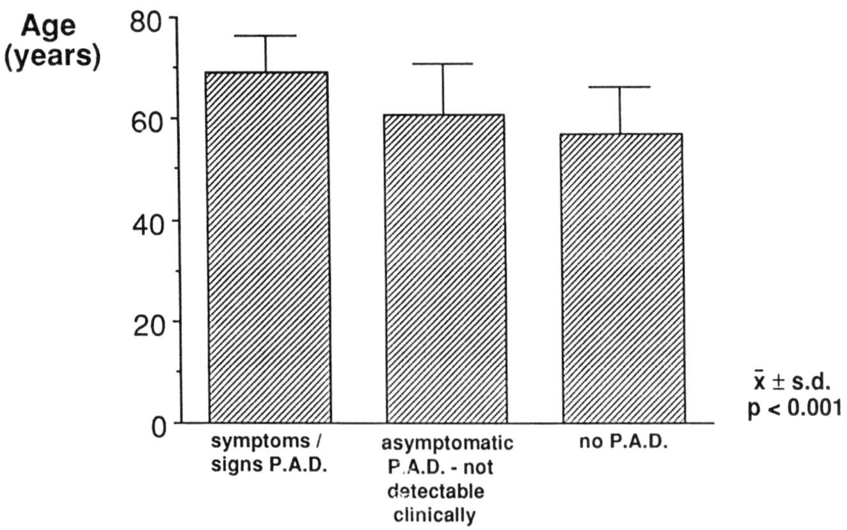

Figure 23.2. Increasing severity of peripheral arterial disease with age in diabetic patients

Occult atherosclerosis in asymptomatic low risk groups

The question remains whether the high prevalence of occult disease seen in arteriopaths, and to a lesser extent in high risk groups, is maintained in a low risk population. Only a few studies have looked at the prevalence of occult atherosclerosis in asymptomatic subjects and many of these have included a few high risk patients in their study population. In these low risk patients the prevalence of occult atherosclerosis appears to be minimal in the young, increasing with age.

The studies investigating silent myocardial ischaemia have used a variety of different methods to investigate cardiac function and have tended to concentrate on the predictive value of the test used rather than on the extent of coronary artery disease *per se*.

To determine the prevalence of occult carotid artery disease in a low risk population we have studied a group of 1300 men working in the transport industry. The subjects, all male, with an age range from 30–75 years were questioned thoroughly and excluded if they had any symptoms of atherosclerosis at all. A Duplex scan of the carotid arteries was performed and stenoses greater than 25% were recorded. The overall prevalence of carotid disease was 6% but this increased markedly with age. No significant disease was detected below the age of 40 and 2.6% of the 40–44 age group subjects had disease compared with 15.2% in the 60–64 year group. Only 13 (1%) had stenoses greater than 50% (Figure 23.3). In a similar study in France,

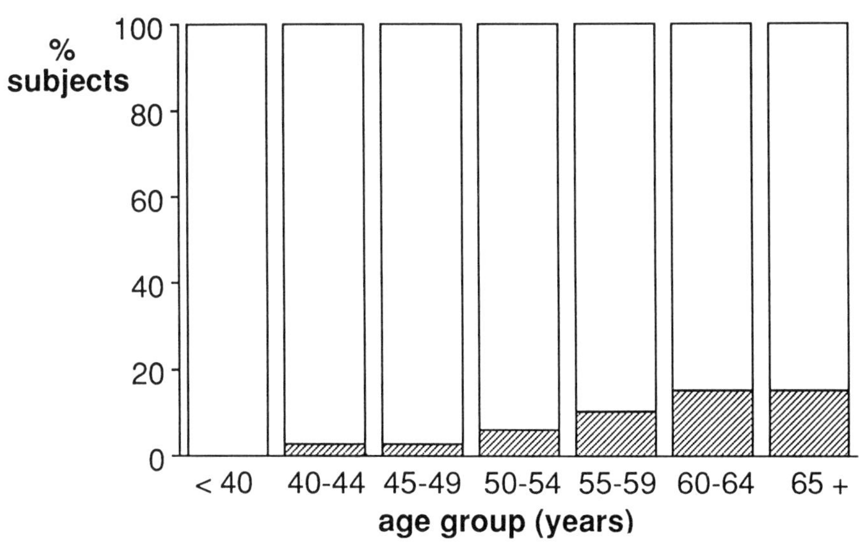

Figure 23.3. Occult carotid artery disease

Josse and co-workers [50] studied 526 volunteers, again with no symptoms of atherosclerosis or high risk factors. In this older group, and using a 15% stenosis to indicate significant disease they reported a 2.4% prevalence in males aged 55–64 years increasing to 30.3% in males aged 75–84 years. Colgan [27] again using 15% stenosis to indicate disease, reported results slightly higher, with an overall prevalence of 17.8%.

The same group of 1300 transport workers were investigated using B-mode ultrasound to detect aortic aneurysms. Only 19 (1.5%) subjects had aortas with a diameter greater than 3 cm and no aneurysms greater than 4 cm were detected. Again, using an older population, Scott and Ashton [25] demonstrated an aortic diameter greater than 3.5 cm in 19 (2.7%) of 753 subjects screened in a general practice. Only 4 (0.6%) had aneurysms greater than 6 cm, and the control groups reported in the previous sections also confirm that the prevalence of aneurysms in a low risk group is low.

Our study of hernia patients suggested that the prevalence of occult peripheral arterial disease in a low risk population was about 10% and this figure is confirmed by Criqui and co-workers [31]. Again, using a stress test they demonstrated large vessel peripheral arterial disease in 11.7% of a population with an average age of 66 years. Intermittent claudication in this group was present in only 2.2% of the men and 1.7% of the women. However, if a stress test is not used much less occult disease is detected. In a younger group, using only a resting ankle-brachial systolic blood pressure index below 0.95 to indicate disease, Walsh and co-workers [22] found occult peripheral arterial disease in only one out of 496 volunteers.

Who should be investigated for occult atherosclerosis?

In summary, the prevalence of occult atherosclerosis is very high in those patients presenting with symptoms of atherosclerosis elsewhere in the arterial tree. The prevalence also appears to be high in asymptomatic subjects already known to be at high risk. In the general low risk population the prevalence is much lower, especially in younger persons.

Only the outcome of occult coronary artery disease has been studied in any depth. The detection of silent ischaemia (rather than the presence or absence of angina) confers a worse prognosis both before and after a myocardial infarction [51, 52] and the prognosis depends upon the severity of the disease detected [53].

Similary, for carotid artery disease and aortic aneurysms the prognosis depends upon the extent of occult disease detected [35, 54]. In the follow-up of occult carotid artery disease the incidence of ischaemic events is higher in patients with a stenosis greater than 80% compared with patients with a stenosis less than 50% and although rupture is usually associated with a larger aneurysm there is evidence that smaller ones rupture too [55–57]. The outcome of asymptomatic peripheral arterial disease is not known.

Who should be investigated depends upon why the subjects are being investigated in the first place. So little is known about the natural history of occult disease that further research into all the different populations is necessary. However, when considering treatment different groups might be targeted.

Prophylactic surgery for all types of occult disease would only be considered for the more severe cases and remains a controversial issue. CABG is commonly performed prior to lower limb revascularisation to reduce the high post-operative mortality due to myocardial infarction [14] but prophylactic carotid endarterectomy and resection of a small aortic aneurysm are much more hotly debated. The morbidity and mortality rates for the prophylactic operations themselves must be considered.

Disease of a less severe nature, often found in low risk groups, might be more amenable to medical treatment. Aneurysm rupture is known to be associated with certain risk factors such as high diastolic blood pressure and obstructive pulmonary disease [55] and the outcome of smaller aneurysms might be affected by intervention at this stage. Similarly, although carotid endarterectomy would not be offered to those with a stenosis of only 25–50%, this might be the group for prophylactic medical therapy.

It remains that the fate of the young man with occult disease in only one site is unknown. Is it the expectation that this disease will remain benign throughout his life and only in rare instances cause trouble, or does this automatically herald full blown atherosclerosis in middle age with all the subsequent surgical consequences and reduced life expectancy?

References

1. Roberts J, Moses C, Wilkins RH. Autopsy studies in atherosclerosis. Circulation 1959; 20:511.
2. Hertzer NR. Fatal myocardial infarction following lower extremity revascularisation – Two hundred and seventy three patients followed six to eleven post-operative years. Ann Surg 1981; 193:492.
3. Hertzer NR, Lees CD. Fatal myocardial infarction following carotid endarterectomy. Ann Surg 1981; 194:212.
4. Hertzer NR. Fatal myocardial infarction following abdominal aortic aneurysm resection – Three hundred and forty three patients followed six to eleven years post-operatively. Ann Surg 1980; 192:667.
5. Crawford ES, Bomberger RA, Glaeser DH *et al.* Aorto-iliac occlusive disease: Factors influencing survival and function following reconstructive operation over a twenty-five year period. Surgery 1981; 90:1055.
6. Kallero KS, Bergquist D, Cederholm C *et al.* Late mortality and morbidity after arterial reconstruction: The influence of atherosclerosis in popliteal artery trifurcation. J Vasc Surg 1985; 2:541.

7. Turnipseed W D, Berkoff H A, Belzer F O. Post-operative stroke in cardiac and peripheral vascular disease. Ann Surg 1980; 192:365.
8. Begg T B, Richard R L. The prognosis of intermittent claudication. Scot Med J 1962; 7:341.
9. Bloor K. Natural history of arteriosclerosis of the lower extremities. Ann Roy Coll Surg Engl 1961; 28:36.
10. Kannel W B, Shurtleff D. The natural history of arteriosclerosis obliterans. Cardiovasc Clin 1971; 3:37.
11. Jelnes R, Gaardsting O, Hougaard Jensen K *et al.* Fate in intermittent claudication: outcome and risk factors. Br Med J 1986; 293:1137.
12. Kallero K S. Mortality and morbidity in patients with intermittent claudication as defined by venous occlusion plethysmography – A ten year follow-up. J Chron Dis 1981; 34:455.
13. Ennix C L, Lawrie G M, Morris G C *et al.* Improved results of carotid endarterectomy in patients with symptomatic coronary disease – An analysis of 1546 consecutive carotid operations. Stroke 1979; 10:122.
14. Hertzer N R, Bevan E G, Young J R *et al.* Coronary artery disease in peripheral vascular patients. A classification of 1000 coronary angiograms and results of surgical management. Ann Surg 1984; 199:223.
15. Hughson W G, Mann J I, Tibbs D J *et al.* Intermittent claudication: Factors determining outcome. Br Med J 1978; i:1377.
16. Dawber T R. The Framingham Study: The epidemiology of atherosclerotic disease. Cambridge, Harvard University Press, 1980.
17. Greenhalgh R M, Laing S P, Ellis M R *et al.* How can we detect early subclinical disease in vascular surgery. In: Issues in current practice, Greenhalgh R M, Jamieson C W, Nicolaides A N (eds). Grune and Stratton 1986; 57.
18. Collin J, Araujo L, Lindsell D. A community screening programme for abdominal aortic aneurysms. Eur J Vasc Surg 1988; 2:83.
19. Vecht R J, Nicolaides A N, Brandao E *et al.* Resting and treadmill electrocardiographic findings in patients with intermittent claudication. Inter Angio 1982; 1:119.
20. Brewster D C, Okada R D, Strauss H W *et al.* Selection of patients for pre-operative coronary arteriography: Use of dipyridamol stress-thallium myocardial imaging. J Vasc Surg 1985; 2:504.
21. Nicolaides A N. The diagnosis and assessment of coronary artery disease in vascular patients. J Vasc Surg 1985; 2:501.
22. Walsh J J, Cofelice M, Lumpkin D *et al.* Is screening for vascular disease a valuable proposition? J Cardiovasc Surg 1988; 29(3):306.
23. Ramsey D E, Miles R D, Lambeth A *et al.* Prevalence of extracranial carotid artery disease: A survey of an asymptomatic population with non-invasive techniques. J Vasc Surg 1987; 5(4):584.
24. Hennerici M, Aulich A, Sandmann W *et al.* Incidence of asymptomatic extracranial arterial disease. Stroke 1981; 12(6):750.
25. Scott R A P, Ashton G L J. Ultrasound screening of a general practice population for aortic aneurysms. Br J Surg 1986; 73:318.
26. Sutton K C, Wolfson S K, Kuller L H. Carotid and lower extremity disease in elderly adults with isolated systolic hypertension. Stroke 1987; 18(5):817.
27. Colgan M P, Strode G R, Sommer J D *et al.* Prevalence of asymptomatic carotid disease – Results of duplex scanning in 348 unselected volunteers. J Vasc Surg 1988; 8(6):674.
28. Hertzer N R, Bevan E G, Young J R *et al.* Incidental asymptomatic carotid bruits in patients scheduled for peripheral vascular reconstruction – Results of cerebral and coronary angiography. Surgery 1984; 96:535.
29. Lederle F A, Walker J M, Reinke D B. Selective screening for abdominal aortic aneurysms with physical examination and ultrasound. Arch Intern Med 1988; 148(8):1753.

30. Allardice JT, Allwright GJ, Wafula JM *et al.* High prevalence of abdominal aortic aneurysm in men with peripheral vascular disease – Screening by ultrasonography. Br J Surg 1988; 75(3):240.
31. Crigui MH, Fronek A, Barnett Connor E *et al.* The prevalence of peripheral arterial disease in a defined population. Circulation 1985; 71(3):510.
32. Perphoniemi V, Gylling H, Salmenkivi K. Peripheral atherosclerosis in familial hypercholesterolaemia. J Intern Med 1989; 225:379.
33. Ruhn G, Evikson U, Olsson AG. Prevalance of femoral atherosclerosis in asymptomatic men with hyperlipoproteinaemia. J Intern Med 1989; 225(5):317.
34. Laing SP. Assessment of symptomatic and asymptomatic peripheral arterial disease using a one-minute exercise test. PhD thesis London University 1984.
35. Moneta GL, Taylor DC, Nicholls SC *et al.* Operative versus non-operative management of asymptomatic high grade internal carotid artery stenosis. Improved results with endarterectomy. Stroke 1987; 18(6):1005.
36. Stavenow L, Karlsson S, Lilja B *et al.* High prevalence of coronary heart disease in patients with intermittent claudication. Acta Chir Scand 1988; 154:447.
37. Collin J. The value of screening for abdominal aortic aneurysm by ultrasound. In: The Cause and Management of aneurysms, Greenhalgh RM, Mannick J (eds.). WB Saunders 1990; 447.
38. Bengtsson H, Ekberg O, Aspelin P *et al.* Abdominal aortic dilatation in patients operated upon for carotid artery stenosis. Acta Chir Scand 1988; 154:441.
39. Bengtsson H, Ekberg O, Aspelin P *et al.* Ultrasound screening of the abdominal aorta in patients with intermittent claudication. Eur J Vasc Surg 1989; 3:497.
40. Lewis RR, Padayachee TS, Arianayagam RP *et al.* Prevalence of severe internal carotid artery disease in hypertensive elderly patients. J Hypertens Suppl 1988; 6(1):833.
41. Lusiani L, Visona A, Castellani V *et al.* Prevalence of atherosclerotic involvement of the internal carotid artery in hypertensive patients. Int J Cardiol 1987; 17(1):51.
42. Allen PM, Gourevitch D, McKinley J *et al.* Population screening for aortic aneurysms. Lancet 1987; II:736.
43. Lindholm L, Ejlertsson G, Forsberg L *et al.* Low prevalence of abdominal aortic aneurysm in hypertensive patients. Acta Med Scand 1985; 218:305.
44. Fredrickson DS, Goldstein JL, Brown MS. The familial hypercholesterolaemias. In: The Metabolic Basis of Inherited Disease. Stanbury JB, Wyngaarden JB, Fredrickson DB (eds.). McGraw Hill Book, New York 1978; 672.
45. Marin-Huerta E, Rayo I, Lara JI. Silent myocardial ischaemia during Holter monitoring in patients with diabetes mellitus. Rev Esp Cardiol 1989; 42(8):519.
46. Krolewski A, Kosinski E, Warram JH *et al.* Magnitude and determinants of coronary artery disease in juvenille-onset Insulin dependent diabetes mellitus. Am J Cardiol 1987; 59:750.
47. Marinelli MR, Beach KW, Glass MJ *et al.* Non-invasive testing vs clinical evaluation of arterial disease. J Am Med Ass 1979; 241(19):2031.
48. Johansen K, Koepsell T. Familial tendency for abdominal aortic aneurysms. JAMA 1986; 256:1934.
49. Bengtsson H, Norrgard O, Angquist KA *et al.* Ultrasonographic screening of the abdominal aorta among siblings of patients with abdominal aortic aneurysms. Br J Surg 1989; 76(6):589.
50. Josse MO, Touboul PJ, Mas JL *et al.* Prevalence of asymptomatic internal carotid artery stenosis. Neuroepidemiology 1987; 6(3):150.
51. Stern S. Clinical outcome of silent myocardial ischaemia. Am J Cardiol 1988; 61(12):16F.
52. Assey ME. Prognosis in stable angina pectoris and silent myocardial ischaemia. Am J Cardiol 1988; 61(12):19F.

53. Cohn PF. Detection and prognosis of the asymptomatic patient with silent myocardial ischaemia. Am J Cardiol 1988; 61(3):4B.
54. Colgan MP, Leahy AL, Grouden MC *et al.* The results of an eight year prospective study of internal carotid artery stenosis in asymptomatic patients. Vascular Surgical Society Presentation, 1989.
55. Cronenwett JL, Murphy TF, Zelenbock GB *et al.* Actuarial analysis of variables associated with rupture of small abdominal aortic aneurysms. Surgery 1985; 98(3):472.
56. Flanigan DP, Quinn T, Kraft RO. Selective management of high risk patients with an abdominal aortic aneurysm. Surg Gynecol Obstet 1980; 150:171.
57. Darling RC. Ruptured arteriosclerotic abdominal arotic aneurysms. A pathologic and clinical study. Am J Surg 1970; 119:397.

24. Prevention of occult atherosclerotic disease

BRENT M. PARKER and VASKAR MUKERJI

The twentieth century has seen an epidemic of cardiovascular disease, much of which is due to atherosclerosis. The major cause of death has become coronary heart disease and cerebral vascular disease [1]. Although atherosclerosis was known in early 1900s it has risen in proportion to other causes of death, especially infectious disease which has declined greatly with the advent of effective therapy. The increase in the incidence of atherosclerosis also parallels the increasing age of the population. In general, there is a correlation between atherosclerosis in one arterial system and atherosclerosis elsewhere in the body [2] (see chapters 7 and 22). For instance, the main cause of death for persons with carotid artery disease is coronary disease [3]. Many patients with abdominal aortic aneurysm have significant coronary disease [4, 5]. Most of what has been written concerning the prevention of atherosclerotic disease has dealt with coronary disease as the prime example. Therefore, in this chapter we will use the information available on coronary disease, highlighting information pertaining to specific other vascular trees when such is available. For this discussion we will not differentiate between occult and clinically apparent atherosclerotic disease since the principles of prevention are the same.

Aetiology of atherosclerosis

It is apparent that prevention of a disease requires knowledge of its aetiology. Unfortunately, the aetiology of atherosclerosis remains speculative. It is known that lipids such as high cholesterol are important in the process [6]. It also appears that damage to the vessel wall may be important [7]. Hypertension may contribute to atherosclerosis in this way. Although the exact origin of atherosclerosis remains uncertain, much has been learned about certain clinical factors which are associated with the presence of

A.-M. Salmasi and A. N. Nicolaides (eds.), Occult Atherosclerotic Disease, 335–347.

atherosclerosis. As the epidemic of atherosclerosis continued and worsened in the 1940s and 1950s, knowledge began to accumulate about associated risk factors. The Framingham Epidemiologic study in Framingham, Massachusetts greatly contributed to our knowledge about the risk factors of atherosclerosis and their importance [8]. The major risk factors identified were: hypertension, cigarette smoking, serum lipid abnormalities and diabetes mellitus. The Framingham data indicated that the presence of hypertension might increase the risk of coronary disease two-fold or three but that grouping of risk factors such as smoking, hypertension, and high cholesterol would increase the risk by over ten-fold [9]. Thus, these risk factors, although not directly aetiologic, seem to be powerful predictors of coronary atherosclerosis.

Importantly, beginning in the late 1950s and early 1960s efforts were made to modify the risk factors [10]. Effective therapy for hypertension became available and was widely applied. The association between smoking and various diseases was recognized and publicized and smoking began to decline. A low cholesterol, low saturated fat diet was advocated by the American Heart Association and others commencing approximately in the mid-1960s. Around this time deaths due to cardiovascular disease which had been climbing progressively showed a definite and continued decline [11]. Although it may never be possible to assign credit for the decline in cardiovascular mortality since new therapies accompanied the risk factor modification and reduction, experts in the field attribute a significant proportion of the decline to changes in lifestyle and modification of risk factors [12].

Individual risk factors

The risk factors for coronary disease have been divided into those which are modifiable and those which are not. The risk factors which are not modifiable include the male sex, increased age, and family history. Males have a much higher incidence of cardiovascular disease and coronary disease and a higher mortality [8]. Beginning at the menopause, the incidence of coronary heart disease in females rises and eventually approximates that of males [8, 13]. Unfortunately, because males have a higher incidence of cardiovascular disease, and because it is easier in clinical trials to show changes in mortality and morbidity in males, there has been no attention to females in risk prevention studies. Thus, the discussion of risk factors that follows will by necessity deal with males. It is certainly possible that what is stated is also true for females, but this must remain speculative.

The cardiovascular mortality rises progressively with increased age [8], hence it would be desirable to have information concerning modification of risk factors in the elderly in terms of the effect on mortality. Unfortunately, such data are generally lacking. For example, there is no evidence concerning cholesterol lowering in patients over the age of 65. The risk factor modification trials have not used elderly patients. There is some evidence concerning smoking and hypertension in the elderly which will be cited as those individual factors discussed below. Although a strong family history of coronary artery disease does indicate an increased risk for another individual in the family, the mechanisms for this association are unclear [14]. It is possible that in some instances this association represents similar lifestyles in family members such as heavy smoking, sedentary activity and a high cholesterol diet. In other families, the association is due to familial lipid abnormalities. For instance, there may be a familial hyperlipidaemia with high serum cholesterol. It also appears that some families have increased risk due to a familial tendency toward a low HDL cholesterol. Unfortunately, this may not be detected if one merely screens the total cholesterol. In families with a history of coronary artery disease before the age of 55, it is clearly indicated to measure the serum fasting lipid profile in other family members. Abnormalities of the lipid profile should be attacked aggressively. In addition, vigorous attempts to prevent or modify other risk factors such as hypertension, cigarette smoking, and the sedentary lifestyle should be undertaken [14].

Cigarette smoking

Cigarette smoking is the most important cause of preventable mortality and morbidity [15]. The association of cigarette smoking to carcinoma of the lung and other cancers and to the chronic obstructive lung disease is unquestioned [15]. There is also no question about the association with atherosclerosis and stroke [16]. The association of cigarette smoking to peripheral vascular disease is strong [17]. These associations may relate to nicotine's known pharmacologic effect of causing arterial vasoconstriction, although the effects of nicotine are numerous and complex. The association to coronary disease is also clear cut [8]. Epidemiologic studies indicate that the young person with coronary artery disease is very likely to be a smoker.

The risk of coronary disease in older patients is approximately 1.5-fold increased in smokers as opposed to non-smokers [8]. Based on the proven association of cigarette smoking to a variety of diseases, public education in the United States began to focus on smoking in the 1960s. As a result, the percentage of the adult males smoking had dropped from approximately 52% to 35% in 1983 [15]. This drop in smoking has been associated with the decline in cardiovascular disease mortality rate and has been felt to be a significant contributor to this decline. It has been estimated that half of the individuals that once smoked have quit. Thus, it is certainly possible for many individuals to give up smoking if they are convinced this is in their best interest. Individuals who stop smoking will have a decrease in risk over a several year period and will approximate the risk of those persons who never smoked [8, 18]. This applies, not only to younger individuals, but to individuals in older age groups [18]. Thus, it does not appear that it is ever too late to stop smoking. Smoking is not only important in primary prevention of coronary disease, that is preventing the disease from developing in the first place, but it is also important in secondary prevention. It has been shown that those individuals who develop a myocardial infarct and who are smokers will live twice as long after the infarct if they stop smoking [19].

The role of physicians and health personnel in helping individuals to stop smoking is important [20]. It is the responsibility of every physician who sees an individual who smokes to point out the risks and to advise stopping. Yet it is distressing how often patients indicate they have never been told that by their physician. A careful smoking history should be part of every encounter and advice to stop smoking should follow. If a patient wishes to stop but is unsure how to do so, or is unsuccessful in attempting to do so, then additional resources should be sought, such as smoking cessation clinics.

Despite the overwhelming evidence concerning the undesirability of smoking, it is a matter of concern that a number of young people continue to take up the habit [15]. This dictates vigorous attempts to help children avoid making the mistake of beginning smoking.

Although, the relationship of pipe and cigar smoking to atherosclerosis is not as strong because less smoke is inhaled, these types of smoking are nevertheless undesirable. For example, pipe smoking is associated with carcinoma of the oropharynx. Pipe and cigar smoking are disagreeable for others, cause passive smoking and should be discouraged.

Hypertension

Hypertension is a major risk factor for a variety of cardiovascular diseases. The incidence of coronary disease is doubled in patients with hypertension, as is the incidence of peripheral vascular disease. Cerebral vascular accidents are increased threefold in hypertensives and congestive heart failure is increased almost five times according to the Framingham data [21]. It has been well established since the landmark cooperative Veterans Administration studies that treating significant hypertension lowers the morbidity and mortality of cardiovascular disease [22]. Initial studies dealt with patients with diastolic pressures over 115 mmHg. However, recent data suggest that treating patients with mild hypertension (diastolic pressures between 90 and 105 mmHg) is also useful [23, 24]. The impact of the treatment of hypertension has been primarily upon cerebral vascular disease and congestive heart failure. The impact upon coronary heart disease incidence and mortality has been minimal [22, 25]. Nevertheless, some recent studies have also demonstrated a decline in cardiac mortality when hypertension is treated [26].

Data on the treatment of hypertension in the elderly have been relatively sparse. However, the European Working Party for Hypertension in the Elderly Study demonstrated a reduced mortality and morbidity in elderly hypertensives who were treated as opposed to a control group [26]. The Hypertension Detection and Follow-up Study also supported therapy in the elderly [24]. Therefore, treatment of hypertension of the elderly appears indicated.

Systolic hypertension with normal diastolic pressures has been termed isolated systolic hypertension. Isolated systolic hypertension has a strong association with cardiovascular mortality and morbidity with a risk that equals or exceeds that of diastolic hypertension [27]. It has been difficult to separate the cause of the increased risk. Is it due to the high pressure itself? Or is it due to the change in the blood vessels which underlies and causes the systolic hypertension? The efficacy of treating systolic hypertension has not been established. Pilot studies have now shown that lowering systolic hypertension with diuretics is feasible and can be done without causing end organ problems [28]. A major study is underway in the United States to ascertain whether treating systolic hypertension in the elderly lowers mortality and morbidity. Results can be expected in several years and will be of great interest and importance.

Mild hypertension can be approached initially with non-pharmacologic methods, such as exercise, low salt diet and behavior modification. In most individuals, it will become necessary to eventually treat with drugs. Many drugs are available and drug therapy should be utilized whenever the diastolic pressure remains above 90–95 mmHg after non-pharmacologic therapy. The choice of drugs depends upon a variety of factors which must be individualized, including cost, patient tolerance, side effects and results. Certain drugs, such as the angiotensin converting enzyme inhibitors and calcium channel blockers among others may be more effective in reversing left ventricular hypertrophy, and for this reason, may be more effective in some individuals [29].

Hypercholesterolaemia

It has been known for over a century that atherosclerotic lesions contain considerable lipid material and that feeding high cholesterol diets to experimental animals, such as rabbits and monkeys, will induce atherosclerosis [30]. Epidemiologic studies have shown that societies with low cholesterol intake in the diet have low average serum cholesterol values and a low incidence of coronary heart disease and atherosclerosis. Societies with high cholesterol diet, such as the western societies, have a high average cholesterol and a high incidence of coronary disease [30]. The Framingham studies and others have shown a clear cut relationship between the serum cholesterol level and the incidence of coronary heart disease [8]. The incidence rises gradually and slowly from the range of 160 to 220 to 240 mg/dL and then sharply increases at levels above 240 mg/dL. There is at least some evidence that the coronary epidemic of the 20th Century has been associated with an increased intake of cholesterol and saturated fats. A concerted physician and public education program by the American Heart Association beginning in the 1950s led to changes in diet in the United States [31]. The average total cholesterol dropped from approximately 230 to 210 mg/dL, as the American Heart Association prudent diet was adopted by many individuals [32]. This drop in cholesterol and change in diet coincided with the decline in the coronary heart disease mortality but data are inconclusive in regards to cause and effect [11].

Data proving that lowering the serum cholesterol will lower coronary heart risk have been difficult to obtain. The Multiple Risk Factor Intervention Trial which utilized a low cholesterol diet among other interventions, did not show a significant decline in cardiovascular mortality after seven years [33]. Clofibrate, a drug to lower cholesterol and triglycerides, was administered in a World Health Organization trial. The cardiovascular mortality was lowered to a modest degree, but there was an increase of cancer in the clofibrate patients, and the overall mortality was higher in the treated patients than in the controls [34]. More recently, two trials using cholestyramine and Gemfibrozil have been reported and touted as showing significant reduction in coronary heart disease mortality and morbidity [35, 36]. The Coronary Primary Prevention Trial reported a 19% reduction in coronary heart disease morbidity or mortality with the use of cholestyramine [35], and the Gemfibrozil Study in Finland reported a 34% reduction in coronary heart disease risk [36]. Despite the claims made for these studies, the results are somewhat disappointing since there was actually only a 1.6% mortality and morbidity reduction in the Coronary Primary Prevention Trial and a 1.4% reduction in the Finnish study [37]. In addition, neither trial demonstrated an overall reduction in mortality. Despite the modest observed benefits, the Coronary Primary Prevention Trial has been used as part of the basis for a National Cholesterol Consensus Conference and a National Cholesterol Education Program in the United States [30]. It was recommended that all persons eat a prudent or low cholesterol, low fat diet. Cholesterol levels as low as 200–240 mg/dL have been defined as the subject for concern. These recommendations have been made based on the conviction of many in the field that this program may do much good and no harm to the population. The critics of the program have been quick to point out the consensus conference was a consensus of believers. Michael Oliver, has called it the 'nonsensus' conference [38]. Critics point out there are no reliable studies showing that diet will lower cardiovascular risk, and they point out that there are no data concerning cholesterol lowering in the elderly or women [39, 40]. They also state that there are no data indicating that lowering cholesterol levels below 240 mg/dL will be useful, since the studies that have shown a small benefit have used an average cholesterol of approximately 290 mg/dL [39, 40, 41]. A Canadian group has recommended higher total cholesterol levels for concern (265 mg/dL) [42]. Iso *et al.* pointed out that low cholesterol levels are associated with an increased incidence of hemorrhagic stroke [43].

Another problem with the National Cholesterol Education Program is the lack of emphasis on the HDL cholesterol. Barr, and Colleagues first described the HDL cholesterol and the fact that low levels were associated with increased risk [44]. Recent studies suggest that the HDL cholesterol is the faction of lipids that is most closely related to cardiovascular disease [45, 46]. Much of the cholesterol screening which has been done does not utilize the HDL cholesterol. It is certainly possible that individuals with low total cholesterol and low HDL are being missed and are at risk. As yet, there are no data to indicate that altering HDL will decrease risk. This is a subject that warrants careful study. HDL cholesterol is lower in men, which may account for some of the increased risk in men. It is lowered by cigarette smoking, and it may be lowered by a low cholesterol diet. For this reason, it is certainly possible that low cholesterol diets may not always be beneficial.

A pending study may give a better perspective on the benefits of lowering total cholesterol. A Scandinavian study with lovastatin, a drug which may lower cholesterol by 30–40% should show significant benefit if lowering cholesterol is indeed as useful as its proponents state. A recent report [47] showed that surgical ileal bypass in hypercholesterolaemia (average cholesterol level 251 mg/dL) in patients after a myocardial infarction can bring up a retardation of progress of coronary artery lesions and reduce mortality. Fish oil, high in omega three fatty acids, has been reported to be beneficial in preventing coronary heart disease. This appears promising but large well-controlled studies are necessary [48]. One of the purported benefits of fish oil is a decreased tendency to coagulation. Studies of the relationship of cholesterol levels to coffee intake have yielded conflicting results [49]. Whatever changes there are, if any, appear to be insignificant.

There remains some controversy over how wide-spread screening for hypercholesterolaemia should be. One can certainly make a case for obtaining a serum cholesterol level in all persons before the age of 20 and periodically thereafter [30]. Nevertheless, the costs and practicality of this measure are a matter of some concern [41, 42]. All authorities would agree that everyone with a positive family history for coronary heart disease should be screened and certainly persons with other risk factors should be tested for hypercholesterolaemia.

At the present time we would recommend that all men should be screened at least once in the late teenage years for hypercholesterolaemia. Those found to have hypercholesterolaemia would need to have follow-up testing and we feel that a prudent low cholesterol diet is justified. An individual with a low serum cholesterol certainly does not need follow a prudent diet if he or she finds it unpalatable. Individuals with serum cholesterol levels of over 250 mg/dL should be treated with diet and if diet fails to lower the cholesterol to below 250 mg/dL drug therapy should be considered. Individuals with cholesterol levels of greater than 300 mg/dL will often need a drug therapy. There are essentially no data after the age of 65 or in women. It would be difficult to justify a low cholesterol diet or drugs for hypercholesterolaemia in patients who are 65 years old or older. It is also uncertain that screening women is useful in the absence of other risk factors [42]. Other concerns about the cholesterol issue include large variability in laboratory results [50], and an overconcern and unnecessary anxiety in some individuals about cholesterol [40].

Diabetes

Diabetes is a major risk factor for atherosclerosis. Although it is an important risk factor for coronary heart disease [8], it is especially important for peripheral vascular disease [51]. In the past it has been assumed that the rigid control of diabetes will slow the onset of vascular complications such as retinopathy, renal failure, coronary heart disease and peripheral vascular disease. However, there is no conclusive proof of this and some patients with relatively mild glucose abnormalities have major vascular problems and complications. To provide an answer concerning the complications of diabetes and diabetes control, there is a multicenter study underway comparing average control to very tight control of diabetes and the development of complications [52]. This should provide answers in this area in a few years.

Sedentary lifestyle

Coincident with the coronary heart disease epidemic there has been a decline in the amount of habitual activity and the exercise required to earn a living. The coronary epidemic coincides with the development of the automobile and other labour-saving devices. Thus, lack of exercise and sedentary lifestyle has been considered as a possible factor in the atherosclerosis problem. A number of studies have looked at the amount of exercise at work or leisure and the incidence of coronary heart disease. Nearly all studies point to sedentary lifestyle as a significant risk factor and a recent review summarizing this information has concluded that sedentary lifestyle should be considered a major risk factor with a relative risk comparable to hypertension, cigarette smoking and hypercholesterolaemia [53]. Paffenbarger *et al.* in a series of studies have provided evidence that those who exercise more have significantly less coronary disease, fewer myocardial infarctions and longer life [54]. There is also experimental evidence concerning exercise. Kramsch *et al.* showed that monkeys fed a high cholesterol diet and divided into an exercise and control group showed a strong difference between the controls which did not exercise and the exercise group [55]. The control group had atherosclerosis whereas the exercise monkeys did not. The amount of exercise generally considered desirable is 20 to 30 minutes of exercise raising the pulse to 70 to 80% of the predicted maximum three times a week. Exercise may exert its beneficial effects in part by enhancing fibrinolysis and in part by favorable lipid changes [53].

Obesity

Obesity may contribute to atherosclerosis by its association with hypercholesterolaemia, hypertension, glucose intolerance, and sedentary lifestyle. In addition, there is some evidence that obesity is a risk factor even if the above mentioned factors are controlled [56]. It has been suggested that obesity is most associated with coronary risk if the excess fat tissue is concentrated in the abdomen [57]. It is clear that significant obesity is undesirable and may contribute to atherosclerosis. Weight reduction and exercise are recommended.

Stress and personality

Stress and personality type are somewhat controversial risk factors. Friedman and Rosen have described increased risk associated with the type A personality; that is the personality with a high degree of aggressiveness, time consciousness and impatience [58]. However, a number of studies have failed to confirm the importance of a type A personality in a variety of settings [59, 60]. Because of this it is not possible to state at the present time that personality and stress are significant risk factors. Perhaps the new emphasis on expressed hostility as a coronary risk factor will prove fruitful [61].

Aspirin

A study in American male physicians has indicated that the administration of low dose aspirin decreases the incidence of first myocardial infarction [62]. The difference achieved statistical significance. Aspirin with or without persantine has also been shown to lower the ratio of reinfarction and mortality after a myocardial infarction [63, 64]. Based on these data, it seems prudent to administer low dose aspirin to middle aged men at risk for coronary heart disease. Data showing benefit in women are lacking for primary prevention.

Intervention trials

Although the individual risk factors are important in the incidence of coronary heart disease and treating hypertension has been beneficial, at least in the prevention of cerebral vascular disease, it has been difficult to show clear-cut benefit in multiple risk factor intervention trials in middle aged men [65]. As mentioned earlier, the Multiple Risk Factor Intervention Trial (MRFIT) did not demonstrate benefit from attempts to decrease cigarette smoking, blood pressure, and cholesterol [33]. It is important, however, to point out that there were changes in the control group in this study and that the study dealt with middle aged men who may have already had significant disease. Intervention trials that showed hopeful results were those of Hjermann *et al.* dealing with cigarette smoking and cholesterol lowering [66], and the Belgian intervention in factories [67]. In the Belgian study, individuals working in factories where advice was given about smoking cessation, hypertension detection and control, diet and exercise had a lower myocardial infarction rate than in control factories without such advice [67]. A study in Rome gave similar results [68].

Based on the available data, Goldman and Cook have concluded that much of the decline of cardiovascular mortality in the past twenty years can be attributed to lifestyle modifications and risk factor alteration [12]. Although much remains to be learned, current evidence supports smoking cessation, control of hypertension, lowering significantly elevated cholesterol levels, good control of diabetes, increased exercise, weight control and the use of aspirin as measures which may be helpful in preventing occult atherosclerosis and its applications.

References

1. Heart Facts. Dallas Texas, American Heart Association, 1983.
2. Taylor PC. Evaluation and surgical management of patients with severe combined coronary artery disease and peripheral vascular atheroschlerosis. Clev Clin Quart 1981; 48:172.
3. Newman DC, Hicks RC. Combined carotid and coronary artery surgery; a review of the literature. Ann Thoracic Surgery 1988; 45:574.
4. Brown OW, Hollier LH, Pairolero PC *et al.* Abdominal aortic aneurysm and coronary artery disease: A reassessment. Arch Surg 1981; 116:1484.
5. Roger VL, Ballard DJ, Hallett JW Jr *et al.* Influence of coronary disease on morbidity and mortality after abdominal aortic aneurysmectomy: A population based study 1971–1987. JACC 1989; 14:1245.

6. Holme I, Solberg L A, Weissfeld L *et al.* Coronary risk factors and their pathway of action through coronary raised lesions, coronary stenoses and coronary death: Multivariate statistical analysis of an autopsy series: The Oslo study. Am J Cardiol 1985; 55:40.
7. Ross R. The pathogenesis of atheroschlerosis – an update. N Engl J Med 1986; 314:488.
8. Castelli W P. Epidemiology of coronary heart disease: The Framingham Study. Am J Med 1984; 76, 2A:4.
9. Coronary Risk Handbook. Estimating risk of coronary heart disease in daily practice, Dallas TX, American Heart Association, 1973.
10. Watkins L O. Why are death rates from coronary heart disease decreasing? Which preventive measures are effective? Postgraduate Medicine 1984; 75:201.
11. Gillium R F, Folsom A R, Blackburn H. Decline in coronary heart disease mortality. Am J Med 1984; 76:1055.
12. Goldman L, Cook E F. The decline in ischaemic heart disease mortality rates: an analysis of the comparative effects of medical interventions and changes in lifestyle. Ann Intern Med 1984; 101:825.
13. Matthews K A, Meilahn E, Kuller L H *et al.* Menopause and risk factors for coronary heart disease. N Engl J Med 1989; 321:641.
14. Barrett-Conner E, Khaw K. Family history of heart attack as an independent predictor of death due to cardiovascular disease. Circulation 1984; 69:1065.
15. Fielding J E. Smoking: Health effects and control. N Engl J Med 1985; 313:491.
16. Abbott R D, Yin Y, Reed D M *et al.* Risk of stroke in male cigarette smokers. N Engl J Med 1986; 315:717.
17. Kannel W B. Cigarette smoking in peripheral arterial disease. Primary Cardiology, March, 1986; 13.
18. Stamler J, Stamler R. Intervention for the prevention and control of hypertension and atherosclerotic diseases: United States and international experience. Am J Med 1984; 76 2A:13.
19. Salonen J T. Stopping smoking and long term mortality after acute myocardial infarction. Br Heart J 1980; 43:463.
20. Cummings S R, Coates T J, Richard R J *et al.* Training physicians in counselling about smoking cessation. A randomized trial of the 'quit for life' program. Ann Intern Med 1989; 110:640.
21. Gordon T, Kannel W B. Predisposition to atherosclerosis in the head, heart and lungs: The Framingham study. JAMA 1972; 221:661.
22. Veterans Administration Cooperative Study Group on antihypertensive agents. Effects of treatment on morbidity in hypertension – results in patients with diastolic blood pressures averaging 115 through 129 mmHg. JAMA 1967; 213:1143.
23. Grimm R H Jr. Should mild hypertension be treated? Early intervention. Medical Clinics of North America 1984; 68:477.
24. Hypertension Detection and Follow-up Program Cooperative Group. Five-year findings of Hypertension Detection and Follow-up Program. JAMA 1979; 242:2562.
25. Medical Research Council Working Party on Mild Hypertension. Coronary heart disease in the medical research council trial of treatment of mild hypertension. Br Heart J 1988; 59:364.
26. Amery A, Brixko P, Clement D *et al.* Mortality and morbidity results from the European Working Party on High Blood Pressure in the Elderly Trial. Lancet 1985; 1:1349.
27. Kannel W B, Dawber T R, McGee D L. Perspectives on systolic hypertension: The Framingham Study. Circulation 1980; 61:1179.
28. Hulley S B, Furberg C D, Gurland B *et al.* Systolic Hypertension in Elderly Program (SHEP), anti-hypertensive effect of chlorthalidone. Am J Cardiol 1985; 56:913.
29. Frohlich E D. Cardiac hypertrophy in hypertension. N Engl J Med 1987; 317:831.

30. The Expert Panel. Report of the National Cholesterol Education Program Expert Panel on detection, evaluation, and treatment of high blood cholesterol in adults. Arch Intern Med 1988; 148:36.
31. Walker WJ. Changing U.S. lifestyle and declining vascular mortality: A retrospective (Editorial). N Engl J Med 1983; 308:649.
32. Abraham S, Rifkind BM, Feinleib M *et al.* Decline in serum cholesterol levels among adults in the United States. (abstract) Circulation 1983; 68:III 179.
33. Multiple Risk Factor Intervention Group. Multiple Risk Factor Intervention Trial. Risk factor changes and mortality results. JAMA 1982; 248:1465.
34. Oliver MF, Heady JA, Morris JN *et al.* A cooperative trial in the primary prevention of ischemic heart disease using clofibrate: Report from the Committee of Principal Investigators. Br Heart J 1978; 40:1069.
35. Lipid Research Clinics Program. The Lipid Research Clinics Coronary Primary Prevention Trial results. Reduction in incidence of coronary heart disease. JAMA 1984; 251:351.
36. Frick MH, Elo O, Haapa K *et al.* Helsinki Heart Study: Primary prevention trial with gemfibrozil in middle aged men with dyslipidemia. N Engl J Med 1987; 317:1237.
37. Weissler AM, Miller BI, Boudoulas H. The need for clarification of percent risk reduction data in clinical cardiovascular trial reports. JACC 1989; 13:764.
38. Oliver MF. Cousensus or nonsensus conference on coronary heart disease. Lancet 1985; 2:1087.
39. Palumbo PJ. National Cholesterol Education Program. Does the emperor have any clothes? (Editorial) Mayo Clin Proc 1988; 63:88.
40. Corday E, Ryden L. Why some physicians have concerns about the cholesterol awareness program. JACC 1989; 13:497.
41. Garber AM. Where to draw the line against cholesterol (editorial) Ann Intern Med 1989; 111:625.
42. Basinski A, Frank JW, Naylor CD *et al.* Detection and management of asymptomatic hypercholesterolemia. A policy document by the Toronto Working Group on Cholesterol Policy. Toronto, Ontario Ministry of Health, 1989.
43. Iso H, Jacobs DR Jr, Wentworth D *et al.* Serum cholesterol levels and six-year mortality from stroke in 350, 977 men screened for the Multiple Risk Factor Intervention Trial. N Engl J Med 1989; 320:904.
44. Barr DP, Russ EM, Eder HA. Protein lipid relationship in human plasma II. In atherosclerosis and related conditions. Am J Med 1951; 11:480.
45. Ginsburg GS, Safran C, Pasternak RC. National Cholesterol Education Program guidelines: The impact of missing HDL. Circulation (abstract) 1988; 78:II 382.
46. Castell, WP, Garrison RJ, Wilson PWF *et al.* Incidence of coronary heart disease and lipoprotein cholesterol levels: The Framingham Study. JAMA 1986; 256:2835.
47. Buchwald H, Varco RL, Matts *et al.* Effect of partial ileal bypass surgery on mortality and morbidity from coronary heart disease in patients with hypercholesterolaemia. Report of the program on surgical control of hyperlipidaemia (POSCH). N. Engl. J. Med. 1990; 323:947.
48. Ballard-Barbash R, Callaway CW. Marine fish oils: role in prevention of coronary artery disease. Mayo Clin Proc 1987; 62:113.
49. Bak AAA, Grobbee DE. The effect on serum cholesterol levels of coffee brewed by filtering or boiling. N Engl J Med 1989; 321:1432.
50. Vermaak WJH. Variability in plasma cholesterol essays. The object that defects the goal (letter) Am J Cardiol 1988; 62:841.
51. West KM. Epidemiology of diabetes and its vascular complications. Elsevier, New York: 1978.

52. Kroc Collaborative Study Group. Blood glucose control and the evolution of diabetic retinopathy and albuminuria. N Engl J Med 1984; 311:365.
53. Powell KE, Thompson PD, Caspersen CJ *et al.* Physical activity and the incidence of coronary heart disease. Ann Rev Public Health 1987; 8:253.
54. Paffenbarger RS, Hyde RT, Wing AL *et al.* Physical activity, all cause mortality and longevity of college alumni. N Engl J Med 1986; 314:605.
55. Kramsch DM, Aspen AJ, Abramowitz BM *et al.* Reduction of coronary atherosclerosis by moderate conditioning exercise in monkeys on an atherogenic diet. N Engl J Med 1981; 305:1483.
56. Hubert HB, Feinleib M, McNamara PM *et al.* Obesity as an independent risk factor for cardiovascular disease: A 26 year follow-up of participants in the Framingham Heart Study. Circulation 1983; 67:968.
57. Larsson B, Svardsudd K, Welin L *et al.* Abdominal adipose tissue distribution, obesity, and risk of cardiovascular disease and death: 13 year follow up of participants in the study of men form in 1913. Br Med J 1984; 288:1401.
58. Friedman M, Rosenman RH. Type A behavior and your heart. New York, Alfred A Knopf, 1974.
59. Ragland DR, Brand RJ. Type A behavior and mortality from coronary heart disease. N Engl J Med 1988; 318:65.
60. Dimsdale JE. A perspective of Type A behavior and coronary disease (editorial) N Engl J Med 1988; 318:110.
61. Williams RB Jr. Refining the Type A hypothesis: emergence of the hostility complex. Am J Cardiol 1987; 60:273.
62. Steering Committee of the Physicians Health Study Research Group. Final report on the aspirin component of the ongoing Physicians Health Study. N Engl J Med 1989; 321:129
63. Klint CR, Knatterud GL, Stamler J *et al.* Persantine-Aspirin Reinfarction Study Part II. Secondary coronary prevention with persantine and aspirin. JACC 1986; 7:251.
64. Harker LA. Clinical trials evaluating platelet modifying drugs in patients with atherosclerotic cardiovascular disease and thrombosis. Circulation 1986; 73:206.
65. Miettinen TA, Huttunen JK, Naukkarinen V *et al.* Multifactorial primary prevention of cardiovascular diseases in middle aged men. JAMA 1985; 254:2097.
66. Hjermann I, Velve BK, Holme I *et al.* Effect of diet and smoking intervention of the incidence of coronary heart disease. Report from the Oslo Study Group of a randomized trial in healthy men. Lancet 1981; 2:1303.
67. Kornitzer M, Dramaix M, Thilly C *et al.* Belgian Heart Disease Prevention Project: Incidence and mortality results. Lancet 1983; 1:1066.
68. Research Group of the Rome Project of Coronary Heart Disease Prevention. Eight year follow-up results from the Rome Project of Coronary Heart Disease Prevention. Prev Med 1986; 15:176.

Subject index

Developments in Cardiovascular Medicine

1. Ch.T. Lancée (ed.): *Echocardiology*. 1979 ISBN 90-247-2209-8
2. J. Baan, A.C. Arntzenius and E.L. Yellin (eds.): *Cardiac Dynamics*. 1980 ISBN 90-247-2212-8
3. H.J.Th. Thalen and C.C. Meere (eds.): *Fundamentals of Cardiac Pacing*. 1979 ISBN 90-247-2245-4
4. H.E. Kulbertus and H.J.J. Wellens (eds.): *Sudden Death*. 1980 ISBN 90-247-2290-X
5. L.S. Dreifus and A.N. Brest (eds.): *Clinical Applications of Cardiovascular Drugs*. 1980 ISBN 90-247-2295-0
6. M.P. Spencer and J.M. Reid: *Cerebrovascular Evaluation with Doppler Ultrasound*. With contributions by E.C. Brockenbrough, R.S. Reneman, G.I. Thomas and D.L. Davis. 1981 ISBN 90-247-2384-1
7. D.P. Zipes, J.C. Bailey and V. Elharrar (eds.): *The Slow Inward Current and Cardiac Arrhythmias*. 1980 ISBN 90-247-2380-9
8. H. Kesteloot and J.V. Joossens (eds.): *Epidemiology of Arterial Blood Pressure*. 1980 ISBN 90-247-2386-8
9. F.J.Th. Wackers (ed.): *Thallium-201 and Technetium-99m-Pyrophosphate. Myocardial Imaging in the Coronary Care Unit*. 1980 ISBN 90-247-2396-5
10. A. Maseri, C. Marchesi, S. Chierchia and M.G. Trivella (eds.): *Coronary Care Units*. Proceedings of a European Seminar, held in Pisa, Italy (1978). 1981 ISBN 90-247-2456-2
11. J. Morganroth, E.N. Moore, L.S. Dreifus and E.L. Michelson (eds.): *The Evaluation of New Antiarrhythmic Drugs*. Proceedings of the First Symposium on New Drugs and Devices, held in Philadelphia, Pa., U.S.A. (1980). 1981 ISBN 90-247-2474-0
12. P. Alboni: *Intraventricular Conduction Disturbances*. 1981 ISBN 90-247-2483-X
13. H. Rijsterborgh (ed.): *Echocardiology*. 1981 ISBN 90-247-2491-0
14. G.S. Wagner (ed.): *Myocardial Infarction*. Measurement and Intervention. 1982 ISBN 90-247-2513-5
15. R.S. Meltzer and J. Roelandt (eds.): *Contrast Echocardiography*. 1982 ISBN 90-247-2531-3
16. A. Amery, R. Fagard, P. Lijnen and J. Staessen (eds.): *Hypertensive Cardiovascular Disease*. Pathophysiology and Treatment. 1982 IBSN 90-247-2534-8
17. L.N. Bouman and H.J. Jongsma (eds.): *Cardiac Rate and Rhythm*. Physiological, Morphological and Developmental Aspects. 1982 ISBN 90-247-2626-3
18. J. Morganroth and E.N. Moore (eds.): *The Evaluation of Beta Blocker and Calcium Antagonist Drugs*. Proceedings of the 2nd Symposium on New Drugs and Devices, held in Philadelphia, Pa., U.S.A. (1981). 1982 ISBN 90-247-2642-5
19. M.B. Rosenbaum and M.V. Elizari (eds.): *Frontiers of Cardiac Electrophysiology*. 1983 ISBN 90-247-2663-8
20. J. Roelandt and P.G. Hugenholtz (eds.): *Long-term Ambulatory Electrocardiography*. 1982 ISBN 90-247-2664-6
21. A.A.J. Adgey (ed.): *Acute Phase of Ischemic Heart Disease and Myocardial Infarction*. 1982 ISBN 90-247-2675-1
22. P. Hanrath, W. Bleifeld and J. Souquet (eds.): *Cardiovascular Diagnosis by Ultrasound*. Transesophageal, Computerized, Contrast, Doppler Echocardiography. 1982 ISBN 90-247-2692-1

Developments in Cardiovascular Medicine

23. J. Roelandt (ed.): *The Practice of M-Mode and Two-dimensional Echocardiography.* 1983 ISBN 90-247-2745-6
24. J. Meyer, P. Schweizer and R. Erbel (eds.): *Advances in Noninvasive Cardiology.* Ultrasound, Computed Tomography, Radioisotopes, Digital Angiography. 1983 ISBN 0-89838-576-8
25. J. Morganroth and E.N. Moore (eds.): *Sudden Cardiac Death and Congestive Heart Failure.* Diagnosis and Treatment. Proceedings of the 3rd Symposium on New Drugs and Devices, held in Philadelphia, Pa., U.S.A. (1982). 1983 ISBN 0-89838-580-6
26. H.M. Perry Jr. (ed.): *Lifelong Management of Hypertension.* 1983 ISBN 0-89838-582-2
27. E.A. Jaffe (ed.): *Biology of Endothelial Cells.* 1984 ISBN 0-89838-587-3
28. B. Surawicz, C.P. Reddy and E.N. Prystowsky (eds.): *Tachycardias.* 1984 ISBN 0-89838-588-1
29. M.P. Spencer (ed.): *Cardiac Doppler Diagnosis.* Proceedings of a Symposium, held in Clearwater, Fla., U.S.A. (1983). 1983 ISBN 0-89838-591-1
30. H. Villarreal and M.P. Sambhi (eds.): *Topics in Pathophysiology of Hypertension.* 1984 ISBN 0-89838-595-4
31. F.H. Messerli (ed.): *Cardiovascular Disease in the Elderly.* 1984 Revised edition, 1988: see below under Volume 76
32. M.L. Simoons and J.H.C. Reiber (eds.): *Nuclear Imaging in Clinical Cardiology.* 1984 ISBN 0-89838-599-7
33. H.E.D.J. ter Keurs and J.J. Schipperheyn (eds.): *Cardiac Left Ventricular Hypertrophy.* 1983 ISBN 0-89838-612-8
34. N. Sperelakis (ed.): *Physiology and Pathology of the Heart.* 1984 Revised edition, 1988: see below under Volume 90
35. F.H. Messerli (ed.): *Kidney in Essential Hypertension.* Proceedings of a Course, held in New Orleans, La., U.S.A. (1983). 1984 ISBN 0-89838-616-0
36. M.P. Sambhi (ed.): *Fundamental Fault in Hypertension.* 1984 ISBN 0-89838-638-1
37. C. Marchesi (ed.): *Ambulatory Monitoring.* Cardiovascular System and Allied Applications. Proceedings of a Workshop, held in Pisa, Italy (1983). 1984 ISBN 0-89838-642-X
38. W. Kupper, R.N. MacAlpin and W. Bleifeld (eds.): *Coronary Tone in Ischemic Heart Disease.* 1984 ISBN 0-89838-646-2
39. N. Sperelakis and J.B. Caulfield (eds.): *Calcium Antagonists.* Mechanism of Action on Cardiac Muscle and Vascular Smooth Muscle. Proceedings of the 5th Annual Meeting of the American Section of the I.S.H.R., held in Hilton Head, S.C., U.S.A. (1983). 1984 ISBN 0-89838-655-1
40. Th. Godfraind, A.G. Herman and D. Wellens (eds.): *Calcium Entry Blockers in Cardiovascular and Cerebral Dysfunctions.* 1984 ISBN 0-89838-658-6
41. J. Morganroth and E.N. Moore (eds.): *Interventions in the Acute Phase of Myocardial Infarction.* Proceedings of the 4th Symposium on New Drugs and Devices, held in Philadelphia, Pa., U.S.A. (1983). 1984 ISBN 0-89838-659-4
42. F.L. Abel and W.H. Newman (eds.): *Functional Aspects of the Normal, Hypertrophied and Failing Heart.* Proceedings of the 5th Annual Meeting of the American Section of the I.S.H.R., held in Hilton Head, S.C., U.S.A. (1983). 1984 ISBN 0-89838-665-9

Developments in Cardiovascular Medicine

43. S. Sideman and R. Beyar (eds.): [3-D] *Simulation and Imaging of the Cardiac System.* State of the Heart. Proceedings of the International Henry Goldberg Workshop, held in Haifa, Israel (1984). 1985 ISBN 0-89838-687-X
44. E. van der Wall and K.I. Lie (eds.): *Recent Views on Hypertrophic Cardiomyopathy.* Proceedings of a Symposium, held in Groningen, The Netherlands (1984). 1985 ISBN 0-89838-694-2
45. R.E. Beamish, P.K. Singal and N.S. Dhalla (eds.), *Stress and Heart Disease.* Proceedings of a International Symposium, held in Winnipeg, Canada, 1984 (Vol. 1). 1985 ISBN 0-89838-709-4
46. R.E. Beamish, V. Panagia and N.S. Dhalla (eds.): *Pathogenesis of Stress-induced Heart Disease.* Proceedings of a International Symposium, held in Winnipeg, Canada, 1984 (Vol. 2). 1985 ISBN 0-89838-710-8
47. J. Morganroth and E.N. Moore (eds.): *Cardiac Arrhythmias.* New Therapeutic Drugs and Devices. Proceedings of the 5th Symposium on New Drugs and Devices, held in Philadelphia, Pa., U.S.A. (1984). 1985 ISBN 0-89838-716-7
48. P. Mathes (ed.): *Secondary Prevention in Coronary Artery Disease and Myocardial Infarction.* 1985 ISBN 0-89838-736-1
49. H.L. Stone and W.B. Weglicki (eds.): *Pathobiology of Cardiovascular Injury.* Proceedings of the 6th Annual Meeting of the American Section of the I.S.H.R., held in Oklahoma City, Okla., U.S.A. (1984). 1985 ISBN 0-89838-743-4
50. J. Meyer, R. Erbel and H.J. Rupprecht (eds.): *Improvement of Myocardial Perfusion.* Thrombolysis, Angioplasty, Bypass Surgery. Proceedings of a Symposium, held in Mainz, F.R.G. (1984). 1985 ISBN 0-89838-748-5
51. J.H.C. Reiber, P.W. Serruys and C.J. Slager (eds.): *Quantitative Coronary and Left Ventricular Cineangiography.* Methodology and Clinical Applications. 1986 ISBN 0-89838-760-4
52. R.H. Fagard and I.E. Bekaert (eds.): *Sports Cardiology.* Exercise in Health and Cardiovascular Disease. Proceedings from an International Conference, held in Knokke, Belgium (1985). 1986 ISBN 0-89838-782-5
53. J.H.C. Reiber and P.W. Serruys (eds.): *State of the Art in Quantitative Cornary Arteriography.* 1986 ISBN 0-89838-804-X
54. J. Roelandt (ed.): *Color Doppler Flow Imaging and Other Advances in Doppler Echocardiography.* 1986 ISBN 0-89838-806-6
55. E.E. van der Wall (ed.): *Noninvasive Imaging of Cardiac Metabolism.* Single Photon Scintigraphy, Positron Emission Tomography and Nuclear Magnetic Resonance. 1987 ISBN 0-89838-812-0
56. J. Liebman, R. Plonsey and Y. Rudy (eds.): *Pediatric and Fundamental Electrocardiography.* 1987 ISBN 0-89838-815-5
57. H.H. Hilger, V. Hombach and W.J. Rashkind (eds.), *Invasive Cardiovascular Therapy.* Proceedings of an International Symposium, held in Cologne, F.R.G. (1985). 1987 ISBN 0-89838-818-X
58. P.W. Serruys and G.T. Meester (eds.): *Coronary Angioplasty.* A Controlled Model for Ischemia. 1986 ISBN 0-89838-819-8
59. J.E. Tooke and L.H. Smaje (eds.): *Clinical Investigation of the Microcirculation.* Proceedings of an International Meeting, held in London, U.K. (1985). 1987 ISBN 0-89838-833-3

Developments in Cardiovascular Medicine

60. R.Th. van Dam and A. van Oosterom (eds.): *Electrocardiographic Body Surface Mapping*. Proceedings of the 3rd International Symposium on B.S.M., held in Nijmegen, The Netherlands (1985). 1986 ISBN 0-89838-834-1
61. M.P. Spencer (ed.): *Ultrasonic Diagnosis of Cerebrovascular Disease*. Doppler Techniques and Pulse Echo Imaging. 1987 ISBN 0-89838-836-8
62. M.J. Legato (ed.): *The Stressed Heart*. 1987 ISBN 0-89838-849-X
63. M.E. Safar (ed.): *Arterial and Venous Systems in Essential Hypertension*. With Assistance of G.M. London, A.Ch. Simon and Y.A. Weiss. 1987 ISBN 0-89838-857-0
64. J. Roelandt (ed.): *Digital Techniques in Echocardiography*. 1987 ISBN 0-89838-861-9
65. N.S. Dhalla, P.K. Singal and R.E. Beamish (eds.): *Pathology of Heart Disease*. Proceedings of the 8th Annual Meeting of the American Section of the I.S.H.R., held in Winnipeg, Canada, 1986 (Vol. 1). 1987 ISBN 0-89838-864-3
66. N.S. Dhalla, G.N. Pierce and R.E. Beamish (eds.): *Heart Function and Metabolism*. Proceedings of the 8th Annual Meeting of the American Section of the I.S.H.R., held in Winnipeg, Canada, 1986 (Vol. 2). 1987 ISBN 0-89838-865-1
67. N.S. Dhalla, I.R. Innes and R.E. Beamish (eds.): *Myocardial Ischemia*. Proceedings of a Satellite Symposium of the 30th International Physiological Congress, held in Winnipeg, Canada (1986). 1987 ISBN 0-89838-866-X
68. R.E. Beamish, V. Panagia and N.S. Dhalla (eds.): *Pharmacological Aspects of Heart Disease*. Proceedings of an International Symposium, held in Winnipeg, Canada (1986). 1987 ISBN 0-89838-867-8
69. H.E.D.J. ter Keurs and J.V. Tyberg (eds.): *Mechanics of the Circulation*. Proceedings of a Satellite Symposium of the 30th International Physiological Congress, held in Banff, Alberta, Canada (1986). 1987 ISBN 0-89838-870-8
70. S. Sideman and R. Beyar (eds.): *Activation, Metabolism and Perfusion of the Heart*. Simulation and Experimental Models. Proceedings of the 3rd Henry Goldberg Workshop, held in Piscataway, N.J., U.S.A. (1986). 1987 ISBN 0-89838-871-6
71. E. Aliot and R. Lazzara (eds.): *Ventricular Tachycardias*. From Mechanism to Therapy. 1987 ISBN 0-89838-881-3
72. A. Schneeweiss and G. Schettler: *Cardiovascular Drug Therapoy in the Elderly*. 1988 ISBN 0-89838-883-X
73. J.V. Chapman and A. Sgalambro (eds.): *Basic Concepts in Doppler Echocardiography*. Methods of Clinical Applications based on a Multi-modality Doppler Approach. 1987 ISBN 0-89838-888-0
74. S. Chien, J. Dormandy, E. Ernst and A. Matrai (eds.): *Clinical Hemorheology*. Applications in Cardiovascular and Hematological Disease, Diabetes, Surgery and Gynecology. 1987 ISBN 0-89838-807-4
75. J. Morganroth and E.N. Moore (eds.): *Congestive Heart Failure*. Proceedings of the 7th Annual Symposium on New Drugs and Devices, held in Philadelphia, Pa., U.S.A. (1986). 1987 ISBN 0-89838-955-0
76. F.H. Messerli (ed.): *Cardiovascular Disease in the Elderly*. 2nd ed. 1988 ISBN 0-89838-962-3
77. P.H. Heintzen and J.H. Bürsch (eds.): *Progress in Digital Angiocardiography*. 1988 ISBN 0-89838-965-8

Developments in Cardiovascular Medicine

78. M.M. Scheinman (ed.): *Catheter Ablation of Cardiac Arrhythmias.* Basic Bioelectrical Effects and Clinical Indications. 1988 ISBN 0-89838-967-4
79. J.A.E. Spaan, A.V.G. Bruschke and A.C. Gittenberger-De Groot (eds.): *Coronary Circulation.* From Basic Mechanisms to Clinical Implications. 1987 ISBN 0-89838-978-X
80. C. Visser, G. Kan and R.S. Meltzer (eds.): *Echocardiography in Coronary Artery Disease.* 1988 ISBN 0-89838-979-8
81. A. Bayés de Luna, A. Betriu and G. Permanyer (eds.): *Therapeutics in Cardiology.* 1988 ISBN 0-89838-981-X
82. D.M. Mirvis (ed.): *Body Surface Electrocardiographic Mapping.* 1988 ISBN 0-89838-983-6
83. M.A. Konstam and J.M. Isner (eds.): *The Right Ventricle.* 1988 ISBN 0-89838-987-9
84. C.T. Kappagoda and P.V. Greenwood (eds.): *Long-term Management of Patients after Myocardial Infarction.* 1988 ISBN 0-89838-352-8
85. W.H. Gaasch and H.J. Levine (eds.): *Chronic Aortic Regurgitation.* 1988 ISBN 0-89838-364-1
86. P.K. Singal (ed.): *Oxygen Radicals in the Pathophysiology of Heart Disease.* 1988 ISBN 0-89838-375-7
87. J.H.C. Reiber and P.W. Serruys (eds.): *New Developments in Quantitative Coronary Arteriography.* 1988 ISBN 0-89838-377-3
88. J. Morganroth and E.N. Moore (eds.): *Silent Myocardial Ischemia.* Proceedings of the 8th Annual Symposium on New Drugs and Devices (1987). 1988 ISBN 0-89838-380-3
89. H.E.D.J. ter Keurs and M.I.M. Noble (eds.): *Starling's Law of the Heart Revisted.* 1988 ISBN 0-89838-382-X
90. N. Sperelakis (ed.): *Physiology and Pathophysiology of the Heart.* (Rev. ed.) 1988 ISBN 0-89838-388-9
91. J.W. de Jong (ed.): *Myocardial Energy Metabolism.* 1988 ISBN 0-89838-394-3
92. V. Hombach, H.H. Hilger and H.L. Kennedy (eds.): *Electrocardiography and Cardiac Drug Therapy.* Proceedings of an International Symposium, held in Cologne, F.R.G. (1987). 1988 ISBN 0-89838-395-1
93. H. Iwata, J.B. Lombardini and T. Segawa (eds.): *Taurine and the Heart.* 1988 ISBN 0-89838-396-X
94. M.R. Rosen and Y. Palti (eds.): *Lethal Arrhythmias Resulting from Myocardial Ischemia and Infarction.* Proceedings of the 2nd Rappaport Symposium, held in Haifa, Israel (1988). 1988 ISBN 0-89838-401-X
95. M. Iwase and I. Sotobata: *Clinical Echocardiography.* With a Foreword by M.P. Spencer. 1989 ISBN 0-7923-0004-1
96. I. Cikes (ed.): *Echocardiography in Cardiac Interventions.* 1989 ISBN 0-7923-0088-2
97. E. Rapaport (ed.): *Early Interventions in Acute Myocardial Infarction.* 1989 ISBN 0-7923-0175-7
98. M.E. Safar and F. Fouad-Tarazi (eds.): *The Heart in Hypertension.* A Tribute to Robert C. Tarazi (1925-1986). 1989 ISBN 0-7923-0197-8
99. S. Meerbaum and R. Meltzer (eds.): *Myocardial Contrast Two-dimensional Echocardiography.* 1989 ISBN 0-7923-0205-2

Developments in Cardiovascular Medicine

100. J. Morganroth and E.N. Moore (eds.): *Risk/Benefit Analysis for the Use and Approval of Thrombolytic, Antiarrhythmic, and Hypolipidemic Agents.* Proceedings of the 9th Annual Symposium on New Drugs and Devices (1988). 1989 ISBN 0-7923-0294-X
101. P.W. Serruys, R. Simon and K.J. Beatt (eds.): *PTCA - An Investigational Tool and a Non-operative Treatment of Acute Ischemia.* 1990 ISBN 0-7923-0346-6
102. I.S. Anand, P.I. Wahi and N.S. Dhalla (eds.): *Pathophysiology and Pharmacology of Heart Disease.* 1989 ISBN 0-7923-0367-9
103. G.S. Abela (ed.): *Lasers in Cardiovascular Medicine and Surgery.* Fundamentals and Technique. 1990 ISBN 0-7923-0440-3
104. H.M. Piper (ed.): *Pathophysiology of Severe Ischemic Myocardial Injury.* 1990 ISBN 0-7923-0459-4
105. S.M. Teague (ed.): *Stress Doppler Echocardiography.* 1990 ISBN 0-7923-0499-3
106. P.R. Saxena, D.I. Wallis, W. Wouters and P. Bevan (eds.): *Cardiovascular Pharmacology of 5-Hydroxytryptamine.* Prospective Therapeutic Applications. 1990 ISBN 0-7923-0502-7
107. A.P. Shepherd and P.A. Öberg (eds.): *Laser-Doppler Blood Flowmetry.* 1990 ISBN 0-7923-0508-6
108. J. Soler-Soler, G. Permanyer-Miralda and J. Sagristà-Sauleda (eds.): *Pericardial Disease.* New Insights and Old Dilemmas. Preface by Ralph Shabetai. 1990 ISBN 0-7923-0510-8
109. J.P.M. Hamer: *Practical Echocardiography in the Adult.* With Doppler and Color-Doppler Flow Imaging. 1990 ISBN 0-7923-0670-8
110. A. Bayés de Luna, P. Brugada, J. Cosin Aguilar and F. Navarro Lopez (eds.): *Sudden Cardiac Death.* 1991 ISBN 0-7923-0716-X
111. E. Andries and R. Stroobandt (eds.): *Hemodynamics in Daily Practice.* 1991 ISBN 0-7923-0725-9
112. J. Morganroth and E.N. Moore (eds.): *Use and Approval of Antihypertensive Agents and Surrogate Endpoints for the Approval of Drugs affecting Antiarrhythmic Heart Failure and Hypolipidemia.* Proceedings of the 10th Annual Symposium on New Drugs and Devices (1989). 1990 ISBN 0-7923-0756-9
113. S. Iliceto, P. Rizzon and J.R.T.C. Roelandt (eds.): *Ultrasound in Coronary Artery Disease.* Present Role and Future Perspectives. 1990 ISBN 0-7923-0784-4
114. J.V. Chapman and G.R. Sutherland (eds.): *The Noninvasive Evaluation of Hemodynamics in Congenital Heart Disease.* Doppler Ultrasound Applications in the Adult and Pediatric Patient with Congenital Heart Disease. 1990 ISBN 0-7923-0836-0
115. G.T. Meester and F. Pinciroli (eds.): *Databases for Cardiology.* 1991 ISBN 0-7923-0886-7
116. B. Korecky and N.S. Dhalla (eds.): *Subcellular Basis of Contractile Failure.* 1990 ISBN 0-7923-0890-5
117. J.H.C. Reiber and P.W. Serruys (eds.): *Quantitative Coronary Arteriography.* 1991 ISBN 0-7923-0913-8
118. E. van der Wall and A. de Roos (eds.): *Magnetic Resonance Imaging in Coronary Artery Disease.* 1991 ISBN 0-7923-0940-5
119. V. Hombach, M. Kochs and A.J. Camm (eds.): *Interventional Techniques in Cardiovascular Medicine.* 1991 ISBN 0-7923-0956-1

Developments in Cardiovascular Medicine

120. R. Vos: *Drugs Looking for Diseases.* Innovative Drug Research and the Development of the Beta Blockers and the Calcium Antagonists. 1991 ISBN 0-7923-0968-5
121. S. Sideman, R. Beyar and A. G. Kleber (eds.): *Cardiac Electrophysiology, Circulation, and Transport.* Proceedings of the 7th Henry Goldberg Workshop (Berne, Switzerland, 1990). 1991 ISBN 0-7923-1145-0
122. D.M. Bers: *Excitation-Contraction Coupling and Cardiac Contractile Force.* 1991 ISBN 0-7923-1186-8
123. A.-M. Salmasi and A.N. Nicolaides (eds.): *Occult Atherosclerotic Disease.* Diagnosis, Assessment and Management. 1991 ISBN 0-7923-1188-4
124. J.A.E. Spaan: *Coronary Blood Flow.* Mechanics, Distribution, and Control. 1991 ISBN 0-7923-1210-4
125. R.W. Stout (ed.): *Diabetes and Atherosclerosis.* 1991 ISBN 0-7923-1310-0

Previous volumes are still available

KLUWER ACADEMIC PUBLISHERS – DORDRECHT / BOSTON / LONDON